THIRD EDITION

Access Device Guidelines

Recommendations for Nursing Practice and Education

D1283302

Editor
Dawn Camp-Sorrell, MSN, FNP, AOCN®

Authors
Diane G. Cope, PhD, ARNP-BC, AOCNP®
Susan A. Ezzone, MS, RN, CNP, AOCNP®
Donna L. Gerber, PhD, RN, AOCN®
Misty Lamprecht, MS, RN, CNS, AOCN®
Debra J. McCorkindale, RN, BSN
Andrea B. Moran, MSN, APRN
Julie G. Walker, MSN, RN, FNP-C
Lois Anaya Winkelman, RN, MS, AOCN®

Reviewers
Amy E. Korinko, RN, BSN, OCN®
Lynn Phillips, RN, MSN, CRNI®
Mary Jo Sarver, MN, ARNP, AOCN®, CRNI®
Cora Vizcarra, RN, CRNI®, MBA

Oncology Nursing Society
Pittsburgh, Pennsylvania

ONS Publishing Division

Publisher: Leonard Mafrica, MBA, CAE
Director of Publications: Barbara Sigler, RN, MNEd
Managing Editor: Lisa M. George, BA
Technical Content Editor: Angela D. Klimaszewski, RN, MSN
Staff Editor: Amy Nicoletti, BA
Copy Editor: Laura Pinchot, BA
Graphic Designer: Dany Sjoen

Library of Congress Cataloging-in-Publication Data

Access device guidelines : recommendations for nursing practice and education / edited by Dawn Camp-Sorrell. – 3rd ed.
    p. ; cm.
Includes bibliographical references and index.
  ISBN 978-1-890504-96-0 (alk. paper)
  1. Nursing. 2. Medical technology. 3. Medical instruments and apparatus. I. Camp-Sorrell, Dawn. II. Oncology Nursing Society.
  [DNLM: 1. Neoplasms–nursing–Practice Guideline. 2. Catheterization–nursing–Practice Guideline. WY 156 A169 2011]
  RT42.A235 2011
  610.28–dc22

                                                                                        2010025391

Publisher's Note

This book is published by the Oncology Nursing Society (ONS). ONS neither represents nor guarantees that the practices described herein will, if followed, ensure safe and effective patient care. The recommendations contained in this book reflect ONS's judgment regarding the state of general knowledge and practice in the field as of the date of publication. The recommendations may not be appropriate for use in all circumstances. Those who use this book should make their own determinations regarding specific safe and appropriate patient-care practices, taking into account the personnel, equipment, and practices available at the hospital or other facility at which they are located. The editor and publisher cannot be held responsible for any liability incurred as a consequence from the use or application of any of the contents of this book. Figures and tables are used as examples only. They are not meant to be all-inclusive, nor do they represent endorsement of any particular institution by ONS. Mention of specific products and opinions related to those products do not indicate or imply endorsement by ONS. Web sites mentioned are provided for information only; the hosts are responsible for their own content and availability. Unless otherwise indicated, dollar amounts reflect U.S. dollars.

ONS publications are originally published in English. Publishers wishing to translate ONS publications must contact the ONS Publishing Division about licensing arrangements. ONS publications cannot be translated without obtaining written permission from ONS. (Individual tables and figures that are reprinted or adapted require additional permission from the original source.) Because translations from English may not always be accurate or precise, ONS disclaims any responsibility for inaccuracies in words or meaning that may occur as a result of the translation. Readers relying on precise information should check the original English version.

Printed in the United States of America

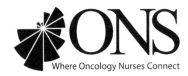

Oncology Nursing Society

Integrity • Innovation • Stewardship • Advocacy • Excellence • Inclusiveness

Contributors

Editor

Dawn Camp-Sorrell, MSN, FNP, AOCN®
Oncology Clinical Instructor
School of Nursing, University of Alabama at Birmingham
Nurse Practitioner
Adult Medical Clinic
St. Vincent's Hospital
Birmingham, Alabama
I. Objectives; II.A. Overview of VADs; II.B. Peripheral IV Catheters (Short Term);
III. Subcutaneous (Hypodermoclysis) Infusion Devices; IX. Ambulatory Infusion Pumps

Authors

Diane G. Cope, PhD, ARNP-BC, AOCNP®
Oncology Nurse Practitioner
Florida Cancer Specialists
Fort Myers, Florida
II.A. Overview of VADs; II.B. Peripheral IV Catheters (Short
Term); II.C. Midline Catheters; XII. Controversial Issues

Susan A. Ezzone, MS, RN, CNP, AOCNP®
(at the time of this writing)
Nurse Practitioner
Arthur G. James Cancer Hospital and Solove Research Institute
Ohio State University Cancer Center
Columbus, Ohio
II.D. Nontunneled Central Venous Lines; II.F. Tunneled Central
Venous Catheters; II.H. Apheresis/Hemodialysis Catheters

Donna L. Gerber, PhD, RN, AOCN®
Clinical Nurse Specialist
University of Texas M.D. Anderson Cancer Center
Houston, Texas
IV. Arterial Access Devices

Misty Lamprecht, MS, RN, CNS, AOCN®
Clinical Nurse Specialist
Arthur G. James Cancer Hospital and Solove Research Institute
Ohio State University Cancer Center
Columbus, Ohio
II.A. Overview of VADs; II.D. Nontunneled Central Venous
Lines; II.F. Tunneled Central Venous Catheters; II.H. Apher-
esis/Hemodialysis Catheters

Debra J. McCorkindale, RN, BSN
RN Senior
Blue Ridge Cancer Care
Roanoke, Virginia
VIII. Implanted Pumps; X. Education and Documentation
Issues for Access Devices

Andrea B. Moran, MSN, APRN
Nurse Practitioner
Neag Comprehensive Cancer Center
University of Connecticut Health Center
Farmington, Connecticut
II.A. Overview of VADs; II.G. Implantable Ports; II.I. Complica-
tions of Short- and Long-Term VADs; XI. Special Consider-
ations for Immunosuppressed Patients

Julie G. Walker, MSN, RN, FNP-C
Advanced Practice Nurse
University of Texas M.D. Anderson Cancer Center
Houston, Texas
V. Intraventricular Access Devices; VI. Epidural and Intrathecal
Access Devices

Lois Anaya Winkelman, RN, MS, AOCN®
Gynecologic Oncology Research Nurse
Rush University Medical Center
Chicago, Illinois
VII. Intraperitoneal Catheters

Reviewers

Amy E. Korinko, RN, BSN, OCN®
Senior Oncology Nurse
UPMC Cancer Centers/Oncology Hematology Association
Washington, Pennsylvania

Lynn Phillips, RN, MSN, CRNI®
Professor Emeritus
Nursing Education Consultant
Butte College
Oroville, California

Mary Jo Sarver, MN, ARNP, AOCN®, CRNI®
Clinical Nurse Specialist/Nurse Practitioner
Northwest Hospital and Medical Center
Seattle, Washington

Cora Vizcarra, RN, CRNI®, MBA
President/Nurse Consultant
MCV and Associates Healthcare, Inc.
Past President
Infusion Nurses Society
Indianapolis, Indiana

Disclosure

Editors and authors of books and guidelines provided by the Oncology Nursing Society are expected to disclose to the readers any significant financial interest or other relationships with the manufacturer(s) of any commercial products.

A vested interest may be considered to exist if a contributor is affiliated with or has a financial interest in commercial organizations that may have a direct or indirect interest in the subject matter. A "financial interest" may include, but is not limited to, being a shareholder in the organization; being an employee of the commercial organization; serving on an organization's speakers bureau; or receiving research from the organization. An "affiliation" may be holding a position on an advisory board or some other role of benefit to the commercial organization. Vested interest statements appear in the front matter for each publication.

Contributors are expected to disclose any unlabeled or investigational use of products discussed in their content. This information is acknowledged solely for the information of the readers.

The contributors provided the following disclosure and vested interest information:

Mary Jo Sarver, MN, ARNP, AOCN®, CRNI®: Eli Lilly and Co., speakers bureau; Genentech, advisory board (Rituxan®)

Table of Contents

List of Abbreviations

APN—advanced practice nurse
BSA—body surface area
CDC—Centers for Disease Control and Prevention
CHG—chlorhexidine gluconate
CNS—central nervous system
CSF—cerebrospinal fluid
CT—computed tomography
CVC—central venous catheter
DEAP—di(2-ethylhexyl) phthalate
D5W—dextrose 5% in water
FDA—U.S. Food and Drug Administration
Fr—French
FUDR—floxuridine
HAI—hepatic artery infusion
HIPEC—hyperthermic intraperitoneal chemotherapy
HSCT—hematopoietic stem cell transplantation
IHI—Institute for Healthcare Improvement

INR—international normalized ratio
INS—Infusion Nurses Society
IP—intraperitoneal
IV—intravenous
MRI—magnetic resonance imaging
NCI—National Cancer Institute
NS—normal saline
PASV—pressure-activated safety valve
PEG—polyethylene glycol
PICC—peripherally inserted central catheter
PO—by mouth
psi—pounds per square inch
SC—subcutaneous
SEP—sclerosing encapsulating peritonitis
tPA—tissue plasminogen activator
TPN—total parenteral nutrition
VAD—vascular access device

Introduction

More than four decades ago, IV drugs could be administered only through short-term peripheral or subclavian access devices. Administration of drugs to other parts of the body such as the epidural or peritoneal spaces was only theorized. After years of improving upon catheters and ports, short-term as well as long-term devices are available to access the venous, intrathecal, arterial, peritoneal, and intraventricular body systems. As a result, complex treatment plans are being developed to increase the patient's overall survival as well as to palliate symptoms, thus improving quality of life.

Evolving technology continuously leads to the frequent introduction of newer access devices and products used with these devices. This technology continues to improve on existing devices to decrease the occurrence of occlusion and infection and increase patient safety. Although basic routine care is common to all devices, each device has specific care requirements. Managing complications of access devices is similar among the different devices, with variations noted. The literature provides numerous studies on caring for and managing complications (see Appendix 1 for Internet resources available). However, evidence on which to base nursing care from these studies is lacking, and controversies still exist concerning the optimal management.

In preparing this revision, an extensive literature search was performed to identify studies published since the 2004 edition of the guidelines. Following is a summary of the search criteria.

Only human, not animal, studies were included in this search. Databases used to search the literature included PubMed, MEDLINE, CINAHL, and the National Guideline Clearinghouse. Subject headings for the searches included *access devices, venous access devices, peripheral IV, subcutaneous devices, hypodermoclysis, apheresis catheters, hemodialysis catheters, nontunneled catheters, central venous lines, temporary venous lines, short-term catheters, long-term catheters, midline catheters, peripherally inserted catheters, tunneled catheters, complications of catheters, infection of catheters, occlusion of catheters, arterial catheters, peritoneal catheters, epidural, intrathecal, Ommaya reservoir, intraventricular catheters, educational needs, staff education, patient education, immunosuppression, myelosuppression, implantable pumps, ambulatory pumps, cost of catheters, maintenance of catheters, indwelling catheters, implantable ports,* and *controversial issues of access devices.* Some of the older references from the previous edition of these guidelines were retained because of their importance to the subject matter.

Few randomized, controlled trials have been conducted on access devices; subsequently, little evidence-based information is available to guide nursing care. Thus, the guidelines developed from this synthesis of literature focus on strict hand washing, strict aseptic technique, and consistent maintenance care. Ongoing surveillance of infection and occlusion rates will help any institution to evaluate its policies and determine whether revisions are necessary.

The Oncology Nursing Society initially developed these guidelines in 1989 to provide recommendations for the application of access device technology within nursing practice. Over the years, these guidelines continue to be updated according to the evidence in practice. For the clinician, the guidelines serve as a basis for providing care to the patient with an access device and in developing policies and procedures in all patient care settings. Nurse educators can use the guidelines in developing access device educational programs. Administrators can use the clinical practicums for competency-based evaluations. The extensive list of controversial issues will be a stimulus to nurse researchers to begin conducting studies to answer these questions. Nursing research is essential to establish scientifically based methods for access device care and the management of complications.

Guidelines for the use of access devices are indispensable in the management of patients with cancer. Modern technology has enhanced the safety and efficacy of administration methods for cancer treatment and supportive care agents. Developing the expertise needed to manage access devices is a continual challenge to healthcare professionals. The intent of these guidelines is to provide the foundation for evidence-based practice that practitioners can use to guide their practice.

It is clear that, despite the lack of evidence-based practice for care of access devices, the patient's quality of life has greatly improved over the past four decades with the advances in access device technology. This edition of *Access Device Guidelines: Recommendations for Nursing Practice and Education* explores the latest technologies, management procedures, and controversies that still exist. Recommendations for management and care are consistent with the literature and are deemed reasonable in the absence of definitive studies.

I. OBJECTIVES

A. Identify the different types of access devices available, their advantages and disadvantages, special features, patient selection criteria, and the use of access devices.

B. Describe anatomic and physiologic parameters influencing the placement and insertion technique of access devices.

C. Describe the maintenance and care of each type of access device.

D. Identify potential complications associated with each type of access device.

E. List nursing interventions for monitoring and treating access device complications.

F. Identify the learning needs of and resources for patients and care providers related to each type of access device.

G. Explore controversial issues associated with access devices.

H. Describe documentation procedures recommended for access devices.

I. Describe educational needs and clinical competency for RNs providing care to patients with an access device.

II. VASCULAR ACCESS DEVICES (VADS)

A. Overview of VADs

1. History: Further development of VADs continues to reduce the risk of accidental needlesticks and increase safety for healthcare personnel. Development and refinement of VADs continues to improve upon infection rates and thrombosis occurrence and enhance patient comfort.

    a) Peripheral: Introduced in 1945 as a plastic catheter to deliver IV solutions (Prue-Owens, 2006; Prunet et al., 2008). Approximately 60% of hospital inpatients have a peripheral IV (Morris & Tay, 2008).

    b) Midline: Midline catheters were first used in the 1950s for surgical patients who required one week of infusion therapy (Anderson, 2004). In the 1980s, the split-away plastic introducer was developed to facilitate midline catheter placement.

    c) Nontunneled central venous catheters, apheresis/hemodialysis catheters (Putigna & Solenberger, 2009)

        (1) Polyethylene catheters were first used for medical catheters in 1945.

        (2) Central venous access was accomplished through the femoral and external jugular vein in 1949.

        (3) In 1952, the subclavian vein was used for central access.

        (4) In 1968, hyperalimentation was given through central access.

    d) Peripherally inserted central catheters (PICCs): Introduced in the 1980s and mainly used for venous access in homecare patients (Bowe-Geddes & Nichols, 2005).

    e) Tunneled (Putigna & Solenberger, 2009)

        (1) Broviac tunneled catheters were first introduced in 1975 for long-term hyperalimentation. Catheter was tunneled within the subcutaneous (SC) tissue to increase the longevity of the catheter and to decrease infection.

        (2) A larger bore catheter, the Hickman catheter, was introduced in 1976 to expand the applications of a tunneled catheter as well as the patient population.

    f) Ports: Developed in the early 1980s to minimize infection risks and reduce care required at the insertion site

2. Definitions

    a) Short term: Catheters inserted for a short period of time, such as up to six weeks (peripheral, midline, nontunneled catheters)

    b) Long term: Catheters inserted for a time greater than six months (PICCs, tunneled, implantable ports)

3. VAD catheter materials and available features (Gallieni, Pittiruti, & Biffi, 2008; Galloway & Bodenham, 2004; Lopez et al., 2009)

    a) Teflon® (DuPont): Material used for peripheral IV devices; not commonly used

        (1) Stiff material that causes damage to the vein intima (inner lining) during insertion

        (2) Best used in short-term devices for less than 96 hours

    b) Polyurethane: Firm, not stiff, material that softens and becomes more pliable in the vein in response to the body core temperature

        (1) Exceptional tensile (physical) strength and flexible endurance that permits the catheter to be constructed with a thinner wall and greater internal diameter for high flow rates

        (2) Smaller external diameter catheters that can be used with less trauma for easier percutaneous insertion and decreased risk of phlebitis and other infectious complications

        (3) Increased biocompatibity within the body and less adherence of fibrin to the catheter material (thromboresistant)

        (4) Used for short-term peripheral devices and long-term devices

    c) Silicone: Flexible material that causes less damage to the intima of the vein on insertion and allows the catheter to float within the vein, which may decrease the risk of thrombosis (Galloway & Bodenham, 2004)

        (1) Requires special insertion technique because of flexibility of material (i.e., peel-away sheaths, Seldinger/modified Seldinger, micropuncture technique)

        (2) Offers increased biocompatibility within the body and less adherence of fibrin to the catheter material (thromboresistant)

        (3) Used for long-term access devices

    d) Antimicrobial coating: Catheter coated with a substance that gives it an anti-infective quality to protect against potential bacterial seeding onto the catheter surfaces (Borschel et al., 2006; Centers for Disease Control and Prevention [CDC], in press; Ramritu et al., 2008)

---

(1) Catheter surfaces are coated, bonded, or impregnated with an anti-infective substance. Agents that have been studied prior to insertion include the following.

　　(a) Antimicrobials: Cephalosporins, penicillin, vancomycin, rifampin, minocycline, miconazole (Fraenkel et al., 2006; Hockenhull et al., 2008, 2009; Niel-Weise, Stijnen, & van den Broek, 2007)

　　(b) Antiseptics: Chlorhexidine, silver sulfadiazine, benzalkonium chloride, silver-platinum-carbon (Kalfon et al., 2007; Khare et al., 2007)

(2) All of these substances have been shown to decrease the incidence of catheter-related bloodstream infections; however, their effectiveness is relatively short term (one to four weeks), and the evidence is contradictory (Borschel et al., 2006; Brun-Buisson et al., 2004; Dunser et al., 2005; Hanna et al., 2004; Leon et al., 2004; Rupp et al., 2005; Yucel et al., 2004). Therefore, more research is indicated to determine if their use could result in decreased costs as related to infection occurrence.

(3) Patients are at risk for allergic reaction to the anti-infective substance.

e) Heparin coating: Catheter coated with heparin prior to insertion to promote biocompatibility within the vein, thus reducing fibrin formation (Anton et al., 2009; Shah & Shah, 2007)

(1) It is thought that heparin will decrease fibrin buildup and thus decrease the occurrence of infection.

(2) Drawbacks associated with heparin-bonded catheters include heparin-induced thrombocytopenia (HIT), in-

creased risk of bleeding, allergic reactions, and increased costs (Anton et al., 2009; Shah & Shah, 2007).

(3) Although more research on heparin coating is needed, limited studies show that heparinization reduces the frequency of catheter-related bloodstream infections at a relatively low cost over a short time period (Shah & Shah, 2007).

f) PASV is a three-way pressure-activated safety valve located in the catheter hub designed to permit fluid infusion and reduce the risk of blood reflux into the catheter lumen during increases in central venous pressure that occur with exercise or involuntary responses, such as coughing.

(1) The three-way safety valve resists fluid or blood backflow, reducing need for clamps and potentially reducing the risk of occlusion and infection.

(2) This unique three-way valve is pressure activated and direction specific and generally eliminates the need for heparin flush (Navilyst Medical, Inc., n.d.).

g) Catheter distal tips are available with a valve or open ended.

h) Radiopaque availability: Common feature of VADs

(1) Assists in confirming placement in the vein under fluoroscopy or radiographically. Catheters are available with radiopaque lateral stripes or dots within the distal tip.

(2) Certain radiologic technologies may need to be implemented to assist with interpretation, such as the use of contrast medium.

i) Catheter sizes are measured in French (Fr) or gauge. French size equals the outside diameter of the catheter in millimeters multiplied by three. Gauge, which ranges from 13 to 28, may indicate inner or outer diameter, with a smaller number indicating a larger size. To minimize the risk of vein stenosis and thrombosis, the smallest diameter required for therapy should be used (Knutstad, Hager, & Hauser, 2003).

4. Costs include insertion kits, the device, the insertion setting (e.g., operating room, bedside, outpatient clinic; interventional radiology), placement verification (chest x-ray or fluoroscopy), and maintenance supplies (Gallieni et al., 2008).

a) Medical supply distributors, home health-care companies, and home infusion services are resources for nursing care, equipment, and supplies in the home setting.

b) Health insurance generally covers insertion expenses. Patients should check with their insurance representative or case managers about reimbursement issues.

c) Maintenance supplies, such as dressing materials, flushing/locking solutions, and syringes, generally are covered. Patients should check with their insurance company about reimbursement issues. Maintenance costs are based on the frequency of care (e.g., daily dressing changes or weekly dressing changes, daily flushing or every-other-day or weekly flushing).

5. Insertion technique: See specific catheter (Institute for Healthcare Improvement [IHI], n.d.; Venkatram, Rachmale, & Kanna, 2009).

a) Care bundles are a group of evidence-based interventions for insertion of VADs.

b) Implementation of the care bundles results in a decrease in infections.

c) Care bundle grouping for insertion includes
   (1) Strict hand hygiene
   (2) Maximal barrier precautions upon insertion
   (3) Chlorhexidine skin cleansing
   (4) Optimal insertion-site selection with avoidance of the femoral vein
   (5) Daily assessment of VAD
   (6) Remove VAD when no longer needed.

6. Maintenance and care of VADs

a) Common maintenance procedures (see Table 1) (Camp-Sorrell, 2007; CDC, in press; Gillies et al., 2003; Infusion Nurses Society [INS], 2006; Lyons, Given, & Marshall, 2008)
   (1) Organize care to minimize entries into the VAD system.
   (2) Maintain strict aseptic technique for all procedures (Olson et al., 2004). Hand hygiene is a vital intervention to reduce healthcare-associated infections (Koff et al., 2009; Morris & Tay, 2008)
   (3) Standardized procedures should be performed by skilled personnel instructed to assess for signs of VAD-related complications, such as pain, redness, swelling, induration, tenderness, fever, chills, and inability to infuse fluid or withdraw blood.

   (4) Secure all tubing connections with Luer locks.
   (5) Avoid use of tape on tubing connections because it has been implicated in the transmission of bacterial contaminates (INS, 2006).
   (6) Change dressing, IV tubing, or protective cap promptly if it becomes wet, soiled, contaminated, or damaged.
   (7) Further research is needed to determine the most effective technique for dressing changes and the use of sterile versus nonsterile gloves during dressing change.
      (a) By definition, *sterile* refers to a condition of being free from living microorganisms or germs.
      (b) *Aseptic* refers to a condition free from septic matter or free from organisms.
      (c) *Clean technique* refers to keeping the area free of debris or organisms.
      (d) No current recommendations exist for which method to use.

b) Site care and dressing management are necessary for infection control and assessment of the VAD exit site, insertion site, and surrounding area. Supplies for site cleansing and dressing changes should be single-use only (Pratt et al., 2007).
   (1) Technique for cutaneous antisepsis: In the past, the generally accepted method for applying skin-cleansing agents was to begin at the catheter exit site and cleanse outward in a circular motion, using care not to return to the clean area with the used sponge or swabstick. However, the manufacturer of ChloraPrep® (CareFusion, Inc.) recommends using a back-and-forth motion for 30 seconds for skin cleansing (see www.chloraprep.com/directions-of-use).

(a) When cleansing the insertion or exit site, use gentle friction for 30 seconds to ensure the disinfectant is absorbed by bacteria in the deeper layers of the skin (Camp-Sorrell, 2007; Morris & Tay, 2008)

(b) Note that alcohol- and iodine-containing products may be contraindicated for use to clean or come in contact with certain catheter materials and some types of protective caps. Contact may weaken or compromise the material over time. Therefore, it is important to obtain specific manufacturer information for each VAD used in a specific practice setting.

Table 1. Common Maintenance Procedures for Vascular Access Devices

Vascular Access Device	Dressing	Flushing*	Cap Change**	Blood Discard
Peripheral and midline (i.e., angiocatheter, butterfly)	Transparent dressing change with IV change. Gauze dressing QOD or PRN if wet, soiled, or nonocclusive.	NS 1–3 ml every 8, 12, or 24 hours	Every week or with catheter change	0.5–1 ml
Central nontunneled (i.e., subclavian)	Dressing change 24 hours after insertion. Transparent dressing every five to seven days. Gauze dressing QOD or PRN if wet, soiled, or nonocclusive.	Heparin 10–100 IU/ml, 3 ml/day or 2 ml/day per each lumen. Valve catheter or closed tip catheter flushed with NS.	Every week or with catheter change	1–2 ml
PICC line	Dressing change 24 hours after insertion. Transparent dressing every five to seven days. Gauze dressing QOD or PRN if wet, soiled, or nonocclusive.	Heparin 10–100 IU/ml, 3 ml/day or 3 ml/day three times a week. Valve catheter or closed tip catheter flushed with NS.	Every week	1–2 ml
Tunneled	Dressing change 24 hours after insertion. Transparent dressing every five to seven days. Gauze dressing QOD or PRN if wet, soiled, or nonocclusive. Once tunnel has healed, no dressing unless immunocompromised.	Heparin 10–100 IU/ml, 3 ml/day; 3 ml every other day; 5 ml three times a week; or 5 ml weekly. Valve catheter or closed tip catheter flushed with NS.	Every week or month	3–5 ml
Implanted port	For continuous access, change noncoring needle and transparent dressing every week or if nonocclusive. Gauze dressing QOD or PRN if wet, soiled, or nonocclusive.	Heparin 100 IU/ml, 5 ml every month or every six to eight weeks and after each use. Valve catheter or closed tip catheter flushed with NS. Flush both lumens.	Every week for continuous access	5 ml
Valve or closed distal tip	See above sections.	NS 5–10 ml weekly or after each use	Every month	3–5 ml
Pheresis	Transparent dressing every five to seven days. Gauze dressing QOD or PRN if wet, soiled, or nonocclusive.	Heparin 1,000–5,000 IU/ml; 1–2 ml/day	Every week	5 ml
Hemodialysis	Transparent dressing every five to seven days. Gauze dressing QOD or PRN if wet, soiled, or nonocclusive.	Heparin 1,000–5,000 IU/ml after each treatment	Every week	5 ml

*VAD should be flushed with 10–20 ml of NS after blood withdrawal. All VADs should be flushed with NS before and after use.

** Change protective cap more frequently if signs of poor integrity of septum from multiple use, signs of blood, precipitate, cracks, leaks, or other defects.

NS—normal saline; PICC—peripherally inserted central catheter; PRN—whenever necessary; QOD—every other day

(2) Cleansing agents (see Table 2): Base protocol and product choices on current research review, patient-specific issues, and catheter materials.

(a) Alcohol: A bacteriocidal that derives its antimicrobial effect by denaturation of proteins. Alcohol should be applied after use of a tincture of iodine but not following use of povidone-iodine solution (INS, 2006).

(b) Iodophors: Complexes that consist of iodine and a carrier that stabilizes the product, thereby reducing skin irritation. Their antimicrobial effect is derived from cell wall penetration, oxidation, and substitution of microbial contents with free iodine. Povidone-iodine (10%) is the most commonly used iodophor. Antimicrobial activity of iodophor occurs during drying; therefore, it must be left on the skin for at least two to three minutes to dry completely. Iodophor has minimal residual effect because free iodine is depleted after drying. Efficacy also is diminished by the presence of organic matter, such as blood or exudates, on the skin.

(c) 2% chlorhexidine gluconate (CHG): Recommended for pre- and post-insertion catheter care (CDC, in press; Danks, 2006; Milstone, Passaretti, & Perl, 2008; Mimoz et al., 2007). CHG is an antimicrobial that derives its activity by causing disruption of microbial cell membranes and precipitation of cell contents. CHG has a strong affinity for the skin, remaining chemically active for at least six hours. Antimicrobial action is rapid, and efficacy is not affected by organic material, such as blood or exudates on the skin.

  i. CHG is superior to alcohol or povidone-iodine in preventing catheter infection (Mimoz et al., 2007; Valles et al., 2008). Meta-analysis of eight studies comparing CHG with povidone-iodine showed that CHG reduced the risk of catheter-related bloodstream infection by 49% (Chaiyakunapruk, Veenstra, Lipsky, & Saint, 2002; Mimoz et al., 2007).

  ii. In 2000 the U.S. Food and Drug Administration (FDA) approved a 2% preparation, which is shown to substantially reduce infections, for use in preoperative skin preparation. It is now recommended for use during venous access device insertion in all patients older than two months of age unless contraindicated.

(d) Persist™ (Becton, Dickinson and Co.) skin preparation: This skin antiseptic allows release of iodine on the skin site for a longer time period to reduce skin irritation and promote antimicrobial action. Persist is a povidone-iodine formulation in an alcohol carrier that was developed as a catheter site antiseptic agent. According to the manufacturer, Persist is as effective as

Table 2. Comparison of Cleansing Agents								
Agent	Mode of Action	Gram +	Gram −	TB	Fungi	Viral	Residual Activity	Duration of Anti-Infective Effect After Application
Alcohol 70%	Denaturation of protein	Excellent	Excellent	Good	Good	Good	None	Brief
Iodophor 10% (povidone-iodine)	Oxidation/substitution by free iodine	Excellent	Good	Good	Good	Good	Minimal	Two hours
Chlorhexidine gluconate 2%	Cell wall disruption	Excellent	Good	Poor	Fair	Good	Excellent	Four to six hours
TB—tuberculosis								

other agents, such as alcohol and povidone-iodine.

(e) Ointments: Routine application of antimicrobial ointment to catheter insertion and exit sites is **not** recommended because of the risk of fungal infections and antimicrobial resistance (CDC, in press; Pratt et al., 2007).

(3) Dressing materials

(a) Gauze and tape: A mesh material traditionally used for dressings that provides no occlusive barrier, acts as a sponge, and is secured in place with various kinds of clean or sterile tape. Gauze dressings are to be changed every 48 hours or when wet, soiled, or the tape is no longer secure (Camp-Sorrell, 2007; CDC, in press; Krzywda & Edmiston, 2002).

(b) Transparent dressing: A semipermeable film with a significant moisture vapor permeability rate that allows for visualization of the VAD exit site but acts as a barrier to extrinsic liquid and microorganisms. Transparent dressings are to be changed every five to seven days or more often, as indicated (CDC, in press; Gallieni et al., 2008). When gauze is placed under a transparent dressing, the dressing type is considered gauze and tape and should be changed every 48 hours.

(c) Securement or stabilization devices: Steri-Strips™ (3M Health Care) or tape can be used to stabilize temporary catheters. Recommend to use securement devices, such as StatLock® (C.R. Bard Inc.), instead of sutures to reduce risk of infection (CDC, in press).

(d) No current recommendations exist for the use of sterile versus nonsterile gloves during dressing changes (CDC, in press; Pratt et al., 2007). Use of a no-touch technique with sterile or nonsterile gloves is recommended to prevent bacterial contamination (Pratt et al., 2007).

(e) No current recommendations exist for the use of a chlorhexidine sponge dressing (Biopatch® Antimicrobial Dressing, Johnson & Johnson). Biopatch is impregnated with chlorhexidine in a sustained-release formulation that is released over 5–10 days. A transparent dressing covers the patch. Studies suggest a decrease in catheter-related infections with CHG-impregnated dressings (Chambers et al., 2005; Ho & Litton, 2006; Ruschulte et al., 2009).

(f) Antimicrobial barrier dressing: Contains silver ions, which provide a sustained release directly into and around the catheter insertion site to reduce infection (Silverlon®, Argentum Medical, LLC). No current recommendations exist for silver dressings.

c) Flushing technique: Flushing is necessary to ensure patency by preventing accumulation of blood and drug precipitates on the catheter lumen. Flushing can prevent fibrin buildup; however, all VADs will accumulate fibrin coating to some extent. Flush vigorously using a pulsatile technique, and maintain pressure at the end of the flush to prevent reflux back into the catheter (Bishop et al., 2007; Camp-Sorrell, 2007; Hadaway, 2006; INS, 2008).

(1) Positive pressure technique is extremely important in preventing the development of fibrin sheaths, leading to withdrawal or infusion occlusions and contributing to the development of venous thrombosis. The following procedures prevent the slight negative pressure on the end of the catheter that results in pulling a small amount of blood into the end of the catheter, where it becomes a fibrin sheath.

(a) Positive pressure is maintained while flushing a VAD by clamping the extension tubing while still flushing the line.

(b) VADs that do not have a clamp may be flushed with positive pressure by withdrawing the syringe from the injection cap while continuing to push fluid through the needle.

(2) Flushing solutions

(a) Heparin sodium (10–5,000 IU/ml) is a sterile solution that inhibits the conversion of prothrombin to thrombin and fibrinogen to fibrin, thus inhibiting coagulation. Higher concentrations, such as 1,000 IU/ml or greater, are used for hemodialysis/apheresis catheters. Heparin is used to prevent fibrin buildup. Some authors have reported that use of heparin may decrease the incidence of catheter-related infections because of decreased risk of thrombus formation (Bishop et al., 2007; CDC, in press). Use of heparin may be contraindicated in patients at risk for heparin-induced thrombocytopenia.

(b) Bacteriostatic 0.9% sodium chloride solution is a sterile solution with approximately the same osmotic pressure and composition as extracellular fluids. Sodium chloride cleans the internal diameter of the catheter from blood or drug.

(3) Syringes/flush systems

(a) Drawing the solution from a vial into a syringe is the least expensive flushing method; however, it may not be appropriate in some patient care settings or for patients with poor eyesight or poor manual dexterity.

(b) Prefilled syringes reduce the risk of touch contamination from preparation and ensure administration of the correct flush and amount.

(c) Single-use flushing systems should be used.

(4) Flushing procedures and protocols

(a) Never use excessive force when flushing VADs. Avoid using a syringe less than 3 ml in size to decrease the pressure on the catheter. Syringe size directly affects the amount of pressure created by the force on the plunger; that is, the smaller the syringe, the greater the pressure in pounds per square inch (psi). The use of high pressure increases the risk of catheter/septum rupture or separation. For example, a 3 ml syringe generates pressure greater than 25 psi, whereas a 10 ml syringe generates less than 10 psi (Hadaway, 2006; INS, 2008). The manufacturer of the individual device determines the maximum pressure that can be exerted on a VAD. (Caution: This does not include physiologic variables that impact pressure, such as fibrin buildup.)

(b) Heparin-locked VADs should be flushed with saline before and after drug administration. If the VAD is being used frequently or locked with a high concentration of heparin, consider withdrawing heparin first to prevent giving therapeutic doses of heparin (Bishop et al., 2007).

(c) VADs with a closed distal tip (Groshong® [Bard Access Systems] valve catheters) or PASV are designed to be flushed vigorously with saline; however, some institutions flush with heparinized saline.

(d) Flush all VADs vigorously using pulsating technique (push-pull motion) with 10–20 ml of normal saline after infusing or withdrawing blood.

(e) Clamps are used as needed when accessing or deaccessing VADs to prevent air embolism or blood backflow.

i. Many VADs have clamps located directly on fortified areas of the catheter.

ii. Never use a hemostat or sharp-edged clamp that could damage or cut the catheter. Toothless plastic clamps should be kept available for emergency use. Scissors should never be used on or near the catheters except for removal of sutures (INS, 2006).

iii. If clamping is not possible, have the patient perform a Valsalva maneuver (forcefully exhale and hold breath) whenever catheter is open to air.

iv. Valved catheters or catheters with PASV do not require clamping if valve is functioning properly. Clamping will damage the catheter.

d) Protective cap: Since 1993, needleless connectors have been available to prevent needlestick injury. In 2000, the Occupational Safety and Health Administration mandated that needleless connectors be used in the clinical setting (Maragakis et al., 2006).

(1) Types of caps: Luer lock, needleless system cap, with or without positive

_____

_____

_____

_____

_____

_____

_____

_____

pressure feature, neutral caps, or antimicrobial coated with silver ions to help prevent microbial contamination

(2) Prior to accessing injection cap, cleanse it vigorously with appropriate cleansing agent (Moran & Camp-Sorrell, 2002). If povidone-iodine is used, it must be allowed to dry for at least two minutes. Controversy exists as to the best type of agent to use.

(3) Studies suggest that the use of a positive pressure device on the hub of a catheter may decrease the incidence of catheter-related thrombus by preventing retrograde flow of blood into the catheter lumen (Rummel, Donnelly, & Fortenbaugh, 2001; Yebenes et al., 2004). Other studies have revealed an increase in catheter-related bloodstream infections after using positive pressure caps (e.g., Maragakis et al., 2006). These authors recommend that infection-control programs carefully evaluate catheter-related infection rates to detect increases in occurrences.

(4) Studies suggest a potential increase in catheter-related infections with some needleless system caps. If a new system is implemented, catheter-related infection rates should be closely monitored. Nurses who use these systems should understand their mechanism and follow manufacturers' recommendations for proper flushing procedure (Hadaway, 2006; Maragakis et al., 2006).

(5) Change the cap every week or when any of the following occur.
   (a) The cap is removed to initiate an infusion or draw blood.
   (b) Blood cannot be completely flushed from the cap after blood withdrawal.
   (c) Signs of blood, precipitate, cracks, leaks, or other defects are noted.
   (d) The septum is no longer intact (e.g., after multiple uses with antibiotics).

e) Techniques for blood withdrawal
   (1) Discard method: This is the most commonly reported method used with the adult population. Blood is withdrawn and discarded prior to sample collection. Discard amounts reported vary from 3–10 ml, with 5–6 ml used most frequently (Adlard, 2008; Camp-Sorrell, 2007).

   (2) Reinfusion method: Instead of discarding the first collected sample, it is saved and reinfused into the patient at the end of sample collection. This method is used in the neonate and pediatric populations to prevent a decrease in blood volume. One study recommended that the discarded blood sample not be reinfused. In a small study of adults, clots were found in the discarded blood samples (Cosca et al., 1998).

   (3) Mixing method: Blood is withdrawn and immediately reinfused into the patient. This method is repeated four times without removing the syringe, and a sample is then taken. The purpose is to minimize blood loss. Studies found no significant errors in laboratory test results or increase in clots when compared to the discard method (Adlard, 2008; Barton, Chase, Latham, & Rayens, 2004).

   (4) Vacutainer method: This method involves inserting a vacutainer into the injection cap to reduce the risk of needlestick and blood contamination when transferring blood to tubes. Vacutainers used with some catheters, such as PICCs or valve catheters, may not yield a blood sample because the pressure may collapse the catheter.

   (5) Syringe method: A syringe is attached directly onto the catheter hub or needleless system, and blood is withdrawn into the syringe. This method may increase the risk of blood and specimen contamination because after blood collection, a needle is placed on the syringe to transfer blood to collection tubes.

   (6) If the VAD is connected to an infusion, discontinue all infusates for at

least one minute before withdrawing the blood sample. Clamp all lumens not being used for blood withdrawal on open-ended catheters.

(7) If laboratory values appear to be grossly inaccurate, redraw a blood sample from a peripheral vein (Bishop et al., 2007).

  (a) Blood coagulation studies should be drawn peripherally unless the catheter is maintained with normal saline, because heparin adheres to the internal catheter lumen and will alter the coagulation results. At some institutions, coagulation levels are drawn after other blood samples are obtained or after discarding 10 ml of blood; however, the literature does not support this practice.

  (b) Some drugs (e.g., aminoglycosides, cyclosporine, gentamicin) can adhere to the catheter wall, which may obscure drug serum level testing (Bishop et al., 2007; Boodhan, Maloney, & Dupuis, 2006). Consider drawing these drug levels peripherally.

f) Routine replacement of administration sets (Scales, 2008)

  (1) Replace IV administration sets every 96 hours (at least 7 days) or with catheter change, except for fluids that enhance microbial growth (i.e., lipids, total parenteral nutrition [TPN], which should be changed daily); this practice is strongly recommended unless catheter-related infection is suspected (CDC, in press; Scales, 2008).

  (2) IV administration sets changed at three days versus four to seven days in 428 low-risk patients (i.e., those not receiving TPN, blood products, or interleukin-2) had no difference in colonization rates (0.4% versus 0.5%) or catheter- or infusion-related bloodstream infections (Raad et al., 2001).

  (3) The only study found to address neutropenic patients reported no difference between IV administration sets changed at 48 versus 24 hours in terms of incidence of colonization or infusion-related septicemia (DeMoissac & Jensen, 1998).

  (4) Tubing used to administer lipids or TPN is replaced every 24 hours after initiation of therapy (CDC, in press).

(5) Tubing for blood and blood components should be changed when the transfusion is complete or every 12 hours.

g) Interventions to reduce the pain of IV insertion and port access should be considered, especially if they increase the chance of success. Interventions include topical anesthetics (see Table 3), injections, and nonpharmacologic techniques.

  (1) An order from a healthcare provider is needed for any pharmacologic interventions. Topical anesthetic may obscure the vein, and vasoconstriction and vasospasm have been associated with topical application.

  (2) Topical anesthetics include creams, patches, gels, and sprays (see Table 3). The majority of studies have been with pediatric populations and insertion of peripheral IVs with favorable response.

Table 3. Topical Anesthetics

Type	Application	Comments
Transdermal cream	Apply thick layer one to two hours prior to device access or IV insertion. Cover with transparent dressing. Remove cream completely, and cleanse site prior to insertion.	May cause localized blisters Small dose absorbed systemically
Transdermal patch	Apply 20–30 minutes prior to insertion.	May cause mild erythema and edema
Intradermal solution (i.e., 1% lidocaine without epinephrine)	With needle bevel up, gently insert needle intradermally above intended insertion site prior to insertion; instill a small amount of solution.	May cause discomfort with needle insertion Monitor for sensitivity to lidocaine.
Electrodes	Apply pads and connect to dose controller to release topical anesthesia in pads.	May cause skin irritation
Topical spray	Holding can several inches away from skin, spray a light mist onto skin and allow to dry prior to insertion.	May cause frostbite reaction

(a) EMLA® (lidocaine 2.5% and prilocaine 2.5%) cream (AstraZeneca, LP) and ELA-Max® (Ferndale Labs) cream significantly decrease pain from venipuncture and IV insertion.

    i. Apply 2.5 g to 4 × 4 cm area for puncture, cover with semipermeable transparent dressing for one to two hours, wipe off, and cleanse site as usual.

    ii. Cream may cause hypersensitivity, inadvertent systemic absorption after prolonged application, and erythema at site.

(b) Numby Stuff® (Iomed Clinical Systems) is a topical, noninvasive delivery system with results found to be superior to other agents.

    i. Iontocaine® (Iomed's brand of lidocaine HCI 2% with epinephrine 1:100,000 topical solution) is used to hydrate the electrode pad.

    ii. Electrode sites are prepared with alcohol skin preparations, and electrodes are applied. The Numby 900 dose controller is attached to the pads. Typical preset dose is 40 mA.

    iii. After delivering the selected current level, the controller automatically turns off. Electrodes are removed, and skin is prepared for device insertion.

(c) Ethyl chloride spray (Gebauer Co.) is a topical anesthetic skin refrigerant causing numbness and lasting only seconds. It may cause frostbite or skin ulceration and is very flammable. Frequent use to access a port on a weekly basis can be a cause of skin breakdown. Port erosion can result (Camp-Sorrell, 2004) (see Figure 1).

    i. Target area and spray three to seven seconds.

    ii. Effect lasts a few seconds to a minute.

(d) Intradermal 2% lidocaine (1–2 ml) injection has been found to be effective, but it may cause erythema at site, inadvertent intravascular injection, pain with injection, or hypersensitivity.

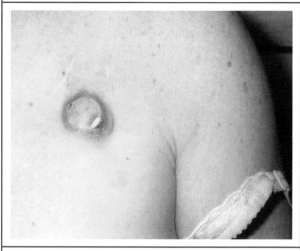

Figure 1. Skin Erosion With an Implanted Port

Note. From "Implanted Ports: Skin Erosion," by D. Camp-Sorrell, 2004, *Clinical Journal of Oncology Nursing, 8,* p. 309. Copyright 2004 by the Oncology Nursing Society. Reprinted with permission.

(e) Topical anesthetic patch (Synera® [70 mg lidocaine/70 mg tetracaine], ZARs, Inc.) has been found to be effective in reducing pain of IV insertion (Sethna et al., 2005).

    i. Transdermal patch (lidocaine 70 mg and tetracaine 70 mg) is applied to the insertion site. When removed from its storage pouch, the patch begins to heat from the heating element, warming the skin after application.

    ii. Patch is applied 20–30 minutes before insertion.

(f) Using music as a distraction can reduce the pain associated with insertion. Other complementary therapy methods, such as acupuncture and hypnosis, also have been suggested.

B. Peripheral IV catheters (short term)

  1. Description and types of catheters (Scales, 2008)

    a) A peripheral IV is used for a short time period (usually less than four days) and involves a short-length catheter (less than three inches) (CDC, in press).

    b) Catheters are defined by their gauge, length, and design.

      (1) Gauges range from 14–28 with single-lumen designs.

      (2) Lengths range from 5/8–2 inches.

(3) Some peripheral IVs are available with a longer stylet and with microbore extension tubing and hub attached. The longer stylet is removed, decreasing the risk of blood contamination or needlestick. Catheters are available with extension tubing attached with Y adapter.

c) Catheter material is made of silicone and polymers, including polyurethane, polyvinyl chloride, and flexane. Latex-free catheters also are available.

d) Specific types of peripheral infusion devices include the following.

(1) Steel-tipped, winged infusion (butterfly) needles

(2) Over-the-needle: Catheter sheath is externally located over the needle stylet.

(3) Through-the-needle: Catheter sheath is located inside the needle stylet.

(4) Needle protection: Shielded butterfly needles, stylet protective devices, and needleless IV access systems are available.

(5) Newer technology provides a closed IV catheter system with dual port extension tubing attached to permit solutions to be administered simultaneously.

(6) To reduce the risk of accidental needlestick injuries, active and passive safety devices have been developed on IV catheters (Lopez et al., 2009; Prunet et al., 2008). Passive safety catheters have an insertion typical of a standard catheter with a protective shield that automatically covers the needlepoint during its withdrawal from the catheter top without any intervention from the nurse inserting the catheter. Active safety requires pressing a button to trigger the withdrawal of the needle in a plastic sleeve using a spring.

(a) During a three-month period, Prunet et al. (2008) evaluated three peripheral catheters (nonsafety catheter, passive safety catheter, and an active safety catheter), examining a total of 759 catheter insertions.

(b) The numbers of failed insertions among the three types of catheters were similar. Insertion of the active safety catheter was found to be the most difficult and caused increased blood exposure to the staff. Needle withdrawal was more difficult with the passive safety catheter.

e) Peripheral IVs are available with radiopaque design.

f) Cost: Catheter is approximately $1–$2.50; insertion kits are available with supplies included at various costs. Example of insertion kit includes gloves, patient label, tape, chlorhexidine pad, 2 × 2 gauze, tourniquet, and transparent dressing for approximately $1.50–$5.

2. Advantages and disadvantages of using a peripheral IV (see Table 4)

3. Patient selection criteria (Polovich, Whitford, & Olsen, 2009; Scales, 2008)

a) Patient's age, in general, does not restrict use of peripheral IV.

b) Indications for peripheral IV include the following.

(1) With adequate vascular integrity, peripheral IVs are recommended for short-duration, nonirritating infusions of less than seven days, which may include antimicrobials, analgesics, blood components, fluid and electrolyte replacement, and nonvesicant chemotherapy. Drugs that cannot be given orally because the molecules are too large to be absorbed or because they are destroyed by digestion are conveniently given by IV.

(2) Peripheral IVs are best used for simple, one-time-use IV therapies, such as administering an IV push of a vesicant or nonvesicant chemotherapy, because the IV is inserted only at the time of therapy and usually is discontinued immediately after the procedure is complete. Sclerosing of veins can occur over time.

(3) Patients with a short life expectancy are candidates for peripheral IVs.

(4) Peripheral IVs are not indicated for continuous vesicant therapy or solutions with a pH less than 5 or greater than 9, or osmolarity greater than 600 mOsm/L.

(5) Using peripheral IVs for blood specimens has mixed recommendations.

(a) The use of peripheral IVs for obtaining blood samples continues to be debated (Prue-Owens, 2006). In general, peripheral IVs flushed with 0.9% normal saline are simple and safe for collecting blood samples, based on the accuracy of sample.

Table 4. Advantages and Disadvantages of Vascular Access Devices

Type of Line	Advantages	Disadvantages
Peripheral IV	• May be inserted by an RN • Can be easy to insert and maintain • Provides quick, simple access to vascular system • May be used in all patient care settings • Involves minimal insertion costs compared to other venous access procedures	• Has a short life span—approximately 72–96 hours (CDC, in press) • May involve discomfort with insertion • Can be difficult to insert and maintain in the very young, older adults, and those with fragile or sclerotic veins • Can be cumbersome and restrictive, especially when inserted near a joint or in a dominant limb • Requires daily care and maintenance • Peripheral vessels can quickly become irritated from infusions of blood components, concentrated dextrose solutions, chemotherapy, and parenteral medications, including antimicrobial agents and electrolyte infusions. • Less desirable access for infusions of vesicant agents (e.g., certain chemotherapy, calcium gluconate), electrolytes, and vasoconstrictors • Could be more costly if used long term, with repeated access, especially in home environment • Frequent site changes can exhaust all suitable peripheral veins.
Midline catheter	• Can be placed at the bedside by a specially trained nurse • Dwell time is one to eight weeks. • Chest x-ray is not required for placement because the tip is not in the central circulation. • Can be used for most IV solutions • Can be removed at the bedside • Relatively economical compared to more permanent lines • Fewer complications than surgically placed devices	• Cannot be used for continuous infusion of vesicants • Not recommended for routine blood draws • Size and flexible nature of the catheter may decrease the ability to draw blood. • Contraindicated for solutions with final concentrations greater than 10% glucose or greater than 5% protein • Patients must have adequate peripheral veins. • Not available as a triple lumen • May cause arm discomfort or immobility • More prone to phlebitis, which may be insertion technique–dependent
Nontunneled central venous line	• May be used to infuse all IV therapies and draw blood • May be inserted at the bedside or in ambulatory surgery using sterile technique • May be inserted without general anesthesia or procedural sedation • May be used to monitor central venous pressure • May be placed in an emergency situation and used immediately • Does not require needle access for use after insertion • Designed for short-term use (up to six weeks) • Available in a variety of gauges and in single, double, and triple lumens • Can be used for multiple, incompatible solutions concurrently (double and triple lumen) • Available antimicrobial-impregnated catheters may decrease risk of infection. • Heparin-impregnated catheters available may decrease risk of venous thrombosis • Catheter valve available, eliminating the need for heparin flush • Power lines available	• Must be placed by a physician. Some states may allow specially trained RNs to insert. • May be associated with discomfort at insertion • More prone to infection because of a lack of tunnel/cuff, the external portion, and insertion at bedside • Requires diligent aseptic care to prevent infection and maintain line function • Placement must be checked with x-ray prior to use. • Not used for long-term venous access • May not be suitable for testing of coagulation studies

(Continued on next page)

Table 4. Advantages and Disadvantages of Vascular Access Devices (Continued)

Type of Line	Advantages	Disadvantages
Peripherally inserted central catheter (PICC)	• May be used immediately after confirmed placement • May be inserted by an RN who has attended an instructional course and has demonstrated clinical competence in insertion technique • Insertion is relatively simple and may be performed at the bedside or in an outpatient setting. • Provides a safe, economical means of vascular access for therapies • Poses no risk of insertion-related pneumothorax or great vessel perforation • Demonstrates lower complication rate than other types of access devices if the device is inserted properly and is well maintained • Available in double or single lumen • Ideal for the very young and older adults because of the small size • Legitimate first choice for venous access in patients who are acutely or critically ill and who need intensive IV therapy and assurance of continuous venous access • Decreases stress exerted on the patient by the reducing number of venipunctures required to administer therapy • Excellent for use in homecare settings, as it decreases the need for unscheduled nursing visits related to site rotation or complications • May be used in all settings for the administration of a variety of IV therapies and to obtain blood samples • Less expensive than nontunneled short-term catheters, long-term catheters, or implanted ports • Power PICC available for contrast injections • Repair kits available	• RN requires educational preparation and attainment of clinical competence. • RN must maintain level of skill and competence. Clinical opportunities for insertion and maintenance of PICC must be available on a consistent basis. • May not be the access device of choice to meet a patient's special needs. PICC should be considered one of several available vascular access devices (VADs) from which to select. • May limit arm movement if inserted in the antecubital area • May not be able to draw blood with small-gauge catheters • Some manufacturers recommend not using 2 French size for red blood cell transfusion. • More expensive than peripheral IVs
Tunneled catheter	• Can be used immediately after placement once radiographic confirmation is made • Preserves peripheral veins • Provides a means for rapid hemodilution of infused solutions • Provides a reliable source of IV access • Designed for long-term IV therapy for frequent venous access and functional for years • Available in single, double, and triple lumens • Provides preattached clamps, except for valved catheters • Tunneling potentially decreases risk of microorganisms entering the venous system because of anatomical distance between insertion and exit sites. • Repair kits for external segments available for tunneled catheters • A variety of sizes available to accommodate pediatric and adult patients • Power lines available	• Requires routine exit-site care • Requires routine flushing of catheter lumens • Poses risk of complications, such as catheter-related infection and thrombosis • Cost of maintenance supplies includes dressings, flushing solutions, injection caps, syringes, and needles. • Body image changes can affect patient. • Insertion is a surgical procedure.

(Continued on next page)

Table 4. Advantages and Disadvantages of Vascular Access Devices *(Continued)*		
Type of Line	**Advantages**	**Disadvantages**
Implanted venous port	• Can be left in place and be functional for many years • Ideal for intermittent access • Less potential for infection than external catheters • No dressing required when the port is not accessed; therefore, ideal for patients with tape sensitivities • Flushing only required every four to eight weeks when not in use • Less potential for catheter to migrate • Can be used to draw blood • Has less effect on body image • Catheter infection may be successfully treated with IV antibiotics, although fungal infections generally require removal of the line (Vescia et al., 2008).	• Insertion is a surgical procedure. • Most expensive VAD to insert • Must be accessed with a needle • Catheter can disconnect from port and migrate, causing extravasation. • Presence of port may interfere with sleep • Over time, buildup of "sludge" (clotted blood, drug precipitates) may collect in port reservoir and decrease flow efficiency. • Requires a trained nurse to access and deaccess • Not available in triple lumen
Temporary apheresis or hemodialysis catheter	• Can be inserted at the bedside when immediate access is required • Can be used immediately after placement • Can be used for both inpatient and outpatient therapy (Exception: temporary femoral catheters usually are not used in outpatients.) • Can be used for IV infusion therapy	• Designed for short-term use • Requires catheter to be reguided frequently, such as every three to four days to every week • Increases incidence of catheter-related infection and sepsis • If inserted into femoral vein, cannot be used for hyperalimentation • Increased risk of catheter displacement because usually not sutured • Often restricted to use for hemodialysis or apheresis only
Tunneled apheresis or hemodialysis catheter	• Can be used immediately after placement • Can be used for both inpatient and outpatient short- or long-term therapy • Provides long-term access for apheresis or hemodialysis • Large internal diameter of catheter provides high flow rate. • Incidence of catheter-related infection is lower than with temporary catheters.	• Insertion is a surgical procedure. • Thrombosis is more likely with polyurethane catheter. • Catheter-related infection or sepsis can occur. • Poor flow may occur because of technique used for catheter placement and rigidity of catheter material, which causes kinking of lumens.

(b) Within certain limitations of infusate, peripheral IVs can be used for blood sampling for many routine tests, including coagulation studies, with reliable results (Prue-Owens, 2006).

(c) No definitive guidelines exist on blood sampling from peripheral IVs; research still needs to be done in this area. Additionally, weighing the benefits and risks of safety, costs, and comfort to the patient may aid in decision making.

c) Vein selection (see Figure 2)

(1) The vein selected should be based on the type of fluid to be infused and the rate and duration of infusion. Ideally, it should not interfere with the patient's comfort or mobility.

(2) Preferred sites

(a) Upper extremity veins in adults; these may include the superficial dorsal and metacarpal veins on the dorsum of the hand as well as the cephalic and basilic veins, and cephalic, basilic, and median veins on the upper arm (see Figure 2).

(b) Hand veins have a lower risk of phlebitis than veins on the wrist or upper arm (CDC, in press; Morris & Tay, 2008).

(c) Select the most distal site possible, but proximal to previous venipuncture.

(3) Sites to avoid (Gabriel, 2008; Morris & Tay, 2008)

    (a) Avoid extremities/sites that have impaired circulation or injury, such as those with lymphedema, postoperative swelling, recent trauma, hematoma, axillary lymph node dissection, local infection, phlebitis, decreased sensation or paresthesia, or open wounds; also avoid extremities where venipuncture has been performed within the last 24 hours, if possible.

    (b) Lower extremities are associated with higher risk of infection than are upper extremities (CDC, in press) and are more likely to develop thrombophlebitis. A physician order is recommended when using a lower extremity, but more importantly, nurses should consult with a physician regarding central line placement or other alternatives prior to using the lower extremity. Replace the lower-extremity IV catheter as soon as it is feasible (CDC, in press).

    (c) Skin changes and changes in the integrity of the vein lumen associated with radiation, prior chemotherapy, or prior IV therapy can make catheter insertion or site care difficult.

    (d) Antecubital veins are not recommended because of the difficulty of detecting infiltration and because they are located on an area of flexion. In an emergency situation, the use of this large vein may be appropriate (Scales, 2008).

    (e) Avoid placing the cannula over a joint such as the wrist or elbow be-

---

Figure 2. Peripheral Venous Anatomy

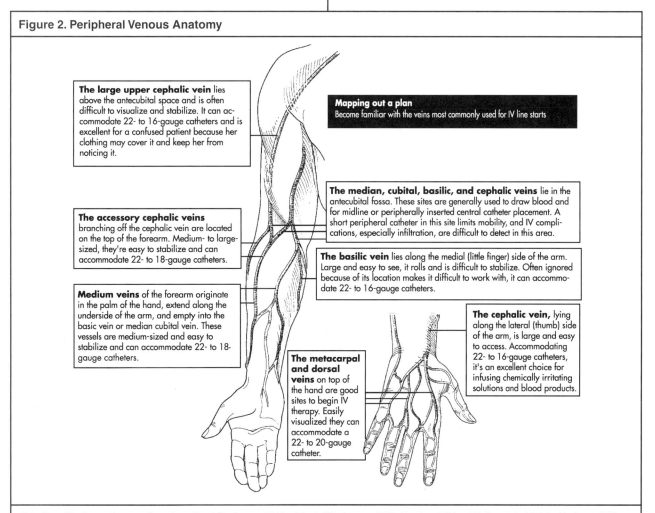

Mapping out a plan
Become familiar with the veins most commonly used for IV line starts

The large upper cephalic vein lies above the antecubital space and is often difficult to visualize and stabilize. It can accommodate 22- to 16-gauge catheters and is excellent for a confused patient because her clothing may cover it and keep her from noticing it.

The accessory cephalic veins branching off the cephalic vein are located on the top of the forearm. Medium- to large-sized, they're easy to stabilize and can accommodate 22- to 18-gauge catheters.

Medium veins of the forearm originate in the palm of the hand, extend along the underside of the arm, and empty into the basic vein or median cubital vein. These vessels are medium-sized and easy to stabilize and can accommodate 22- to 18-gauge catheters.

The median, cubital, basilic, and cephalic veins lie in the antecubital fossa. These sites are generally used to draw blood and for midline or peripherally inserted central catheter placement. A short peripheral catheter in this site limits mobility, and IV complications, especially infiltration, are difficult to detect in this area.

The basilic vein lies along the medial (little finger) side of the arm. Large and easy to see, it rolls and is difficult to stabilize. Often ignored because of its location makes it difficult to work with, it can accommodate 22- to 16-gauge catheters.

The cephalic vein, lying along the lateral (thumb) side of the arm, is large and easy to access. Accommodating 22- to 16-gauge catheters, it's an excellent choice for infusing chemically irritating solutions and blood products.

The metacarpal and dorsal veins on top of the hand are good sites to begin IV therapy. Easily visualized they can accommodate a 22- to 20-gauge catheter.

Note. From "An Expert Answers Questions About Starting an I.V. Line," by A. Ellenberger, 1999, *Nursing, 29*(3), p. 57. Copyright 1999 by Lippincott Williams & Wilkins. Reprinted with permission.

cause the movement of the joint may produce mechanical phlebitis and increase kinking of the catheter (Scales, 2008).

 (f) If possible, avoid venipuncture or IV insertion on extremities of a mastectomy site (Poage, Singer, Armer, Poundall, & Shellabarger, 2008).

d) Catheter or device selection (Scales, 2008)

 (1) Use the smallest-gauge device and shortest length that will successfully deliver the prescribed therapy at the desired rate.

 (2) Select catheter based on intended purpose, expected length of therapy, viscosity of fluid, fluid components, and condition of vein.

 (3) Avoid use of steel needles for administration of fluids and medications that may cause tissue necrosis if extravasation occurs (CDC, in press); limit use of steel needles to short-term or single-dose administration or one-time infusion and IV push only.

 (4) Considerations for gauge selection include the following (Scales, 2008).

  (a) 16–18 gauge for major surgery

  (b) 18–20 gauge for rapid infusion of IV fluids, blood components, or viscous medications

  (c) 20 gauge for most IV applications and for blood products

  (d) 22–24 gauge with ¾-inch catheter for older adult and pediatric patients. Short length and small gauge is less traumatizing, reduces irritation, and permits better blood flow; 24 gauge can infuse up to 250 ml of fluid per hour.

 (5) Obese patients with veins deep in the SC tissue may need slightly longer peripheral IV catheters, or a PICC may be considered as the catheter of choice.

 (6) Risk of chemical phlebitis (irritation of the vein wall by medications) is reduced with good blood flow past the cannula to disperse the drug into the bloodstream.

4. Overview of insertion techniques (Gabriel, 2008; Morris & Tay, 2008; Scales, 2008)

 a) Perform patient assessment and preparation before the procedure; consider any special needs regarding age, physical condition, or type of fluid being infused. Explain the insertion procedure to the patient, and answer any questions the patient and significant others may have.

 (1) Older patients have fragile veins and less SC support tissue because of thinning of the skin.

 (2) Use minimal tourniquet pressure over clothing or no tourniquet with older adults. Venous distention may take longer because of slower venous return.

 (3) Children's veins are smaller in diameter and may be covered by a layer of SC fat, which can make veins difficult to access.

 (4) Access sites for infants and toddlers may include the scalp and feet. Older children usually use the hands and arms.

 b) Consider interventions to reduce the pain of IV insertion, especially if they increase the chance of success. Interventions include topical anesthetics, injections, and nonpharmacologic techniques.

 (1) An order from a healthcare provider is needed for any pharmacologic intervention.

 (2) Topical anesthetics include creams, patches, gels, and sprays (see Table 3).

 (3) Dry heat has been found to be successful in IV insertion when compared to moist heat (Fink et al., 2009). Dry heated towels were used to wrap the upper extremity in a sample of 136 patients with hematologic cancer. Dry heat was more likely than moist heat to result in successful IV insertion on the first attempt and was more comfortable.

 c) Wash hands: Good hand hygiene and standard precautions are used for insertion and IV maintenance; a new pair of disposable, nonsterile gloves are used in conjunction with a "no-touch" technique for peripheral IV insertion.

 (1) With no-touch technique, the planned IV insertion site is not palpated after skin cleansing, unless sterile gloves are worn.

 (2) Aseptic no-touch technique aims to prevent microorganisms on hands, surfaces, or equipment from being introduced to the IV insertion site.

 (3) Wash hands before and after IV catheter insertion and dressing change (CDC, in press).

d) Organize equipment (see Appendix 2 for peripheral IV clinical practicum).

    (1) Prepare IV fluid, attach administration set, and prime if peripheral IV is to be connected to continuous fluids.

    (2) If using peripheral IV for bolus medication administration, prepare IV medication and check for accuracy.

    (3) If using peripheral IV as a saline lock, obtain protective cap and normal saline flush.

e) Examine veins on both extremities by visual inspection and palpation, keeping in mind the purpose of the IV therapy and any physical limitations of the patient, such as a stroke limiting the use of an arm or the side of an axillary node dissection. Assess distal veins, and then move proximally.

    (1) The Vein Entry Indicator Device (VEID™, Vascular Technologies) has been used with success in infants and children who can be technically challenging with small vein size (Simhi, Kachko, Bruckheimer, & Katz, 2008). VEID attaches to the distal end of an IV cannula with a standard Luer connection. An audible sound indicates when the needle penetrates the blood vessel, which reduces the risk of going through the vein.

    (2) Other techniques used to locate and insert a peripheral IV include ultrasound guidance, which requires special training.

f) Place tourniquet 5–6 inches above insertion site. Tourniquet should obstruct the venous flow, not the arterial flow. Check presence of distal pulse, and if not felt, loosen the tourniquet. Tourniquets are for single use.

    (1) Select site. To assist in palpating a vein lightly, tap the vein, apply local warming, or have the patient hang arm downward (Simhi et al., 2008).

    (2) Remove tourniquet for patient's comfort.

    (3) If a large amount of body hair is present at the insertion site, clip the area. Avoid shaving, which can increase irritation and risk of infection (INS, 2006).

g) Select appropriate IV needle or catheter. Administer local anesthetic as needed (see Table 3).

h) Cleanse site and allow it to dry before inserting catheter (see Table 2). Chlorhexi-dine 2% is recommended for skin cleansing prior to IV insertion (Morris & Tay, 2008; Pratt et al., 2007). If patient is known to have an allergy to chlorhexidine, 70% alcohol or povidone-iodine can be used. Allow to dry before inserting the catheter.

i) Reapply tourniquet, and put on disposable gloves.

j) Perform venipuncture. Insert needle at 15°–30° angle with bevel up distal to actual site of venipuncture.

k) Look for blood return through tubing of butterfly needle or catheter, which indicates that needle has entered the vein. A butterfly needle may be taped in place at this time or threaded into the vein. An IV catheter should be threaded in its entirety into the vein and the stylet removed.

l) Release tourniquet, and attach catheter to infusion set or syringe.

m) Flush the catheter free of blood while holding the IV catheter or needle in place. Watch insertion site during initial flush to assess the integrity of the vein. Edema or pain/discomfort at the site indicates an infiltration or ruptured vein. If this occurs, remove the IV and restart it elsewhere.

    (1) If the IV must be restarted, use the other extremity or select a site proximal to the previous venipuncture.

    (2) When administering a vesicant chemotherapy agent, select a site on the opposite extremity, if possible.

n) Secure IV catheter or needle with tape or a securement or stabilization device, and apply occlusive dressing over the insertion site. Do not put tape directly over the insertion site (Frey & Schears, 2006).

    (1) Use of transparent, semipermeable dressings is recommended and results in significantly fewer dislodged catheters, with a trend toward reduced phlebitis and infiltration compared to gauze dressings.

    (2) StatLock, a securement device, significantly reduced dislodgment episodes and increased dwell times of peripheral IVs.

        (a) Three securement methods were evaluated to determine which method could extend the average peripheral IV time.

        (b) The study demonstrated the following methods to secure the catheter: nonsterile tape, which resulted in a peripheral short catheter

survival rate of 8%; HubGuard®
(Centurion Medical Products),
which resulted in a 9% rate; and
StatLock, which resulted in a 52%
rate (Smith, 2006).

(c) Other securement devices are
available (Frey & Schears, 2006;
Smith, 2006).

(3) For extremely short dwell times, less
than 30 minutes during a procedure,
micropore tape could be used, but it
should be clean and not in contact with
the insertion site.

o) No more than two attempts at cannulation
per nurse per patient should be done to
avoid unnecessary trauma to the patient. If
possible, use the opposite arm to select a
vein. If not possible, select a site proximal
to the first venipuncture (INS, 2006; Lavery
& Smith, 2007; Polovich et al., 2009).

p) Document the number of attempts, location, type of catheter, gauge of catheter,
dressing type, securement, and patient's
response after procedure is completed.

5. Removal technique: Change peripheral catheter every 72–96 hours or earlier for signs of
phlebitis or infiltration (CDC, in press; Gabriel, 2008; Lavery & Smith, 2007; Scales, 2008).
Catheter should be removed when no longer
required for therapy.

a) Verify order for removal and indication.
b) Explain procedure to patient.
c) Place patient in chair or bed to stabilize extremity.
d) Inspect general condition of catheter pathway.
e) Discontinue all infusions into the device.
f) Put on gloves; remove dressing; and observe site for any pain, edema, redness, or
discharge.
g) Change gloves; pull catheter out in the same
angle of insertion while stabilizing the skin
and vein with sterile gauze.

h) If removal of catheter is indicated for infection, send catheter tip for culture per order (INS, 2006).

i) Apply constant, firm pressure to exit site
until bleeding stops (longer in patients with
coagulopathies or on anticoagulants). Apply dressing or adhesive bandage, and monitor as necessary.

j) Instruct patient/caregiver to report any discomfort or signs of bleeding, bruising, redness, swelling, or drainage.

k) Inspect device for defects. Report any defects to the manufacturer and regulatory
agencies. Examine distal tip for signs of
jagged, uneven edges suggestive of breakage.

l) Document observations and actions.

6. Maintenance and care (ASHP Commission on
Therapeutics, 2006; CDC, in press; Gabriel,
2008; Prue-Owens, 2006; Scales, 2008) (see
Table 1 for common maintenance procedures)

a) Inspect catheter insertion site and palpate for
tenderness daily through the intact dressing
(CDC, in press). Manipulation of the catheter should be kept to a minimum to prevent mechanical phlebitis (Scales, 2008).

b) All catheters inserted under emergency conditions are replaced within 48 hours when
adherence to aseptic technique cannot be
ensured (CDC, in press).

c) Routine replacement of catheters: A new
catheter is placed in another site, and old
catheter is removed.

(1) Replacement of peripheral IV catheters
every 72–96 hours is strongly recommended to prevent phlebitis and catheter-related infections, as well as patient discomfort. This recommenda-
tion is based on experimental, clinical,
or epidemiologic studies with a strong
theoretical rationale (CDC, in press).

(2) Although the incidence of thrombophlebitis and bacterial colonization of
catheters has been reported to increase
when catheters are left in place for more
than 72 hours (CDC, in press), several studies have shown no difference
in complication rates with extended
dwell times.

(a) In a study of the use of 665 catheters in 451 patients, the rate of phlebitis was 19.7% without a demonstrated increased risk for catheters
remaining in place after three days
(Bregenzer, Conen, Sakmann, &
Widmer, 1998).

(b) In a study of 722 patients, restarting the IV after 72 hours did not reduce the risk of complications when compared to continuing the original catheter (Homer & Holmes, 1998).

(c) No difference in phlebitis rates was shown for dwell times of 72 hours versus 96 hours in a study involving 2,503 catheters (3.3% and 2.6%, respectively) (Lai, 1998).

(d) When 34 catheters were left in place for more than 72 hours (73–120 hours), no phlebitis was detected (White, 2001).

(e) Of 1,161 catheters examined in another study, the overall phlebitis rate was 3.7%. It was recommended that if phlebitis is not present at 72 hours, continued assessment of the site may be more cost-effective and cause less discomfort for the patient than restarting the peripheral IV (Powell, Tarnow, & Perucca, 2008).

d) Dressing: Change transparent dressing when catheter is changed providing the dressing is intact, clean, and dry. Change gauze and tape dressing every two days or as needed if wet, soiled, or nonocclusive. Dressing changes require an aseptic no-touch technique.

e) Flushing: 0.9% normal saline 1–3 ml every 8, 12, or 24 hours when device is not in use to maintain patency (ASHP Commission on Therapeutics, 2006)

f) All devices added onto the catheter should be Luer lock, including needleless connectors, stopcocks, short extensions, filters, injection caps, and multisite connectors.

(1) Connections should be used only when necessary, as these are entry portals for infection.

(2) Devices should be changed when IV catheter is changed or when no longer intact.

(3) All IVs and equipment should be labeled with date and time to serve as a reminder of the need to change.

(4) Needleless connectors allow for IV administration without the use of a needle, thus reducing the risk of needlestick. These devices also ensure the IV system remains closed. These devices can be left in place until the catheter is changed (Scales, 2008).

g) Blood specimens: Blood discard of 0.5–1 ml; obtain specimen and flush with 3 ml of normal saline. With different brands of peripheral IVs, saline locks, and extension sets, standardization of the amount of blood discard and flush is difficult. Prior to policy development, the dead space volume of the products used must be known.

h) Bolus injections: Cleanse injection cap, allow solution to dry, infuse over a short period of time (usually 3–5 minutes), and flush with 1–3 ml of normal saline.

i) Intermittent infusions: Used for drugs that require dilution or slow administration. Cleanse injection cap, allow solution to dry, infuse over specified time, and flush with 1–3 ml of normal saline.

j) Continuous infusions: Most common method of administering IV fluids, drugs, and IV nutrition

7. Complications (Lavery & Smith, 2007; Polovich et al., 2009)

a) Insertion complications include bleeding, vein injury, nerve injury, infiltration, phlebitis, and thrombosis.

b) Risk of vein injury from catheters can result in pain, tenderness, edema, redness (vasodilation), thrombosis, sclerosis, and infiltration.

c) Prevention of the most common complication, phlebitis, is related to having sufficient vessel size to accommodate the catheter and allow hemodilution, having a nontraumatic insertion, and infusing nonirritating solutions.

(1) Phlebitis most commonly occurs with prolonged dwell time and from mechanical or chemical irritation; risk increases with age and with irritating infusates (Powell et al., 2008; Scales, 2008).

(2) Signs and symptoms are pain, erythema, and edema.

(3) Older patients may not experience pain from phlebitis or infiltration because of a decrease in sensory perception; monitoring for complications through observation is important.

d) Infiltration is a common complication.

(1) Signs and symptoms include leaking fluid around insertion site, cool and pale skin, possibly decreased infusion rate, and skin tightness or discomfort.

(2) Assess for infiltration by occluding the vessel at the tip of the catheter with

digital pressure. If the infusion continues, the fluid is probably infiltrating.

(3) Use of appropriately sized syringes will prevent vein rupture or infiltration with IV push administration or a vacuum on blood aspiration.

  (a) The larger the syringe, the less pressure is generated when force is applied; the larger the syringe, the more force is required to create a vacuum. Thus, less force is generated in either infusion or aspiration with larger syringes, thereby reducing or preventing complications.

  (b) A 1 ml syringe is not recommended for use with peripheral IV catheters. A 3 ml size is recommended for all flushing and administration of medications.

e) Infection

(1) Infection can occur through a peripheral IV by the external catheter upon insertion, the interior of the catheter, contamination of connectors, or repalpation of a proposed puncture site prior to IV insertion or by contaminated infusion (Lopez et al., 2009; Morris & Tay, 2008).

(2) Peripheral IVs rarely are associated with bloodstream infections.

(3) The reported rate of bloodstream infections attributed to peripheral IVs is 0.5% per 1,000 catheter days (Maki, Kluger, & Crnich, 2006).

(4) Use strict aseptic technique for insertion and maintenance care.

8. For a practicum on peripheral IV insertion and care, see Appendix 2.

9. Education and documentation (see Section X)

C. Midline catheters

1. Description and types

a) Catheter material: Silicone or polyurethane (Hadaway, 2010)

b) Available as radiopaque, latex free, or with closed-valve tip

c) Available in single and double lumens

d) Range from 2 Fr (23 gauge) to 6 Fr (18 gauge)

e) Range from 3–8 inches in length

f) Prime volume of 0.5–1.5 ml

g) Considered a peripheral line because the tip is not located in the central circulation

h) Considered a midline when the catheter terminates at the axillary vein in the up-

per arm (Gallieni et al., 2008; Polovich et al., 2009)

  i) Approximate cost: $75

2. Advantages and disadvantages: See Table 4.

3. Patient selection criteria

a) Patients with limited peripheral veins for venous access

b) Patients with need for venous access for a limited length of time (one to four weeks)

c) Patient or caregiver is willing and able to understand and follow instructions on how to properly care for the device in the home setting.

d) IV therapy planned is appropriate for midline catheter. Contraindicated IV fluids include (Perucca, 2010)

(1) Continuous infusion of vesicants

(2) Solutions with glucose concentration greater than 10%

(3) Solutions with protein concentration greater than 5%

(4) Solutions with osmolarity greater than 600.

e) Patient preference for this type of device over more permanent devices

f) Limited life expectancy of the patient

g) For patients scheduled to receive IV therapy for more than a week, a plan should be followed to maximize comfort and preserve the integrity of the veins.

h) An extremity affected by a mastectomy, lymph node dissection, or lymphedema is not appropriate for midline catheter insertion (Hadaway, 2010).

4. Insertion technique

a) Insert in an antecubital vein terminating in the upper arm or axilla (see Figure 2). Appropriate veins include

(1) Basilic

(2) Cephalic

(3) Median cubital.

b) Determine if the patient is a suitable candidate for a midline catheter based on patient selection criteria and patient's willingness to care for and protect a catheter.

c) Explain the procedure to the patient and answer any questions the patient or significant others may have.

d) Organize equipment and wash hands.

e) Examine veins on both extremities, taking into account the purpose of the IV therapy, the most comfortable exit site for the patient, and any physical limitations the patient may have, such as stroke or lymphedema, that could limit the use of one arm.

f) Use local anesthetic (topical, injectable) per institutional policy and patient preference. Be aware that anesthetic may obscure the vein secondary to vasoconstriction and vasospasm. An order from a healthcare provider is needed (see Table 3).

g) Place the line per manufacturer's guidelines for the type of catheter being used; the nurse inserting should be trained for the individual product.

h) Anticipate insertion site to be 1–1.5 inches above or below antecubital fossa. Extend patient's arm, and abduct the arm at a 45° angle.

i) Place tourniquet 5–6 inches above insertion site at the mid-upper arm area. Tourniquet should obstruct venous, not arterial, flow. Check presence of distal pulse. Remove tourniquet for patient's comfort.

j) Clip the area if a large amount of body hair is present at insertion site. Avoid shaving, which can cause increased irritation and risk of infection.

k) Cleanse site, and allow to dry. Reapply tourniquet. Apply sterile gloves. Drape arm with sterile drapes for sterile field. Flush catheter with 0.9% sodium chloride solution.

l) Stabilize vein below access site with nondominant hand. Perform venipuncture by inserting needle at a 15°–30° angle with bevel up distal to actual venipuncture site.

m) Look for blood return through tubing of catheter, which indicates that the needle has entered the vein. Advance to length of needle, and remove tourniquet.

n) Once venipuncture is complete, retract the needle into the needle safety tube on the external end of the catheter. The tip of the catheter is advanced slowly for several inches to the desired initial length through the introducer. Remove guidewire slowly while stabilizing midline catheter at insertion site. Remove introducer, and break away or peel away from catheter by pulling apart at wings. Flush with normal saline.

o) Secure IV catheter with tape, stabilizing device, or securement device, and apply dressing over insertion site.

p) The dressing should be changed 24 hours after insertion to assess for complications, and then per protocol for transparent film or gauze dressing.

q) Because a midline catheter is not considered a central catheter, x-ray verification of tip placement is not indicated.

r) Document insertion, including type of line used, length of catheter, and patient tolerance.

5. Removal technique
   a) Verify order for removal and indication.
   b) Explain the procedure to the patient and answer questions.
   c) Place the patient in a reclining position.
   d) Inspect the general condition of the catheter.
   e) Discontinue all infusions into the device.
   f) Put on gloves, remove dressing, and observe site for redness, swelling, bruising, or drainage.
   g) If drainage is present, send swabs for culture with provider order.
   h) Change gloves.
   i) Grasping device by the hub, pull slowly and steadily until completely removed from patient.
   j) If infection is suspected, send catheter tip for culture.
   k) Apply constant firm pressure to the exit site until the bleeding has stopped (longer in patients with coagulopathies or decreased platelet count). Apply sterile occlusive dressing, and monitor for bleeding or drainage.
   l) Measure catheter for appropriate length and catheter integrity. Examine distal tip for jagged edges that would suggest breakage. If found, report to physician.
   m) Document length of catheter on removal, action, and patient response.

6. Maintenance and care (see Table 1) (Gorski & Czaplewski, 2004)
   a) Dwell time: One to eight weeks
   b) Dressing: Transparent dressing changed every seven days. Gauze and tape dressing changed every two days or as needed if wet, soiled, or nonocclusive.
   c) Flushing: Normal saline 1–3 ml every 8, 12, or 24 hours

d) Cap change: Every week or with catheter change

e) If the catheter is used for blood draw: Discard 0.5–1 ml of blood, obtain specimen, and flush with 3 ml normal saline.

7. Complications: See Sections II.B and II.I.

8. Education and documentation: See Section X.

9. Special considerations for pediatrics

a) Available in 24- and 22-gauge sizes

b) Lengths range from 3–6 inches.

c) Patients who need venous access for a limited length of time (approximately one to eight weeks)

d) Appropriate for administration of IV fluids, blood products, and medications

e) Midline catheter insertion sites include the basilic and cephalic vein in the upper extremity, the saphenous and femoral vein in the leg with the tip below the groin and away from flexion areas, and the temporal scalp vein or the external jugular.

10. Special consideration for older adults (Moureau, 2008): Avoid tourniquet use in older adults with fragile veins and thin skin.

D. Nontunneled central venous lines

1. Description and types

a) Catheter material: Silicone or polyurethane

b) Available options: Latex free, radiopaque, antimicrobial impregnated, and heparin impregnated (Gallieni et al., 2008)

c) Range from 14–24 gauge in single-lumen and multilumen designs

d) Distal tip openings are open or valved (Groshong-type).

e) Distal tip openings on multilumen catheters may be side-by-side or staggered.

f) Power line available to allow for power injection of contrast media at an infusion rate of 5 ml/s.

2. Advantages and disadvantages: See Table 4.

3. Patient selection criteria

a) Size of patient/vein may determine the gauge of catheter and number of lumens used. Catheters of the smallest gauge necessary for indicated therapy should be placed to decrease the incidence of venous thrombosis (Gallieni et al., 2008).

b) Patients receiving short-term treatment (up to six weeks) with no need for extended therapy anticipated (Gabriel, 2008)

c) Patients with poor peripheral venous access

d) Patients who require treatment with fluids that are hyperosmolar, alkaline, or acidic (Gabriel, 2008)

e) Patients who require frequent venous access for infusion or blood specimens

f) Poor surgical candidates for long-term catheter placement

g) Critically ill patients requiring multilumen access or central venous pressure monitoring (Gabriel, 2008)

4. Insertion location (see Figure 3). Healthcare professionals specifically trained can insert. Refer to individual state board of nursing for regulations.

a) Preferentially, use the right internal jugular vein as the entry site because it follows a fairly straight course to the subclavian. A triangle of landmarks (clavicle and the two heads of the sternocleidomastoid muscle) identifies the insertion site.

b) Cannulate the subclavian vein on the left side, if possible, because it has a smooth curve to the superior vena cava without an acute turn.

c) If the right internal jugular is not available, the left internal jugular, the external jugular, or the subclavian veins may be used (Weigand & Carlson, 2005). The following conditions may require use of the affected side, or even femoral placement of the central venous catheter (Gabriel, 2008).

   (1) Enlarged axillary or subclavian nodes

   (2) Tumor mass

   (3) Previous surgery or radiotherapy to the axillary or subclavian area

   (4) History of previous thrombosis

   (5) Presence of cardiac pacemaker

d) Femoral insertion with the tip in the inferior vena cava is possible but has an increased risk of infection and thrombotic complications (Marschall et al., 2008).

5. Insertion techniques (Marschall et al., 2008; Weigand & Carlson, 2005)

a) Perform a preplacement assessment of the patient to determine if a nontunneled catheter is appropriate, based on patient selection criteria.

b) Explain the insertion procedure to the patient and answer any questions the patient or significant others may have. Ensure that informed consent is obtained. Determine if the patient has allergies to iodine or tape products, and inform the practitioner placing the line.

c) Position the patient

   (1) Usually, the patient is placed in a 15°–25° Trendelenburg position, which distends the vein selected for cannula-

Figure 3. Venous Anatomy

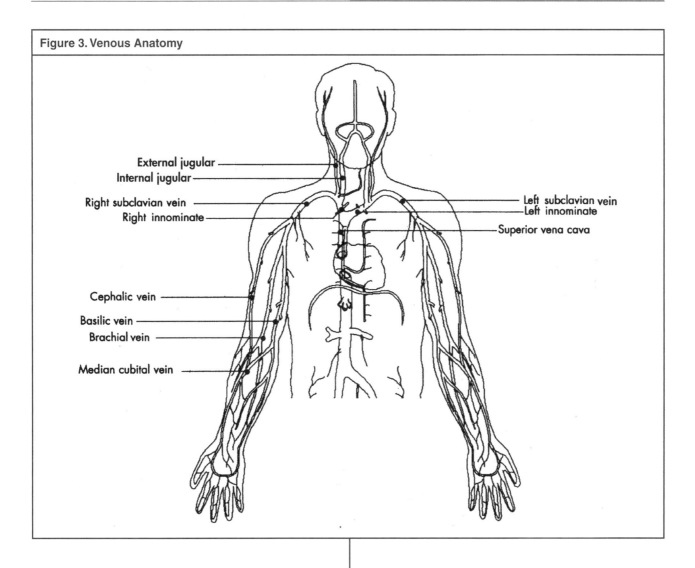

External jugular

Internal jugular

Right subclavian vein

Right innominate

Left subclavian vein

Left innominate

Superior vena cava

Cephalic vein

Basilic vein

Brachial vein

Median cubital vein

tion and decreases the risk of air embolism.

  (2) If the internal jugular is to be used, the patient's head should be turned to the opposite side of the catheterization to decrease contamination and make the site more accessible.

  (3) A rolled towel may be placed beneath the patient's neck and shoulders to increase venous distention.

d) Use of maximal sterile barrier precautions, including mask, cap, sterile gown, and sterile gloves, by all practitioners involved with the insertion procedure and draping of the patient with a large drape are essential to reduce infection risk.

e) Prepare the insertion site with a chlorhexidine-based cleansing agent, provided the patient is older than two months of age (see Table 2) (Marschall et al., 2008). If necessary, clip (do not shave) long hair to decrease contamination.

f) Use local anesthetic to decrease insertion discomfort (see Table 3).

g) Use of ultrasound guidance for cannulation has been shown to reduce complications, the number of failed attempts, and the time required for insertion (Gallieni et al., 2008; Hind et al., 2003). Insert needle percutaneously into the vein with a stylet and guidewire, using the clavicle as a guide.

  (1) When a flashback is observed in the syringe, the syringe is removed, and a guidewire is advanced into the vein. The guidewire should not be advanced farther than 18 cm in order to minimize complications.

  (2) The catheter is advanced over the guidewire into the subclavian vein until it reaches the superior vena cava.

  (3) The guidewire is removed.

h) Flush each lumen with saline.

i) Avoid suturing; secure catheter with tape, securement device, or stabilization device, and then apply an occlusive dressing over the exit site (CDC, in press).

    (1) SecurAcath™ (Interrad Medical) utilizes a very small anchor that deploys under the skin to hold catheter in place.

    (2) Newer method for holding nontunneled catheters in place without suturing

  j) Obtain radiographic confirmation before therapy is initiated to determine proper placement and location of the tip, and to detect pneumothorax, although there is a low incidence of complications following subclavian or nontunneled central line placement (Gabriel, 2008). Tip placement should be in the distal third of the superior vena cava.

  k) Allow a healthcare provider to verify the proper position in the superior vena cava; then the line may be used immediately for infusion.

  l) Document length of catheter, presence of blood return, and condition of patient.

6. Removal of device

  a) Nontunneled lines are removed when therapy is completed, when the line is no longer functional because of thrombus or mechanical failures, or when the line is infected.

  b) Routine replacement of a nontunneled central catheter should not be performed (CDC, in press).

  c) Verify order for removal and indication.

  d) Note the length of the catheter on insertion.

  e) Explain the procedure to patient.

  f) Place patient in a reclining position.

  g) Inspect the general condition of the catheter.

  h) Discontinue all infusions into the device.

  i) Put on gloves, remove dressing, and inspect exit site for redness, pain, swelling, exudate, or other problems.

  j) Change gloves and remove sutures, if present.

  k) Have patient perform Valsalva maneuver (Weigand & Carlson, 2005). Performing the Valsalva maneuver decreases the risk of air embolism during catheter removal. The maneuver is contraindicated in patients with increased intracranial pressure and those who are intubated.

    (1) Instruct patient to take a deep breath and hold it.

    (2) Patient should "bear down" for 10 seconds.

    (3) Patient then exhales.

  l) Grasp the hub of the nontunneled catheter, and gently and steadily retract catheter until completely removed from patient.

  m) Apply constant, firm pressure to the exit site until bleeding stops (longer in patients with coagulopathies or decreased platelet count). Apply sterile, occlusive dressing, and monitor patient for discomfort, bleeding, bruising, redness, swelling, or drainage. Advise patient and family to report any of these signs.

  n) Visually inspect VAD for appropriate length and defects, such as holes, tears, or jagged edges suggesting breakage. If length is shorter than expected or the edges appear broken, notify the physician.

  o) Document observations, actions, and patient teaching.

7. Maintenance and care (see Table 1)

  a) Dwell time: Short-term catheters, approximately up to six weeks

  b) Dressing: Dressing changed 24 hours after insertion

    (1) Transparent dressing changed every five to seven days

    (2) Gauze and tape dressing changed every two days or as needed if wet, soiled, or nonocclusive

  c) Flushing: Heparin 10–100 IU/ml: 2–3 ml/day per each lumen. May heparin lock after use for intermittent infusions after flushing with normal saline.

  d) Cap change: Every week or if no longer intact

  e) For blood specimens: Discard 1–2 ml of blood; flush with 10–20 ml of normal saline.

8. Complications (see Section II.I): Potential complications related to central line removal include venous air embolism, dyspnea, pain, bleeding from the insertion site, and arrhythmias (Weigand & Carlson, 2005).

9. Education and documentation: See Section X.

10. For a practicum on short-term venous catheter care, see Appendix 3.

E. PICCs
1. Description and types (Hagle, 2007)
   a) Catheter material: Silicone, polyurethane, or elastomeric hydrogel
   b) Range from 16–28 gauge in single- and double-lumen designs; pediatric sizes range from 24–28 gauge in single- and double-lumen designs.
   c) Lengths range from 15–27 inches.
   d) Prime volume of 0.5–1.5 ml
   e) PowerPICC® (C.R. Bard, Inc.) catheters are now available for the delivery of power injection flow rates required for contrast-enhanced injections.
   f) PICCs are available with PASV on 3 Fr catheters.
   g) Radiopaque is available for PICCs.
   h) Cost: Approximately $714–$985, excluding cost of radiology confirmation
2. Advantages and disadvantages: See Table 4.
3. Patient selection criteria (Gallieni et al., 2008; Hagle, 2007)
   a) Patients without accessible peripheral vessels or with a minimal number of adequate vessels available for use in the administration of therapy for moderate duration (three to six months); however, the FDA has approved the use of PICCs for up to 12 months (Gallieni et al., 2008). There is no established dwell time (the maximum expected duration considered appropriate for a given type of device) for PICCs (CDC, in press).
   b) Patients who are in need of vesicant or irritating medication infusions
   c) Patients who are in need of hyperosmolar solution infusions, such as TPN
   d) Patients who prefer this type of device over other VADs that may be equally appropriate for the situation
   e) In the home setting, patients who have a family member or significant other who can properly care for the device
   f) For patients scheduled to receive IV therapy for more than five days, a plan should be followed to maximize comfort and preserve the integrity of the veins.
4. Insertion techniques (Hagle, 2007): Appropriate tip location for a PICC is the distal third of the superior vena cava (Gallieni et al., 2008; Hamilton, 2006). Only healthcare professionals who have successfully completed a PICC insertion course should insert PICCs. This course is beyond the scope of these guidelines.
   a) Insert PICCs via the vein (see Figure 4).
      (1) Cephalic
      (2) Accessory cephalic
      (3) Basilic
      (4) Median cubital
      (5) Pediatric considerations for insertion: Conscious sedation may be considered (Mickler, 2008; Pettit, 2007).
         (a) Three months of age: Superficial temporal, posterior auricular, saphenous, or median cubital veins
         (b) Four months of age until ambulatory: Saphenous, cephalic, basilic, or median cubital veins
         (c) Ambulatory child: Basilic, cephalic, brachial, or median cubital veins
      (6) Special considerations for insertion in older adult patients (Moureau, 2008): Avoid tourniquet use in those with fragile veins and thin skin.
   b) Perform a preplacement assessment of the patient to determine if a PICC is appropriate.
   c) Choose appropriate PICC size (diameter) for solution to be administered. Use the smallest acceptable catheter diameter to decrease incidence of thrombophlebitis (INS, 2006).
   d) Explain the insertion procedure to the patient and answer any questions the patient or significant others may have. Ensure that informed consent is obtained.
   e) Gather all necessary supplies, including any IV administration sets and medications or IV fluids to be used.
   f) Wash hands with a cleansing agent.
   g) Examine patient's arms and select the best vein for cannulation.
      (1) Avoid veins that are sclerotic on inspection and palpation.
      (2) Select patient's nondominant arm, if possible.
      (3) Avoid extremities that may have compromised circulation, such as those with the presence of lymphedema or venous congestion secondary to superior vena cava syndrome.
      (4) If possible, the basilic vein would be the best choice, as it is the straightest and has the most direct route to the central venous system (Hagle, 2007).
      (5) The cephalic vein is the second choice because its abrupt angle that joins to the axillary vein makes advancement

Figure 4. Peripherally Inserted Central Catheter Placement

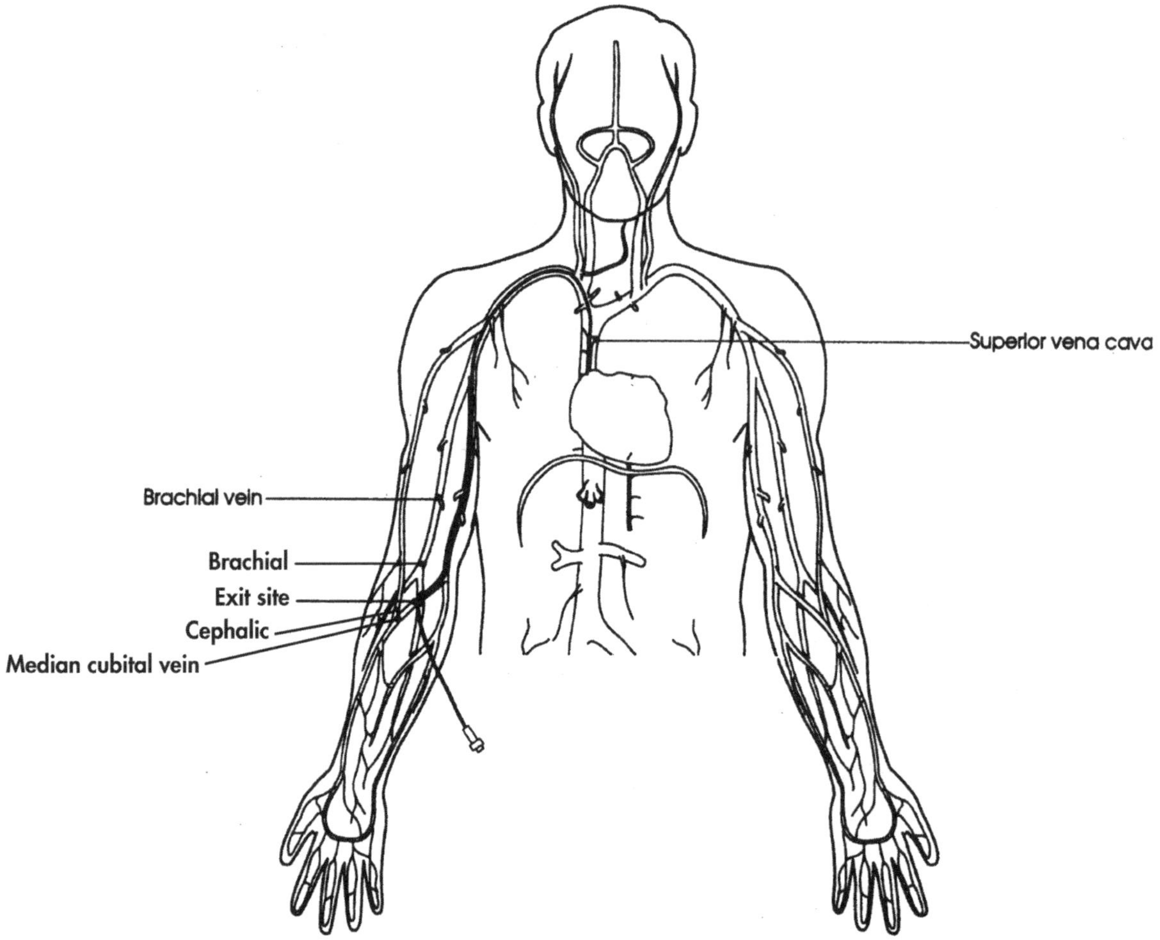

of the line more difficult. Position the patient's arm at a right angle to the body to assist with insertion (Bullock-Corkhill, 2010).

h) Consider the use of a local anesthetic (topical cream or intradermal injection, see Table 3) to reduce the pain associated with insertion (Bullock-Corkhill, 2010). An order is needed from a healthcare provider with prescriptive authority.

i) Use a measuring tape to determine appropriate catheter length by measuring from the point of venipuncture, over the course of the selected venous pathway, across the shoulder to the right side of the sternal notch, and down to the third intercostal space. The tip of the catheter should rest in the superior vena cava (see Figure 4). Add 2.5 cm (1 inch) onto this measurement to account for the length of the catheter outside of the insertion site.

j) Open the PICC tray and, following sterile technique, add additional supplies. The general insertion procedure may vary according to the type of PICC being used. The RN needs to be familiar with the product selected and follow the manufacturer's directions.

k) Position the patient's arm at a 45°–90° angle from the body, below heart level, to aid in vein engorgement.

l) Perform catheterization with full sterile technique, including surgical hand scrub, mask, sterile gown, gloves, drapes, and appropriate cleansing agents (Bullock-Corkhill, 2010; INS, 2006).

m) Place sterile waterproof drape under patient's arm.

n) Cleanse the area and allow it to air-dry before initiating cannulation.

o) Fill two syringes with normal saline. Use one syringe to prime extension tubing that may be needed during the procedure.

p) Place fenestrated sterile drape (a sterile drape with an opened center) over the arm, leaving the insertion site exposed.

q) Prepare the catheter.

    (1) Measure the length of catheter needed, using the sterile measuring tape.

    (2) Pull the guidewire back ½ inch from this distance.

    (3) Trim the catheter with sterile scissors according to the manufacturer's recommendation. Some PICC manufacturers do not recommend trimming the catheter. Others recommend trimming at a 45° or 90° angle. Groshong PICCs are trimmed proximally and not at the distal tip.

r) Apply tourniquet approximately 4 inches above selected site. Check distal pulse to ensure that arterial circulation has not been compromised. Change sterile gloves.

s) While stabilizing the vein, perform venipuncture. Note blood return, which indicates introducer location inside the vein.

t) Release tourniquet, and continue to advance the catheter according to the PICC insertion technique.

    (1) Peel-away sheath technique: Venipuncture is made with a needle/sheath device. After the stylet is removed, the catheter is threaded into the vein, and the sheath/cannula is removed down to the hub of the catheter. Wings of the sheath/cannula are cracked, and the two sections are pulled apart and away.

        (a) Advantages: Risk of catheter damage is low, a variety of gauge sizes are available, and it can be performed virtually without blood spills.

        (b) Disadvantages: A larger introducer unit is required, as is the acquisition of a new skill (peeling away a sheath). It has a higher incidence of thrombophlebitis than the modified Seldinger method and may cause more bleeding around the exit site during the first few hours after insertion.

    (2) Over-wire Seldinger method: Venipuncture is made with a smaller-gauge steel needle. Blood is obtained in the attached syringe. The syringe is removed, and a guidewire is threaded through the needle into the vein. The needle and cannula are removed, and a peel-away sheath is threaded down to the skin over the guidewire introducer. The guidewire is removed and the catheter is advanced, stabilized, and the sheath removed and torn away.

        (a) Advantages: Requires smaller venipuncture, a variety of gauge sizes are available, and the risk of catheter damage is eliminated.

        (b) Disadvantages: It is a more complex technique, the need for a minor surgical incision may limit its insertion in particular settings and by certain clinicians, and insertion costs more than other methods.

    (3) Placement of PICCs is guided with the use of ultrasound. Positioning systems are available to identify the placement of PICCs.

        (a) The VasoNova™ Vascular Positioning System™ assists in accurate placement of a PICC. The technology uses Doppler technology with internal physiologic parameters to accurately guide PICCs into superior vena cava. Using this navigation system reduced supply and labor costs because of accuracy in insertion (Naylor, 2007).

        (b) The Sherlock™ II tip location system is designed for use with Bard Access Systems PICCs (C.R. Bard, Inc.). This system detects slight magnetic fields generated by the preloaded stylet to guide catheter into position. Audible or visual signals indicate the location of tip position.

        (c) Locater systems help to reduce risks associated with blind placement.

u) Attach prefilled syringe, and flush with normal saline. Ensure adequate blood return. Primed extension tubing may be attached at this time.

v) After securing the catheter hub with tape, SteriStrips, or stabilizing or securement device, flush with heparin solution.

w) Apply dry, sterile gauze above insertion site, and place an occlusive dressing over the insertion site and external part of the catheter up to the hub. Change dressing 24 hours after initial insertion (likely to have bloody drainage), and apply only a transparent dressing. Several manufacturers have developed PICC line securing devices.

x) Radiographic confirmation must be performed to ensure correct placement. Some institutions may require that the guidewire be left in place to aid in PICC line verification during radiographic study because the small size of PICCs makes radiographic visualization difficult but possible. Extreme caution should be used during the radiographic study to prevent catheter puncture. Guidewires should not be left in place for a long period of time.

5. Removal technique: Ensure removal is in the scope of practice from individual state board of nursing.

a) Verify order for removal of catheter.

b) Gather materials needed: measuring tape, alcohol pad, gauze, and tape.

c) Wash hands, and don nonsterile gloves.

d) Remove existing dressing. Remove contaminated gloves and replace.

e) Grasp PICC at the insertion site and slowly pull outward, about one inch, pulling parallel to the skin.

f) Release it and grasp again at insertion site, continuing to pull the PICC out in short increments.

g) When PICC is completely removed, place gauze over the site and apply light pressure until bleeding stops, then apply occlusive dressing. Change dressing in 24 hours and observe site. Apply dressing if needed.

h) Observe catheter tip for integrity, and measure length and compare it to the length documented at insertion.

i) Problems with removal
  (1) Venospasm
    (a) If you sense resistance during removal, stop. Reposition the arm and attempt to remove it again.
    (b) If resistance continues, apply warm compress to upper arm for 15–20 minutes and attempt gentle removal again.
    (c) If the catheter has been removed far enough so that you can apply a tourniquet above the area containing the catheter, apply the tourniquet to the arm, and attempt removal again.
    (d) If resistance is still present, apply gauze and tape dressing to insertion site and leave alone for 12–24 hours and attempt removal again.
  (2) Thrombosis
    (a) Will cause the PICC to eventually lodge in the lumen of the vessel as you attempt removal
    (b) If during removal you are only able to pull the PICC out four inches or less, stop.
    (c) Because you do not know whether this is caused by venospasm or thrombosis, use interventions recommended for venospasm.
    (d) If these attempts fail, notify physician for possible radiologic studies to rule out thrombus.
  (3) Catheter fracture
    (a) Catheters may be damaged prior to removal or may become damaged if excessive force is applied during the removal process.
    (b) If the catheter breaks during removal but is still long enough to be pulled, clamp the catheter and continue removal.
    (c) If the catheter breaks at the insertion site, clamp it and apply a tourniquet around the upper arm in an attempt to prevent migration of the fragment. The tourniquet should not impede the arterial flow; check radial pulse.
    (d) Notify the physician immediately, as a cut-down procedure will be needed to extract the catheter.
    (e) If a complete fracture occurs within the vein above the insertion site, immediately apply the tourniquet at the highest point on the arm.
    (f) The fragment can become an embolus. Place patient in Trendelenburg position, and contact the physician immediately. Observe for

shortness of breath, tachycardia, confusion, pallor, or hypotension. The fragment will need to be removed by an interventional radiologist, thoracic surgeon, or vascular surgeon.

6. Maintenance and care (see Table 1) (Bowe-Geddes & Nichols, 2005; Gorski & Czaplewski, 2004)
   a) Dwell time: Approximately 12 months
   b) Dressing: 24 hours after insertion. Transparent dressing changed every five to seven days. Gauze and tape dressing changed every two days, or as needed if wet, soiled, or nonocclusive. See Figure 5.
   c) Flushing: Heparin 10–100 IU/ml: 3 ml/day or 3 ml/day three times a week
   d) Cap change: Every week
   e) For blood specimens: Discard of 1–2 ml of blood, flush with 10 ml normal saline
7. Complications: See Section II.I.
8. Education and documentation: See Section X.
9. For a practicum on long-term VAD insertion and care, see Appendix 4.
F. Tunneled central venous catheters (CVCs)

Figure 5. Peripherally Inserted Central Catheter Line

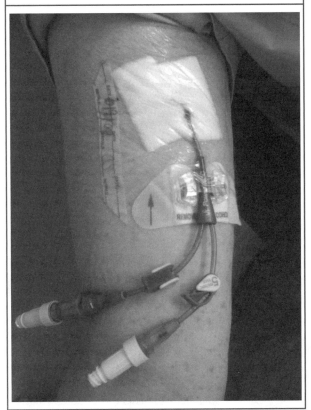

1. Description and types
   a) Catheter material: Polyurethane, silicone, a combination of the two, or Bio-Flex® catheter (Medical Components, Inc.)
   b) Lengths range from 35–100 cm (29.5–42.7 inches).
   c) Range from 2.7–12.5 Fr in single-, double-, and triple-lumen designs
   d) Internal diameters range from 0.5–1.6 mm.
   e) Prime volume of 0.15–2 ml
   f) Flow rate ranges from 49 ml/hr to approximately 3,500 ml/hr.
   g) Types of catheter cuffs
      (1) Dacron® (DuPont) cuff: Positioned in the SC tunnel 1–2 inches from the exit site
         (a) The cuff allows fixation of the catheter to the SC tissue by becoming enmeshed with fibrous tissue, thus promoting the securing of the catheter. However, this does not guarantee that dislodgment will not occur.
         (b) The cuff potentially minimizes risk of ascending infection from the exit site into the tunnel (CDC, in press).
      (2) Antimicrobial VitaCuff® (Vitaphore Corp.)
         (a) The device potentially creates another physical barrier for migration of bacteria.
         (b) The device releases an antimicrobial agent for approximately four to six weeks or until the catheter is embedded into tissue.
      (3) Radiopaque catheters: Tunneled catheters such as Groshong, Hickman, and dialysis/apheresis catheters visualized on radiographic imaging
   h) Types of catheters
      (1) Open-ended distal tip catheters: Require clamping for connection of IV tubing or syringes
      (2) Closed-ended distal two-way pressure-sensitive valve tip catheters
         (a) Catheters are available with PASVs located in the catheter hub.
         (b) Clamping is not required because the valve remains closed except during infusion and aspiration.
      (3) Power Hickman catheter available, allowing injection of contrast media for scans at maximum rate 5 ml/s and 300 psi limit.

2. Advantages and disadvantages: See Table 4.
3. Patient selection criteria: May be used in any patient population that requires long-term IV access, such as hematopoietic stem cell transplant (HSCT) recipients, those with hematologic disease, or those with malignant diseases requiring IV chemotherapy that will result in a prolonged nadir of blood counts.
4. Insertion technique: Surgical procedure by surgeon or interventional radiologist after informed consent is obtained
   a) Select the vein according to the individual patient's anatomic structure, type and purpose of catheter, and the vessel used. The most common veins used for insertion include the following (see Figure 3).
      (1) Subclavian vein
      (2) Internal or external jugular vein
      (3) Cephalic vein
      (4) Femoral vein
   b) Perform percutaneous insertion (Biffi et al., 2009).
      (1) It is the most common insertion technique using the subclavian or internal jugular vein. Once the vein is cannulated, the guidewire is advanced into the vein.
         (a) A pull-apart sheath introducer is threaded over the guidewire.
         (b) The guidewire is removed, and the catheter is advanced through the introducer into the vein.
         (c) The catheter is tunneled through the SC tissue. The tunnel is created from the vein entry site to the exit site. With the anterograde technique, the catheter is pulled from the exit site through the tunnel to the vein entry site and trimmed. With the retrograde technique, the catheter is pulled from the vein entry site to the exit site and trimmed.
      (2) The exit site depends on male and female anatomy; however, usually it is above the nipple line midway between the sternum and clavicle.
   c) Perform the cut-down insertion (Biffi et al., 2009).
      (1) The procedure greatly reduces risk of hemothorax or pneumothorax.
      (2) This technique is more time-consuming and difficult to perform than other methods.
      (3) The procedure requires more manipulation of the skin and SC tissue, thereby increasing the infection rate.

      (4) The veins used include the axillary, external jugular, internal jugular, cephalic, and subclavian.
   d) Verify catheter position by radiographic imaging.
   e) Secure catheter with sutures.
      (1) Exit-site sutures remain in place until healing occurs, which can range from 10 days to 6 weeks or longer if immunosuppression is present.
      (2) Sutures are removed after healing to prevent irritation and infection at the exit site.
      (3) In some cases (e.g., the use of apheresis catheters), sutures are left in place until the catheter is removed because of the risk of catheter dislodgment caused by the external weight of the catheter.
5. Removal technique: RNs may be able to remove tunneled catheter, depending on their specific State Board of Nursing Practice Act.
   a) Verify order for removal and indication.
   b) Note length of catheter on insertion.
   c) Explain procedure to the patient.
   d) Place the patient in reclining position.
   e) Inspect general condition of catheter and tunneled pathway.
   f) Discontinue all infusions into the device.
   g) Put on gloves, remove dressing, and observe site for edema, erythema, or other problems.
   h) Change gloves and remove sutures as needed.
      (1) Have the patient perform Valsalva maneuver.
      (2) Grasp the hub of the VAD and gently and steadily retract catheter until completely removed.
   i) Send catheter tip for culture with provider order if the VAD removal indicates infection.
   j) Apply constant firm pressure to exit site until bleeding stops (longer in patients with coagulopathies or patients on anticoagulant therapy). Apply occlusive dressing. Change in 24 hours and assess site. Some institutions use triple-antibiotic gauze or petroleum jelly gauze when dressing is applied to prevent air from entering SC space.
   k) Instruct patient or caregiver to report any discomfort or signs of bleeding, bruising, erythema, edema, and drainage.
   l) Inspect device for appropriate length and for defects. Report any defects to the manufacturer and regulatory agencies. Examine

distal tip for signs of jagged, uneven edges suggestive of breakage.

m) Document observations, patient tolerance, and actions.

n) Contact a physician immediately if difficulty occurs in retrieving the cuff or with removal of catheter.

o) If tunnel infection is suspected, a cut-down procedure may be performed to remove the cuff, based on physician preference.

p) If there is a question of incomplete catheter removal, call the physician immediately. A chest x-ray or cathetergram is recommended.

6. Maintenance and care (see Tables 1 and 2)

a) Dwell time: Several years

b) Dressing: Dressing changed 24 hours after insertion.

   (1) Transparent dressing changed every five to seven days. Gauze and tape dressing changed every two days or as needed if wet, soiled, or nonocclusive.

   (2) Once healed, tunneled catheters may go without a dressing unless the patient is immunocompromised (Olson et al., 2004).

   (3) Instruct patients with external catheters who shower or swim to completely cover exit site and external catheter with a waterproof covering (e.g., AquaGuard®, Cenorin, LLC). Some physicians prefer that patients with external catheters refrain from swimming because water can contain virulent organisms. Little information is available in the literature on swimming with external catheters and the increased risk of infection.

c) Flushing: Heparin 10–100 IU/ml: 3 ml/day or 3 ml/day every other day or 5 ml three times a week or 5 ml weekly. Groshong: 5–10 ml normal saline every week.

d) Cap change: Every week or month depending upon use

e) For blood specimens: Discard 3–5 ml of blood, obtain specimen, and flush with 10–20 ml of normal saline.

7. Complications: See Section II.I and Tables 5 and 6 (Green, 2008; Hamilton, 2006).

8. Education and documentation: See Section X.

9. For a practicum on long-term venous device care, see Appendix 4.

Table 5. Venous Access Device Insertion Complications

Complication	Etiology	Symptoms	Clinical Intervention
Air embolism (Lyons et al., 2008; Mirski et al., 2007)	Occurs when intrathoracic pressure becomes less than atmospheric pressure at the open needle or catheter	Sudden respiratory difficulty, tachypnea; cyanosis; chest pain; apnea; hypotension; cardiac arrest; aphasia; seizures; hemiplegia; coma; a churning sound heard over the pericardium on auscultation, produced by the presence of air and blood in the right ventricle	Clamp catheter proximal to any breaks or leaks noted; place patient on left side in Trendelenburg position; administer 100% oxygen; attempt to aspirate air from vascular access device.
Brachial plexus injury (Karakaya et al., 2000; Porzionato et al., 2003)	Occurs when advancing catheter into jugular vein. This process can also injure the phrenic and laryngeal nerves.	Tingling of fingers, pain shooting down arm, paralysis	Observe symptoms, which usually resolve in minutes to several hours after insertion; administer analgesics as necessary. If symptoms persist, remove vascular access device.
Carotid artery puncture	Occurs when artery is punctured during percutaneous internal jugular vein catheterization	Rapid hematoma formation; internal or external bleeding at insertion site; pallor; weak pulse; tachycardia; stroke; hypotension; upper airway impingement if trachea is compressed	Remove needle or catheter; apply local pressure; perform chest x-ray; observe site and patient closely for several hours.
Cardiac tamponade (Ahmed et al., 2009; Askegard-Giesmann et al., 2009)	Results from cardiac compression of fluid accumulated within the pericardial sac, exerting increased pressure around the heart that restricts blood flow in and out of the ventricles. Occurs when catheter causes cardiac perforation.	May occur hours or days after insertion; anxiety; tachypnea; mild dyspnea to severe respiratory distress; light-headedness; restlessness; confusion; chest discomfort (fullness, heaviness); cyanosis; face and neck vein distention; decreased heart sounds; hypotension; tachycardia	Remove catheter and perform pericardial aspiration. May require surgery to perform pericardial window and placement of drainage tubes.

(Continued on next page)

Table 5. Venous Access Device Insertion Complications *(Continued)*

Complication	Etiology	Symptoms	Clinical Intervention
Catheter embolism (de Graff et al., 2006; Mirza et al., 2004; Surov et al., 2008)	May occur when catheter is pulled back and sheared off through inserting needle; catheter rupture; or pinch-off syndrome	Chest pain, cardiac arrhythmias	If in the periphery, apply tourniquet, ensuring not to occlude arterial pressure; obtain stat radiology consult to determine strategy for fragment removal.
Catheter tip malposition (Trerotola et al., 2007)	Occurs when catheter tip is misdirected on insertion. Malposition of catheter can cause cardiac perforation, tamponade, venous thrombosis, or cardiac arrhythmias (especially ventricular). Inadvertent catheter placement into other veins (e.g., azygos, brachiocephalic, jugular)	Withdrawal occlusion; sluggish infusion; patient reports tingling sensation and gurgling sounds in neck; arm/shoulder pain; chest pain; cardiac arrhythmias; cardiac arrest	Confirm placement; reposition catheter using fluoroscopy or guidewire exchange; remove catheter.
Exit-site bleeding/hematoma	Caused by introducer sheath larger than catheter left in place or traumatic insertion. Patient may have coagulopathies or thrombocytopenia or be on anticoagulants.	Oozing or frank bleeding from the exit site sometimes persisting for several hours; discoloration or bruising; may result in compartment syndrome (large pooling of blood) in extreme cases (i.e., in the antecubital fossa, a triangular space exists where blood can accumulate, forming a compartment) (Udy et al., 2009)	Apply local pressure; change dressing as needed; drain compartment; observe area frequently; remove catheter if necessary. Apply Gelfoam® (Pfizer Inc.) or fibrin to stop or decrease bleeding.
Pneumothorax, hemothorax, chylothorax, or hydrothorax (McGee & Gould, 2003; Vahid, 2006)	Caused by air, blood, lymph, or infusion fluid in the pleural cavity due to pleura, vein, or thoracic duct injury during catheter insertion	Chest pain; tachypnea; dyspnea; decreased breath sounds; shift in location of heart sounds; cyanosis; decreased cardiac output	Perform chest x-ray and discontinue infusions; administer oxygen; prepare for needle aspirations and chest tube drainage. Perform thoracotomy for repair if necessary.
Subclavian artery damage	Occurs when advancing needle is directed laterally to the subclavian vein and the subclavian artery is penetrated; can result in arterial embolism	Rapid hematoma formation; internal or external bleeding at insertion site; pallor; weak pulse; tachycardia; hypotension; upper airway impingement if trachea is compressed	Remove needle/catheter; apply local pressure; perform chest x-ray; and observe patient and site closely for several hours.

Table 6. Treatment of Device Occlusions

Occlusion	Treatment Protocol*
Blood/fibrin	Instill tPA 2 mg/2 ml sterile water, wait 30–120 minutes, and aspirate. Repeat if unsuccessful. Remove device if unable to resolve occlusion.
Mineral precipitate	Instill hydrochloric acid 1 ml of 0.1 N equal to internal volume of vascular access device (VAD), wait 20 minutes, and aspirate. Repeat if unsuccessful. Remove device if unable to resolve occlusion.
Medication precipitate	Instill sodium bicarbonate of 8.4% solution (1 mEq/ml) equal to internal volume of VAD. Wait 20 minutes. Aspirate and repeat if unsuccessful. Remove device if unable to resolve occlusion.
Lipids	Instill 70% ethanol (ethyl alcohol) equal to internal volume of VAD. Wait one to two hours. Repeat if necessary. Remove device if unable to resolve occlusion.
	Infuse sodium hydroxide (soda lye, NaOH) 0.1 N 10 ml at 1 ml/hr, then quick flush with 20 ml 0.9% sodium chloride. Repeat if necessary. Remove device if unable to resolve occlusion.
Venous thrombosis	Administer anticoagulation therapy with heparin, low-molecular-weight heparin, or infusion of fibrinolytic agent.

* Use a syringe 3 ml or larger to instill medication.

MEq—millequivalent; tPA—tissue plasminogen activator

Note. Based on information from Bader et al., 2006; Cummings-Winfield et al., 2008; Kerner et al., 2006; Liu et al., 2004.

G. Implanted venous ports (see Figure 6)
 1. Description and types (Gallieni et al., 2008; Vescia et al., 2008)
  a) All ports are designed with a portal body and a catheter.
   (1) The portal body consists of a septum and reservoir within the portal housing.
    (a) The portal body is made of plastic, titanium, polysulfone, or a combination of materials.
    (b) The portal body has two to eight suture holes to stabilize the port in the port pocket.
    (c) Portal bodies are available in standard height and low profile for smaller chests and/or peripheral placement, measuring from 9.8–17 mm.
    (d) The weight of the portal body ranges from 4.8–34 g.
    (e) The diameter of the portal body ranges from 16.5–40 mm.
    (f) Port systems ("power ports") have been introduced to allow for power injection of contrast material. Using at least a 10 ml syringe, the port can withstand infusions at a rate of up to 5 ml/s at a maximum of 300 psi (Bard Access Systems, 2007b; Navilyst Medical, Inc., n.d.). Maximum pressure for non-power ports is 40 psi.
    (g) The Vortex Port® system (Angio-Dynamics, 2009) employs a rounded inner portal body and placement of the catheter on the portal body to encourage a circular flow of fluid through the portal body. The chaotic flow through the portal body potentially decreases outflow obstruction and infections by minimizing the collection of blood and other matter in the portal body (Goossens et al., 2008; Stevens et al., 2000).
   (2) The septum is made of densely compressed silicone.
    (a) Each septum can withstand 1,000–3,600 punctures, depending on the device and the size of the noncoring needle used (Hayden & Goodman, 2005).
    (b) The septum of a peripheral port can withstand up to 500 punctures with a 22-gauge needle (Smiths Medical, 2005a).
   (3) Inside the portal body is a reservoir with a volume of 0.2–1.47 ml.
  b) The catheter is available preattached to the portal body or separate from the portal body. The catheter is attached at the time of insertion with a locking device.
   (1) Catheters range in length from 19.7–35.4 inches and in sizes from 4–12 Fr. Catheters are available with an open end, a valve distal end, or PASV (Navilyst Medical, n.d.). PASV technology also is located at the portal body and catheter connection in open-ended catheter ports.
   (2) Various locking devices are available to connect the unattached catheters to the portal body during insertion, including locking collars, bayonet locks, and locking sleeves.
   (3) A needle guard is present on the catheter and portal body connection to protect the catheter from accidental needle puncture when the port is accessed.
   (4) Ports are available in single- and double-lumen designs with catheters made of silicone or polyurethane.
  c) Radiopaque
   (1) Many portal bodies have some component of radiopacity to confirm catheter locking mechanism is intact, and the catheter itself is often radiopaque to confirm tip placement. However, ports often are designed to cause minimal interference with diagnostic testing.

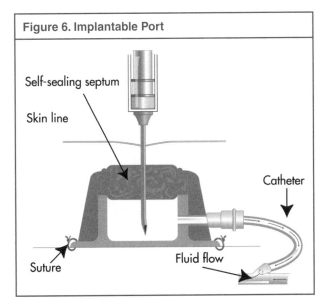

Figure 6. Implantable Port

Self-sealing septum

Skin line

Catheter

Suture

Fluid flow

(2) Some portal bodies have radiopaque identifiers that when imaged can confirm the presence of a flipped portal body.

(3) Certain radiologic technologies may need to be implemented to assist with interpretation, such as the use of contrast medium.

d) A peripheral port also is available for placement proximal or distal to the antecubital fossa. The portal body is approximately half the size of a standard port with a longer catheter (open-ended, valve-ended, or PASV). Peripheral ports are only available as single lumens.

e) Cost of implanted port includes insertion kits, the device, use of operating room or interventional radiology suite, placement verification (chest x-ray or fluoroscopy), and maintenance supplies for therapy at home.

f) Insertion expenses generally are covered by health insurance. Patients should check with their insurance representative or case manager about reimbursement issues.

2. Advantages and disadvantages (see Table 4)

3. Patient selection criteria
   a) Patients who require intermittent IV therapy
   b) Patients who are unwilling to care for an external line
   c) Patients who are unable to care for an external line because of poor vision, poor dexterity, inability to comprehend, or lack of caregiver
   d) Patients with a very active lifestyle, including swimming and outdoor activities
   e) Peripherally placed ports are an option in patients with chest pathology or those patients in whom obesity would make it difficult to access a chest-placed port.
   f) Adequate antecubital veins are necessary for peripheral port placement.

g) Patients with poor peripheral access and ongoing IV needs

h) Poor candidates for port placement:
   (1) Patients who are extremely obese, because the port must be sutured to the muscle and under the adipose layer, making it difficult to locate and access the port septum. Also, the port can migrate further in SC tissue.
   (2) Patients who find needlesticks extremely traumatic
   (3) Patients with open chest wounds, tumor involvement of the chest wall, or radiation fibrosis, because ample chest area is required

4. Insertion techniques
   a) Ideally, the nurse should assist in determining the optimum location for the portal body (Hayden & Goodman, 2005).
      (1) The portal body should be located over a rib for stability.
      (2) Placing the port over the sternum in obese patients assists in locating and accessing the port.
      (3) In women, the port should not lie under a bra strap or edge; therefore, the woman should be sitting and clothed when placement is determined.
      (4) Consider the activity level of the patient.
      (5) Avoid placement in the axilla, breast tissue, or soft tissue of the abdomen to avoid access problems.
      (6) A preferred site and an alternate site should be marked for the surgeon.
      (7) A peripheral port is placed below or above the antecubital fossa to minimize range of motion impairment.
   b) After giving consent, the patient is taken to the operating room or interventional radiology. The procedure may be performed under straight local anesthesia, a local with the addition of sedation, or general anesthesia. Insertion may be performed under fluoroscopy to facilitate correct tip placement.
   c) The catheter is placed using the cut-down technique or the percutaneous method.
      (1) Preattached catheters are measured and cut from the distal end.
      (2) Separate catheters are inserted and then may be cut at the proximal (portal body) end.
   d) If portal body is separate, the catheter is connected per manufacturer's instructions based on the type of locking mechanism.

e) An incision is made to create a port "pocket," preferably in a previously determined location.
- (1) The portal body is placed over a bony area for stabilization, under the adipose layer, and sutured to the fascia layer.
- (2) The suture line should not be over the top of the port septum to maintain the integrity of the suture line (Hayden & Goodman, 2005).

f) Following closure of the port pocket, the port is accessed using a noncoring needle, and the system is flushed to ensure patency and blood return.
- (1) If the port is to be used immediately, the needle should be left in place and dressed occlusively, as postoperative edema and tenderness of the incision make postsurgical access more difficult (Ozdemir et al., 2009).
- (2) If the port is not used immediately, the needle is removed and a dressing applied over the port pocket incision and the catheter entry site.
- (3) Ideally, the port should not be accessed for several days to allow edema and tenderness to resolve. If it needs to be used sooner, instruct the patient to apply an ice pack to minimize edema. If the port is used immediately, the patient may not be able to report pain or burning for several hours related to the type of local anesthetic used. Take care and ensure a blood return if administering a vesicant, hyperosmolar agent, or solution with pH less than 5 or greater than 9.
- (4) When a peripheral port is placed, that arm should not be used to obtain blood pressure and should not be used for peripheral blood drawing or infusions of IV solutions except through the port (Smiths Medical, 2005a).

g) Radiographic imaging is obtained following insertion to determine tip placement in the distal third of the superior vena cava and to assess for complications of insertion.

5. Access and deaccess procedures (see Appendix 5 and Figure 7)
- *a)* Implanted ports must be accessed with a special noncoring needle (see Figure 6).
  - (1) A specially designed needle tip separates the silicone septum, preventing

"coring" of the diaphragm, which could lead to debris in the reservoir and ultimate degradation of the integrity of the septum.
- (2) An offset bevel allows the tip of the needle to be flush with the bottom of the reservoir without impeding the flow of solution.
- (3) Noncoring needles are available in a variety of sizes and configurations.
  - *(a)* Length varies from 0.5–2 inches.
  - *(b)* Most commonly used gauge is 19–22.
  - *(c)* Straight needles are available for flushing with immediate deaccessing or bent at a 90° angle for intermittent or continuous infusions.
  - *(d)* Needles are available with various types of short pieces of extension tubing attached with and without clamps.
    - i. Wings may or may not be attached to the hub for easier access and stabilization of the needle to the chest.
    - ii. The extension tubing may have a Y-site.
  - *(e)* Power needles are available for power ports.
  - *(f)* Huber needles are available with a built-in safety system to prevent

Figure 7. Port Access

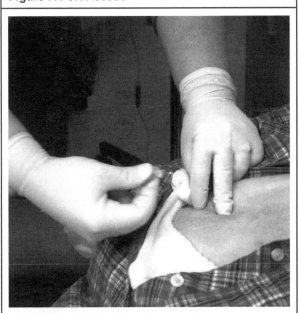

Note. Photo courtesy of Hematology Oncology Associates of Alabama, LLC. Used with permission.

accidental needlestick. When the needle is removed from portal system, the needle is covered with a safety mechanism (SafeStep®, C.R. Bard, Inc.).

b) To decrease discomfort during needle access, the patient may be offered topical anesthetic with a physician's order (see Table 3).

c) Port access procedure
(1) Wash hands. Prior to each access, the site should be examined for complications, including examination of the veins of the ipsilateral chest and neck, which might reveal venous thrombosis, erythema, drainage, or leakage.
(2) Palpate the outline of the portal body.
(3) Wash hands. Apply gloves. Cleanse port site with chlorhexidine for 30 seconds and allow to dry.
(4) Administer topical anesthetic, if ordered. Stabilize portal body with one hand. Insert Huber needle into septum with the other hand until portal backing felt.
(5) Ensure patency by blood return. If no blood return, use interventions to assess port patency.
(6) Stabilize port with tape, securement device, or stabilization device. Apply dressing. For short-term use, such as for outpatient treatment, gauze and tape could be used after stabilizing needle.

d) Port deaccess procedure
(1) Wash hands and apply gloves.
(2) Remove dressing and inspect site. Remove gloves.
(3) Wash hands. Apply gloves. Flush device with 20 ml normal saline followed by heparin flush.
(4) Stabilize port with one hand, and remove needle with the other hand. Maintain positive pressure while deaccessing by flushing the catheter while withdrawing the needle from the septum.
(5) Apply bandage or dressing.

e) When not in use, implanted ports must be accessed and flushed every four to eight weeks to maintain patency. However, no evidence exists to support the optimal frequency for maintenance flushing (Gholz, Whitehill, & Franer, 2009; Kefeli et al., 2009; Kuo et al., 2005).

6. Port removal technique
a) Procedure can be performed in the operating room or in an outpatient setting.
b) A cut-down procedure is used to remove the port from the port pocket.
c) The catheter is removed by pulling outward. The port pocket incision is reclosed with sutures or Steri-Strips.

7. Maintenance and care (see Table 1) (Camp-Sorrell, 2007; CDC, 2002; Gillies et al., 2003; INS, 2006; Lyons et al., 2008)
a) Dressing materials used during continuous port infusions
(1) Gauze and tape: Changed every 48 hours or when wet, soiled, or no longer occlusive
(2) Transparent dressing: Changed every five to seven days or more often, as indicated
(3) An occlusive dressing should be changed along with the needle once weekly, unless soiled, wet, or no longer intact.
(4) An occlusive dressing should be applied to any port site when the needle is to be left in; however, for short-term infusions, a light dressing may be used in place of an occlusive dressing if desired. More research is needed to determine the type of dressing needed for short-term infusions. The important aspect is to ensure the needle is secure in the portal septum with tape, Steri-Strips, and a securement or stabilization device. If the needle does not lie securely to the skin, padding (such as gauze) is needed to fully secure the needle into the septum.
b) Flush each port lumen (i.e., double-lumen ports). Flushing technique: Every four to eight weeks with 5 ml heparin solution (100 IU/ml) when not in use. Flush with 10–20 ml after infusing medications or withdrawing blood (Gholz et al., 2009; Kefeli et al., 2009; Kuo et al., 2005).
c) Blood withdrawal: Remove and discard 5–10 ml of blood. Draw specimen. Flush with 10–20 ml of normal saline.
d) Change port needles every week per manufacturer. Frequency to replace is an unresolved issue (CDC, in press).

8. Complications: See Section II.I and Tables 5 and 6.

9. Education and documentation: See Section X.

10. For a practicum on implanted port care, see Appendix 5.

H. Apheresis/hemodialysis catheters
1. Description and types (Otto, 2005)
    a) Temporary nontunneled catheters constructed of silicone or polyurethane material, or a combination of both, provide access for apheresis or hemodialysis.
        (1) Open-ended catheter requires clamping during IV access for connection of IV tubing or syringes.
        (2) Catheter length ranges from 12–40 cm, with an outer diameter ranging from 10–18.5 Fr and an internal diameter ranging from 1.5–2 mm.
        (3) Available in single- and double-lumen designs.
        (4) Priming volume of catheter is 0.8–1.5 ml, allowing a flow rate of 300–400 ml/hr or greater.
    b) Tunneled catheters constructed from silicone provide long-term access for apheresis or hemodialysis (Bard Access Systems, 2007a).
        (1) Open-ended catheter requires clamping during IV access for connection of IV tubing or syringes.
        (2) Available with Dacron or antimicrobial cuff.
        (3) Ointments containing polyethylene glycol (PEG) should not be placed on these catheters. PEG causes the polyurethane catheter material to become opaque, swell, and crack. PEG is a common ingredient in many antimicrobial ointments.
        (4) Catheters range from 8.4–11.5 Fr in lengths of 5.4–18 inches.
        (5) Available in single-, double-, and triple-lumen designs. The third lumen of the triple-lumen design is a smaller lumen.
2. Advantages and disadvantages: See Table 4.
3. Patient selection criteria are based on type of therapy or indications for use.
    a) Patients who require apheresis of blood components, including stem cells, to be used with HSCT. A temporary catheter may be used for collection of stem cells from allogeneic donors who have poor peripheral venous access.
    b) Patients who require leukapheresis
    c) Patients who require plasmapheresis
    d) Patients who require hemodialysis for management of acute and chronic renal failure
    e) Patients who may need venous access for continuous arterial venous hemodialysis, ultrafiltration, or continuous veno-venous hemodialysis
4. Insertion techniques: See Section II.D for nontunneled catheters or Section II.F for tunneled catheters.
5. Removal techniques: See Section II.D for nontunneled catheters or Section II.F for tunneled catheters.
6. Maintenance and care (see Section II.D and Tables 1 and 2)
    a) Dwell time: Several years for tunneled, and short-term for nontunneled (approximately seven days)
    b) Dressing: Dressing changed 24 hours after insertion.
        (1) Transparent dressing changed every five to seven days. Gauze and tape dressing changed every two days or as needed if wet, soiled, or nonocclusive.
        (2) Once site is healed, tunneled catheters may go without a dressing unless patient is immunocompromised.
        (3) Instruct patients with external catheters who shower or swim to completely cover exit site and external catheter with waterproof covering (e.g., Aqua-Guard). Some physicians prefer that patients with external catheters refrain from swimming because water can contain virulent organisms. Little information is available in the literature on swimming with external catheters and the increased risk of infection.
    c) Flushing
        (1) If frequent use of the catheter is indicated, change the heparin flush concentration to 1,000 IU/ml and flush every day or after use. If the heparinized saline is not aspirated and discarded, monitor coagulation levels (i.e., partial thromboplastin time) because this amount of heparin may lead to therapeutic serum levels.

(2) Some institutions require a physician order if the catheter is to be used for reasons other than hemodialysis or apheresis.

(3) Typical flush includes heparin 1,000–5,000 IU/ml after each treatment; 1–2 ml/day.

(4) Hemodialysis/apheresis catheters should be flushed after use for hemodialysis or apheresis.

d) Cap change: Every week depending on use or if cap is not intact

e) Blood specimens: Discard 5 ml of blood, obtain specimen, and flush with 10–20 ml of normal saline after blood withdrawal.

7. Complications: See Section II.I and Tables 5 and 6.

8. Education and documentation: See Section X.

I. Complications of short- and long-term VADs

1. Prevention of complications (CDC, in press; IHI, n.d.)

a) Central venous catheterization should be performed only when the potential benefits appear to outweigh the inherent risks of the procedure.

b) Catheter tip should *not* be placed in or allowed to migrate into the heart. The distal tip of a CVC (other than short-term peripheral catheters and subclavian catheters) should be placed in the superior vena cava at the junction of the right atrium. Placement too high in superior vena cava increases the risk for thrombus or migration of catheter tip. Tip too low in right atrium can trigger dysrhythmias (Bishop et al., 2007; Gallieni et al., 2008).

c) Catheter tip position should be confirmed using x-ray or another imaging modality, such as cathetergram or ultrasound, and be rechecked if symptoms of malposition or no blood return is present. Some clinicians have suggested that catheter placement be checked by chest x-ray every three months (Aitken & Minton, 1984; Gallieni et al., 2008; Kerner, Garcia-Careaga, Fisher, & Poole, 2006).

d) Central venous catheterization must be performed by trained personnel who are knowledgeable in anatomic landmarks, safety techniques, sterile barrier precautions, and potential complications. Users in training must be supervised closely by qualified personnel to ensure their technical expertise before independent performance of these procedures. Ongoing monitoring of experienced trainees should be undertaken to ensure continued competence.

e) Those placing VADs should be familiar with the specific equipment used as well as with the proper selection of insertion site, vein site, and catheter type, size, and length. Except in emergencies, catheterization should be performed with full aseptic technique, which includes hand washing, sterile gloves, mask, hat, gown, drapes, and proper skin antiseptic (Pratt et al., 2007).

f) Those caring for patients with indwelling VADs should be well informed of the appropriate care and associated complications of VADs.

g) Manufacturers should include specific labeling to address the potential complications of VAD use. Therefore, users should read all manufacturer labels, instructions, and warnings because they contain important and useful information for the safe and effective use of the catheter.

h) Catheters placed in less-than-sterile fashion should be replaced as soon as medically permissible.

2. Insertion complications (Gallieni et al., 2008): See Table 5.

3. Postinsertion complications/interventions

a) Catheter migration (DeChicco et al., 2007)

(1) Etiology: Catheter tip migrates spontaneously from the superior vena cava because of a change in intrathoracic pressure related to coughing, sneezing, or vomiting; forceful flushing; vigorous upper extremity movements; or accidentally by patient or caregiver pulling on catheter (DeChicco et al., 2007; Pikwer, Baath, Davidson, Perstoft, & Akeson, 2008).

(2) Symptoms: May include change in ability to infuse fluids or withdraw blood; increased external catheter length; and patient report of tingling sensation or gurgling in neck, arm or shoulder pain, vague back discomfort, swelling, chest pain, or arrhythmia.

(3) Diagnostic tests such as x-ray or cathetergram if catheter tip malposition is suspected

(4) Clinical interventions to reposition catheter tip or flipped port (Guth, 2001;

Thalhammer, Jacobi, Balzer, & Vogl, 2002)

    (a) Use patient positioning to redirect catheter.

    (b) Employ fluoroscopic catheter guidance to redirect catheter.

    (c) Nontunneled VADs: Perform partial catheter withdrawal or guidewire catheter exchange. The potential exists for complications, such as shearing the catheter or reintroducing infectious organisms.

    (d) Power flushing for PICCs

    (e) Remove catheter.

    (f) Surgically reposition port in pocket.

  (5) Ports can flip in the SC tissue and need to be surgically corrected (see Figure 8).

b) Pinch-off syndrome (D'Silva, Dwivedi, Shetty, & Ashare, 2005; Jensen, 2008; Mirza, Vanek, & Kupensky, 2004; Nuss, Cole, Le, Orsini, & Harned, 2008; Surov et al., 2008)

  (1) Definition: The anatomic, mechanical compression of a catheter as it passes between the clavicle and first rib at the costoclavicular space

  (2) Etiology: When percutaneously placed too medially, the catheter travels through the costoclavicular space next to the subclavian vein rather than inside it, therefore becoming vulnerable to compression with shoulder movement. Catheter fracture is defined as the complete or partial breakage of a VAD catheter internally with migration of the distal catheter fragment, usually into the right ventricle or pulmonary artery.

  (3) Symptoms of pinch-off: Difficulty infusing fluids or withdrawing blood, able to infuse or withdraw with patient repositioned such as raising arms or changes in shoulder position, lying supine

  (4) Symptoms of fracture: Arrhythmia, extra heart sound, palpitations, extravasation, shortness of breath, unable to draw blood

  (5) Diagnostic tests

Figure 8. Rotation of Port

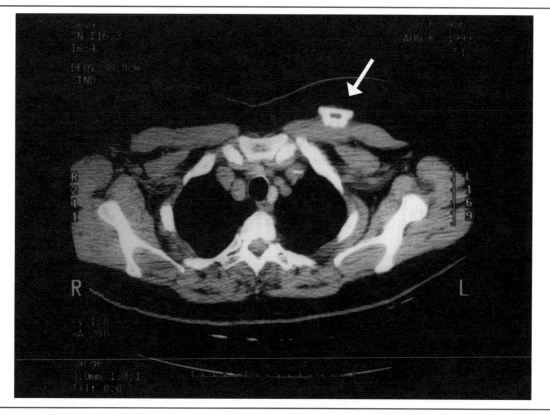

(a) Early radiographic (chest x-ray) detection of catheter compression is vital to prevent catheter fracture. For accurate imaging, patient should be upright with arms at side.

(b) If there is radiographic confirmation of pinch-off with luminal narrowing, the catheter should be removed and reinserted appropriately (Kerner et al., 2006; Mirza et al., 2004).

(6) Prevention

(a) To prevent pinch-off syndrome, the catheter should be inserted laterally to the midclavicular line. This places the catheter inside the subclavian vein, instead of next to the vein, through the clavicle and first rib.

(b) Pinch-off syndrome can be assessed intraoperatively following insertion of a long-term VAD by fluoroscopically evaluating the catheter during movement of the ipsilateral shoulder to evaluate narrowing of the catheter lumen (Mirza et al., 2004).

(c) Heavy lifting should be minimized if pinch-off has been identified. Case reports exist of fractures occurring within weeks of lifting weights.

(d) If fracture occurs (see Figure 9), embolized fragment removal should be attempted in interventional radiology (Mirza et al., 2004).

(7) Monitoring for pinch-off syndrome

(a) Surveillance x-rays should be used immediately following insertion of a catheter and at regular intervals in the first six months following insertion (such as months 1, 3, and 5) (Mirza et al., 2004). No studies confirm frequency of surveillance or the type of imaging study to be performed.

(b) If pinch-off syndrome is suspected or confirmed, the catheter should be removed immediately because of the high risk of catheter embolization.

c) Occlusions (partial/total): See Table 6.

(1) Etiology (Bader, Balke, Jonkers-Schuitema, Tas, & Sauerwein, 2006; Camp-Sorrell, 2007; Couban et al., 2005;

Figure 9. Port Fracture With Leakage (Arrow) of Dye

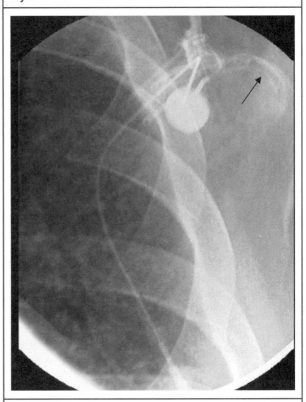

Note. Image courtesy of the Carole and Ray Neag Comprehensive Cancer Center, University of Connecticut Health Center. Used with permission.

Hadaway, 2006; Kerner et al., 2006; Lyons et al., 2008; Shah & Shah, 2007)

(a) Intraluminal blood/fibrin forms within the catheter lumen, resulting in partial or complete occlusion.

(b) Precipitates or lipid deposits occur from infusion of incompatible solutions or inadequate flushing resulting in drug crystallization.

(c) Fibrin tail or sheath (see Figure 10) occurs when fibrin adheres to the tip of the catheter and external surface, acting as a one-way valve permitting infusion but not withdrawal of blood.

(d) Mural thrombosis occurs when the fibrin from the catheter surface binds with fibrin from a vessel wall injury and forms a venous thrombus.

(e) Occlusions also can result from the port needle not being in the proper position.

(2) Risk factors: Normal physiologic clotting response, type of malignancy (such as solid tumor of the lung), thrombogenic composition of VAD, location of catheter tip (increased risk of thrombosis if catheter tip is located proximal to lower third of superior vena cava) (Blom, Doggen, Osanto, & Rosendaal, 2005; Couban et al., 2005; Kuter, 2004; Lyons et al., 2008); infusion of incompatible solutions, drug crystallization, and inadequate routine flushing (Hadaway, 2006; Kerner et al., 2006).

(3) Prevention
  (a) Adequate catheter flushes with normal saline and locking with low-dose heparin solution both routinely and after catheter use can aid in preventing occlusions.
  (b) Systemic anticoagulation remains a controversial method of minimizing catheter occlusions because of the risk of complications. Oral low-dose warfarin (1 mg/day) has been shown to decrease the rate of catheter-related thrombosis but may increase the patient's risk of bleeding (Akl et al., 2008; Couban et al., 2005; Kuter, 2004; Young et al., 2009). Currently, routine use of systemic anticoagulation is not recommended (Geerts et al., 2008; Pratt et al., 2007).
  (c) Routine locking with thrombolytics such as high-dose heparin and tissue plasminogen activator (tPA) requires more research (McGill, Spero, Sysak, Sandroni, & Marcus, 2008; Moran & Ash, 2008; Ragni, Journeycake, & Brambilla, 2008).
    i. Alteplase (recombinant tPA, Cathflo® Activase®, Genentech, Inc.) has been proved safe and effective for the prevention of fibrin buildup that may lead to catheter dysfunction. tPA degrades fibrin clots as well as fibrinogen and other plasma proteins by activating plasminogen to the active enzyme plasmin (Bamgbola, del Rio, Kaskel, & Flynn, 2005; Blaney et al., 2006; Davies, Casey, Li, Crowe, & McClelland, 2004; Fisher, Deffenbaugh, Poole, Garcia, & Kerner, 2004). tPA currently is the

Figure 10. Catheter With Fibrin Tail

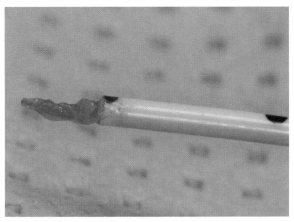

Fibrin tail with "initial" attachment on the outside of catheter, allowing for "trap door" effect and demonstration of partial withdraw occlusion; ability to flush easily but no blood return when attempting to aspirate.

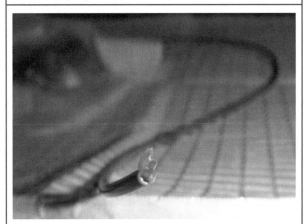

Fibrin tail with attachment on the inner aspect of catheter; however, this is a triple-lumen catheter, and it demonstrates that close proximity of lumens can be occluded with single fibrin buildup.

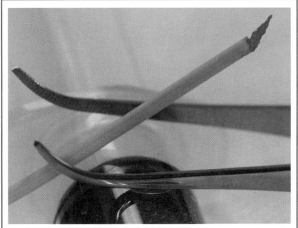

Fibrin tail and the extent of "clot burden" extend approximately 4 cm inside the catheter.

Note. Photos copyright by Penny Offer, CRNI. Used with permission.

most commonly used agent to treat catheter occlusion.

ii. Reteplase and tenecteplase, recombinant forms of tPA, currently are available only for treatment of myocardial infarction. With more research, these agents may be alternative treatments for catheter clearance (Liu, Jain, Shields, & Heilbrun, 2004).

iii. Urokinase is an enzyme produced by the kidneys and found in the urine that converts plasminogen to plasmin. This action degrades fibrin clots as well as fibrinogen and other plasma proteins. Maintenance use has been shown to decrease the rate of occlusion from fibrin buildup (Molinari et al., 2004; Svoboda et al., 2004). Urokinase currently is being marketed in large vials only and is indicated for pulmonary emboli.

(4) Symptoms (Camp-Sorrell, 2007; Kerner et al., 2006)

(a) Partial: Inability to withdraw blood but able to infuse; difficulty withdrawing blood and infusing fluids; ability to infuse or withdraw dependent on patient position

(b) Total: Inability to withdraw blood or infuse fluid

(c) Venous thrombosis: Pain or edema in neck or upper extremities

(d) Edema distal to insertion site (possible with PICCs and superior vena cava syndrome)

(5) Diagnosis of occlusion

(a) Diagnosis of thrombin complications may be based on symptoms.

(b) Diagnosis of lipid deposits or precipitates may be based on drug regimen.

(c) Cathetergram or dye study can be used to image the tip of the catheter and to assess for backtracking of fluids.

(d) Doppler ultrasound may be used to diagnose venous thrombosis. Use with catheters with total occlusion.

(e) Chest x-ray visualizes the catheter and tip to assess for migration or pinch-off syndrome.

(6) Clinical interventions: Intraluminal blood or fibrin, precipitates, and lipid deposits; see Table 6 for treatment (Bader et al., 2006; Cummings-Winfield & Mushani-Kanji, 2008; Kerner et al., 2006). Use 3 ml or larger syringe to instill medication. Nonpharmacologic methods include the following.

(a) Flush the catheter with normal saline gently using the push-pull method.

(b) Reposition the patient.

(c) Ask the patient to cough and deep breathe.

(d) Perform fibrin sheath removal with a snaring or stripping procedure to remove fibrin sheath from catheter tip in interventional radiology (Reddy, Lang, Cutts, Loh, & Rosen, 2007).

(7) Additional references related to catheter occlusion include Bowers, Speroni, Jones, and Atherton, 2008; Linenberger, 2006; Rosenthal, 2002; Rosovsky and Kuter, 2005; Smith, 2008; and Thibodeau, Riley, and Rouse, 2007.

d) Infection: VAD-related infections are costly and potentially life threatening; however, the definition, pathogenesis, diagnosis, and treatment of VAD-related infections lack standardization.

(1) Definitions most commonly used (Bishop et al., 2007; Camp-Sorrell, 2007; CDC, in press; Mermel et al., 2009; Pratt et al., 2007; Moran & Camp-Sorrell, 2002; Tilton, 2006; Vescia et al., 2008; Worthington & Elliott, 2005)

(a) Local VAD infection: Infection occurs at insertion site, port SC pocket (of a totally implanted intravascular device), or tunnel (along the SC track of the catheter).

    (b) Systemic VAD infection: Most serious type of infection; catheter-related septicemia, semiquantitative or quantitative catheter culture, and blood cultures are positive for the same species with a negative infusate culture; no evidence of another source for the septicemia is disclosed by clinical or microbiologic data.

  (2) Etiology

    (a) Contamination during VAD insertion; colonization of skin at VAD insertion site, exit site, port pocket, or tunnel (CDC, in press; Esteve et al., 2007; Tilton, 2006; Vescia et al., 2008; Worthington & Elliott, 2005)

    (b) Patient neutropenic when VAD was inserted

    (c) Contamination of infusate or any other infusion system components

    (d) Hematogenous seeding of microorganisms from an infection in a remote site within the body

    (e) Physical condition of the patient: Increased risk of infection in immunocompromised patients, patients with advanced age, comorbid conditions, severe illness, and prolonged hospitalizations (Maki & Crnich, 2003)

    (f) Catheter hub contamination during manipulation

    (g) Catheter material upon which bacteria adheres to the surface

    (h) Adherence of bacteria to a fibrin sheath and/or thrombosis, producing an "extracellular slime" that protects the organism from antibodies (Aslam, 2008; Safdar & Maki, 2006)

    (i) Inappropriate use of needleless connection systems (Esteve et al., 2007; Hadaway, 2006; Yebenes & Serra-Prat, 2008; Yoshida et al., 2008).

    (j) Use of parenteral nutrition (Opilla, 2008)

    (k) Use of chemotherapeutic agents that may irritate/extravasate resulting in local/cutaneous infection (Chang, Tsai, Huang, & Shih, 2003)

    (l) The most commonly occurring organisms (Camp-Sorrell, 2007; CDC, in press; Opilla, 2008; Vescia et al., 2008; Worthington & Elliott, 2005)

      i. Coagulase-negative staphylococci

      ii. *Staphylococcus aureus*

      iii. *Candida* species

      iv. *Corynebacterium* species

      v. *Klebsiella* and *Enterobacter* species

  (3) Prevention (Eggimann et al., 2005; IHI, n.d.; INS, 2006; Marschall et al., 2008; Mermel, 2007; Misset et al., 2004; Pratt et al., 2007; Pronovost, 2008)

    (a) Incorporation of central line bundle into maintenance and care

      i. Frequent hand washing before and after all VAD care

      ii. Maximal barrier precautions upon insertion

      iii. Chlorhexidine skin antisepsis

      iv. Optimal catheter site selection

      v. Daily review of line necessity with prompt removal of unnecessary lines

      vi. Alcohol hub decontamination before each hub access

    (b) Consistent maintenance procedures using strict aseptic technique

    (c) Routine surveillance for infection rates

    (d) Patient and caregiver education

    (e) Administration of preplacement antibiotic is not effective in preventing catheter-related infection (CDC, in press; Penel & Yazdanpanah, 2008; van de Wetering & van Woensel, 2007).

    (f) Monitor patients with comorbid diseases such as diabetes or chronic obstructive pulmonary disease or those on corticosteroid therapy closely for infection because these conditions can predispose a patient to infection (Conly, 2005).

  (4) Symptoms (see Figure 11)

    (a) Local: Swelling, tenderness, erythema, induration, cellulitis, and drainage with positive culture

    (b) Systemic: Fever, chills, diaphoresis, fatigue, arthralgias, weakness, hypotension, tachycardia, hyperventilation, mental status chang-

Figure 11. Infected Port Line

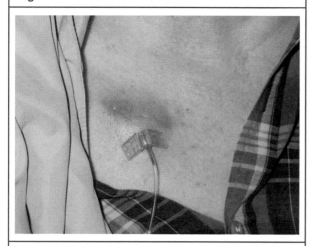

Note. From "Maintenance of Venous Access Devices in Patients With Neutropenia," by A.B. Moran and D. Camp-Sorrell, 2002, *Clinical Journal of Oncology Nursing, 6,* p. 128. Copyright 2002 by Oncology Nursing Society. Reprinted with permission.

es, abdominal pain, vomiting, and diarrhea

(5) Diagnosis of infection (Catton et al., 2005; Gallieni et al., 2008; Mermel et al., 2009; Moran & Camp-Sorrell, 2002; Raad et al., 2004; Tanguy, Seguin, Laviolle, Desbordes, & Malledant, 2005; Worthington & Elliott, 2005)

(a) Exit-site infection is diagnosed by cultures (swab) obtained from exudate noted at the exit site. Can occur either with or without a synchronous bloodstream infection.

(b) Blood cultures taken from the VAD and peripherally are used to diagnose systemic infections.

(c) Cultures can be interpreted either paired (positive versus negative), by measuring the time it takes for a culture to become positive, or quantitatively (compares the number of organisms found in each culture); a VAD culture showing more than 100 colony-forming units/ml is considered a positive culture.

(d) VAD catheters positive for bacteremia or fungemia and with no other source of infection found are considered positive for VAD infection.

(e) Cultures can be obtained from suspected infusate.

(f) Definitive diagnosis of catheter-related infection generally is made by identification of infectious or-

ganism from explanted catheter tip culture (Worthington & Elliott, 2005).

(6) Clinical interventions (Marschall et al., 2008; Raad, Hanna, & Maki, 2007; Vescia et al., 2008)

(a) Daily documentation of site assessment with local inspection and light palpation of exit site, tunnel, or port pocket. Immunocompromised patients may not demonstrate symptoms of infection because of a decrease in the number of white blood cells. If infection is suspected in a port, it is recommended not to access it because of the potential to introduce microorganisms into the bloodstream. However, it may be necessary to access a suspicious port to obtain blood cultures upon a physician order (Camp-Sorrell, 2007).

(b) Local infection: Culture exit-site drainage. Apply sterile gauze and tape dressings daily, apply warm compresses, and administer PO/IV antibiotics as ordered for 10–14 days. If symptoms do not resolve within 48–72 hours after initiating antibiotics, remove VAD (Kuizon, Gordon, & Dolmatch, 2001). The use of antibacterial ointment remains controversial (CDC, in press; Lok et al., 2003; McGee & Gould, 2003).

(c) Systemic infection: Obtain blood cultures from device and from the peripheral circulation; culture infusate, and consider obtaining cultures from port pocket (Mermel et al., 2009).

(7) If catheter-related bloodstream infection is suspected, it is recommended that two blood cultures be obtained. One culture is drawn from the catheter, and one culture is drawn from a peripheral venipuncture site and labeled accordingly (Krzywda & Edmiston, 2002). Care should be given to use strict aseptic technique, as one contaminant can produce a false-positive result. Developing a consistent protocol or set of guidelines for blood culturing when catheter-related bloodstream infection is suspected can result in rapid isolation and detection of microorganisms, which will en-

sure prompt and appropriate treatment (Penwarden & Montgomery, 2002).

(a) More research is needed to determine if blood should be discarded prior to withdrawing the blood specimen for the culture. If the infusate or solution within the internal lumen of the catheter is thought to be contaminated, no blood should be discarded.

(b) More research is needed on how to prepare the access site prior to obtaining blood for cultures. Chlorhexidine has shown effectiveness as a cleansing agent.

(c) Accessing a port that appears to be infected is controversial. It may be necessary to access it to determine the organism within the port system.

(8) Treatment (Mermel et al., 2009)

(a) Administer IV antibiotics. For multilumen catheters, rotate the lumens for antibiotic administration to ensure that all of the lumens are treated.

(b) Antibiotic lock technique involves instilling 1–2 ml of high-concentration antibiotic solution into the catheter lumen, allowing the antibiotic to dwell for a period of time, and then withdrawing the antibiotic (Mermel et al., 2009; Rijnders, Van Wijngaerden, Vandencasteele, Stas, & Peetermans, 2005; Safdar & Maki, 2006; Yahav et al., 2008).

(c) Questions still remain, including the appropriate antibiotic concentration, duration of treatment, and instillation time.

(d) The use of antibiotic-lock flushes (e.g., vancomycin) remains controversial because of the risk of allergic reaction and formation of resistant organisms (CDC, in press; Safdar & Maki, 2006).

(e) If thrombus-related infection is present, consider thrombolytic or anticoagulant therapy concurrently with antibiotics to prevent further clotting and to lyse the existing clot because the residual clot may harbor microorganisms, resulting in recurrent infection.

(f) Perform surgical stripping of thrombus from vein if traditional

measures are not effective (Reddy et al., 2007).

(g) If a nontunneled catheter is involved, a guidewire exchange of catheter is contraindicated because the infection could be reintroduced into the bloodstream (CDC, in press). However, some reports exist of successful management of tunneled catheters by guidewire exchange (Casey et al., 2008).

(h) If the patient remains symptomatic 24–48 hours after initiation of antibiotics, remove the VAD.

(i) Catheter removal usually is warranted for the following (Bishop et al., 2007; Mermel et al., 2009; Raad et al., 2007; Vescia et al., 2008).

   i. Persistent or recurrent tunnel infection after antibiotic therapy for three to four weeks

   ii. Fungus, gram-negative bacilli, enterococcus, or yeast infection

   iii. Continuation of signs and symptoms of infection despite antibiotic therapy

   iv. Confirmed VAD-related sepsis

(j) Catheters not removed after confirmed VAD-related infection have a higher risk of recurrent VAD infection.

e) Damaged catheter

(1) Etiology: Catheter dislodged from port septum; external portion of catheter sheared or fractured by powerful flush; catheter cut with scissors or clamps; disruption of skin integrity over port exposing portal body through the skin (Gallieni et al., 2008)

(2) Symptoms: Visible leak, moist dressing, pain, edema, visible port body

(3) Diagnostic tests: Chest x-ray or cathetergram to visualize catheter

(4) Clinical interventions (Gallieni et al., 2008)

(a) If a catheter is separated from a port body or internally damaged, the VAD must be removed. Repair is possible if damage or separation occurred with a two-piece attachable design (e.g., implantable ports).

(b) If nontunneled catheter is damaged, replace it using an over-the-

guidewire exchange. Some external portions of PICCs can be repaired with the manufacturer's repair kit.

    (c) If the external portion of a tunneled catheter (single- or multi-lumen design) is damaged, catheter can be repaired using the manufacturer's repair kit.

    (d) If port body becomes exposed through the skin, the port should be removed.

f) Extravasation (Polovich et al., 2009)

    (1) Etiology: Peripheral vein wall puncture, administration of a vesicant in a vein below a recent venipuncture, inadequately secured IV catheter, incomplete port needle insertion, dislodged needle from port septum, separation of catheter from port body, deeply implanted port, damaged long-term catheter in the SC tunnel, catheter tip migration outside venous system and backtracking of drug along tunnel resulting from a fibrin sheath (Hadaway, 2004; Rosenthal, 2007; Schulmeister, 2007, 2008)

    (2) Prevention

      (a) Select a needle length that will be adequate to pierce septum and secure in port septum.

      (b) Decrease the likelihood of needle dislodgment from ports by needle stabilization and using nonsiliconized, noncoring needles for access (Schulmeister & Camp-Sorrell, 2000).

      (c) Frequently check VAD exit site and for a blood return during vesicant administration.

      (d) Teach the patient to report any symptoms.

    (3) Symptoms (see Figure 12): Redness, edema, pain, burning, and absence of blood return during or following infusion, difficulty infusing solution, leaking around the IV catheter or implanted port

    (4) Clinical interventions: Stop infusion; aspirate residual drug from the IV device or port needle using a 3 ml syringe; remove IV or port needle; assess site of suspected extravasation; estimate amount of extravasated drug; give antidote if indicated; apply cold or heat as indicated; determine cause;

Figure 12. Doxorubicin-Associated Extravasation

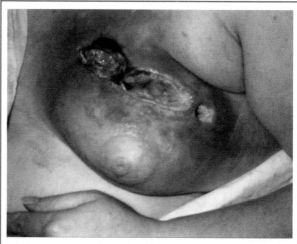

Photo a: Ulceration 8 weeks after doxorubicin administration

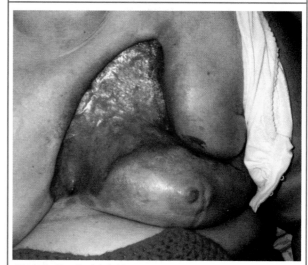

Photo b: Surgical debridement

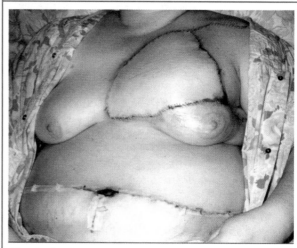

Photo c: Surgical resection 12 weeks post initial extravasation

Note. From "Chemotherapy Extravasation From Implanted Ports," by L. Schulmeister and D. Camp-Sorrell, 2000, *Oncology Nursing Forum, 27,* p. 535. Copyright 2000 by Oncology Nursing Society. Reprinted with permission.

notify physician; observe site regularly; measure and photograph site; and document (Schulmeister, 2007).

    (5) Avoid giving vesicants through a VAD without a blood return. Catheter must be confirmed to be in correct position, intact, and patent (Camp-Sorrell, 2007; Schulmeister, 2008).

        (a) Have the patient change positions, and flush catheter in attempt to obtain blood return.

        (b) Flush catheter with push-pull technique.

        (c) Try to declot catheter if clot is suspected.

        (d) Confirm placement and intactness by cathetergram or Doppler.

        (e) Obtain physician order to use catheter if needle is correctly in place and catheter patency is confirmed.

        (f) Ensure that the patient is informed of symptoms of extravasation.

g) Phlebitis (Rosenthal, 2006)

    (1) Etiology

        (a) Mechanical irritation or injury to vein wall, which may occur from insertion or by the presence or movement of catheter within the vein

        (b) Chemical irritation from high acidity (vancomycin, amikacin) or alkalinity (sodium bicarbonate, ampicillin) of solution, from irritant drugs, and from infusates high in osmolality, such as parenteral nutrition

        (c) Chemical irritation during insertion of catheter before cleansing solution is allowed to dry

    (2) Symptoms: Redness, swelling, induration, pain, tenderness, presence of venous cord

    (3) Clinical interventions

        (a) Rest and elevate extremity and apply warm compresses to affected area several times per day.

        (b) If symptoms do not resolve in 48–72 hours, catheter may have to be removed.

h) Infiltration (INS, 2006)

    (1) Etiology: The inadvertent leakage of a nonvesicant medication into the tissue surrounding a venous access device

    (2) Symptoms

        (a) Diminished flow rate of infusate as fluid accumulates in SC tissue

        (b) Coolness of skin, edema, pain or discomfort at infiltration site, leaking fluid at site, no blood return from device

    (3) Clinical interventions

        (a) Prevention: Early recognition of potential infusion complication, sequencing medications appropriately (i.e., vesicants first), and diligent monitoring of venous access sites and devices

        (b) Remove device.

        (c) Evaluate for extent of infiltration using standardized measurement of infiltration scale.

        (d) Monitor site of infiltration for further complications, including nerve damage or compartment syndrome.

        (e) Educate the patient to notify caregiver of signs of difficulty with infusion.

III. SUBCUTANEOUS (HYPODERMOCLYSIS) INFUSION DEVICES

A. History (Justad, 2009; Lybarger, 2009; Walsh, 2005)

1. Term *hypodermoclysis*, meaning a washing out beneath the skin, also is used to described SC infusion.

2. Hypodermoclysis was first used in the 1940s for pediatric dehydration. By the 1950s, hypodermoclysis was disfavored because of reports of shock and deaths caused by severe osmotic shifts resulting from therapy. However, these complications were found to be the result of improper technique, inappropriate fluids, excessive fluid volumes, and rapid infusion rates.

3. SC analgesia infusions were first introduced in England in 1979. Shortly afterward, the practice began in the United States.

4. SC therapy has been recognized as a cost-effective means of delivering medication fluid. Unfortunately, SC therapy does not generate an increased acuity level and often is not reimbursed.

B. Description of SC infusion therapy and types of devices

1. SC infusions provide continuous prolonged or short-term administration of parenteral drugs or fluids into the loose connective tissue underlying the dermis (Justad, 2009; Walsh, 2005), which consists of large blood vessels, nerves, and adipose tissue. A short-length catheter or needle is used for several days, although with repeated access, infusions may last weeks or months.

2. Fluid is absorbed into the intravascular compartment by a combination of perfusion, diffusion, hydrostatic pressure, and osmotic pressure.

3. Several specific types of devices are used.

   a) Similar peripheral IV devices are used for SC infusions as well as specific SC products.

      (1) Small-gauge, short-length, metal butterfly needles: Use only 25 or 27 gauge.

      (2) Small-gauge, short-length catheter

          (a) Either over-the-needle or through-the-needle catheter

          (b) Use only 24-gauge, ¾-inch catheter.

   b) Use of the catheter instead of a butterfly needle is recommended because of the longer life and reduced risk of needlestick injury, although shielded butterfly needles are available.

   c) Commercially available SC infusion sets are available, such as the ClearView™ Sub-Q™ infusion set (Norfolk Medical). This 27-gauge, 90° needle is situated on a clear, flexible anchoring disk. The manufacturer offers a variety of needle and tubing lengths to meet patient needs. The "Skippy Disk" sets are designed for pediatric patients with a smaller ½-inch disk and 27-gauge needle.

   d) Aqua-C™ (Norfolk Medical) hydration system also is available. The set provides all supplies needed to administer SC infusion.

4. Approximate cost: Includes needle ($0.50–$1.50), extension tubing ($1.50–$5), dressing supplies ($2–$5), administration set ($5–$8), and medication

C. Advantages and disadvantages of SC infusions (see Figure 13)

D. Patient selection (Fonzo-Christe, Vukasovic, Wasilewski-Rasca, & Bonnabry, 2005; Hunter, 2008; Khan & Younger, 2007; Lybarger, 2009; Walsh, 2005)

1. Patient age: Generally not restrictive

2. Mainly used in geriatric and palliative medicine; however, is suitable in hospital and home-care situations

3. Can be administered by family members or a nurse at home

Figure 13. Advantages and Disadvantages of Subcutaneous Infusions

Advantages
- Simple insertion by RN at any time
- Low maintenance
- Low cost
- Easily accessible supplies
- Less painful insertion than peripheral IV
- Slightly less likely than IV administration to cause fluid overload
- Suitable for home care and long-term care but can be used in any setting
- Less risk of systemic adverse effects (septicemia, respiratory depression)
- Caregivers can administer
- No complications of thrombophlebitis or thrombosis

Disadvantages
- Limited volume for rapid fluid replacement
- Small volume available for continuous administration
- Limitations on administration of specific fluids
- Local reactions may occur but generally are no more frequent than with peripheral IVs
- Recommended to use volumetric controlled pump for infusions
- Not appropriate for emergencies
- Potential for site abscess or cellulitis formation

4. Indications for SC infusion
   a) When an oral or transdermal route is inappropriate or ineffective (e.g., bowel obstruction, intractable nausea or vomiting, dysphagia, malabsorption, inadequate oral fluid intake secondary to confusion or infection in older adults)
   b) If the patient has poor peripheral veins (e.g., obese, older adult, or very young patients, those whose veins have been overused)
   c) When a single-lumen, long-term VAD is being used for other incompatible IV therapy
   d) For patients with delirium, confusion, stupor, or other mental status changes for which oral administration is contraindicated because of aspiration risk
5. Purpose of SC infusion
   a) Pain management
      (1) For acute pain management when vascular access is difficult (e.g., patients with sickle-cell disease who are in pain crisis) (Justad, 2009)
      (2) For chronic pain management when oral or transdermal route is not available, transdermal route is not tolerated, and there are no other indications for IV therapy (Justad, 2009)
      (3) Short-term, self-limiting SC infusion system with a local anesthetic directly into the incision site for operative and postoperative pain (beyond the scope of these guidelines)
   b) Reduction or alleviation of intractable nausea and vomiting
   c) Hypercalcemia treatment
   d) Iron chelation: For iron removal from transfusional iron overload or hemochromatosis
   e) Fluid replacement: For short-term, reversible fluid deficits when fluid replacement is not an emergency and is less than 3,000 ml/24 hr (Remington & Hultman, 2007)
   f) Infusion of amino acid solution to limit malnutrition (Lybarger, 2009)
   g) Infusion of immune gamma globulin
E. Contraindications (Fonzo-Christe et al., 2005; Lybarger, 2009; Walsh, 2005)
   1. If patient has generalized edema, poor peripheral circulation, or minimal SC tissue, although cachexia is not an absolute contraindication for SC infusion
   2. When rapid control of severe pain or frequent boluses or changes are needed
   3. If patient has a bleeding or coagulation disorder
   4. When rapid infusion or more than 3,000 ml/24 hr are required
   5. In emergency situations such as circulatory failure, severe electrolyte imbalance, and severe dehydration
F. Patient setting
   1. Patients may receive SC infusions in any setting—acute care, home care, long-term care, intermediate care, or hospice (Remington & Hultman, 2007).
   2. SC infusions are particularly well suited for non-acute care sites because of the ease of maintenance and restarts, low probability of systemic complications, reduced pain on insertion, and decreased number of injections required.
   3. Continuous SC infusion is shown to be as effective as IV therapy, more cost-effective, and a safe option for homecare delivery (Justad, 2009).
G. Insertion procedure (Fonzo-Christe et al., 2005; Hunter, 2008; Justad, 2009; Khan & Younger, 2007; Lybarger, 2009; Walsh, 2005) (see Appendix 6 for clinical practicum)
   1. Infusion sites include anterior chest wall, upper abdomen, anterior or lateral aspects of thighs, above the scapula on the back, and outer upper arm.
      a) For ambulatory patients, the upper chest area (subclavicular area) is recommended because it allows full range of movement.
      b) The upper abdomen is best for patients with little peripheral SC tissue, such as with cachectic patients.
      c) Access site should have intact skin and be located away from bony prominence and patient's umbilical area to ensure adequate adipose tissue (INS, 2006).
      d) Rotate sites when changing the needle, although it may remain in the same region.
      e) The interscapular or subscapular region can be useful for confused patients who may attempt to remove the device.
   2. Procedure
      a) Explain purpose of infusion, rationale for type of infusion, and procedure to the patient and family/significant others.
      b) Select site. Maintain strict aseptic technique.
      c) Prepare site with cleansing agent (chlorhexidine 2%). Allow to dry (see Table 2).
      d) Use smallest gauge needle/catheter available (e.g., 25 or 27 gauge).
      e) Attach tubing and infusion bag with fluids or medication; prime set.
      f) Put on gloves. Stabilize tissue with free hand, holding hand flat in a natural posi-

tion, or pinch skin slightly. Local anesthetic may be used (see Table 3).

  g) Insert needle with bevel down at about a 20°–30° angle almost up to hub.

    (1) Other authors have recommended a 45°–60° insertion angle (Anderson & Shreve, 2004; Walsh, 2005).

    (2) The angle of the needle depends on the amount of fatty tissue and SC tissue available and whether the tissue is held flat or pinched. When minimal SC tissue is available, the smaller angle is recommended to ensure correct placement.

    (3) When the needle is beveled, it is placed bevel down so that the fluid is infused into the SC tissue and to promote absorption.

  h) Secure wings or hub with tape or with a securement or stabilization device.

  i) Check for blood return (i.e., lower unclamped solution bag or pull back on syringe). There should be *no* blood return, although an air bubble may be seen.

    (1) If blood is seen in tubing, clamp tubing and remove needle.

    (2) Repeat procedure using new needle at an adjacent site.

    (3) If no blood is seen, clamp tubing.

  j) Attach tubing to pump, set correct rate, unclamp tubing, and turn pump on.

  k) Cover with semipermeable, transparent dressing. Secure tubing to either dressing or skin.

H. Maintenance and care (Justad, 2009; Khan & Younger, 2007)

1. Observe site every eight hours for local irritation or leakage, and assess the patient's comfort with infusion placement and infusion rate.

2. Recommendations for catheter or needle replacement vary. Catheters and needles may be replaced every three days; every five days; weekly; if bruising, erythema, or other signs of local irritation or infection appear; or if the site is painful to the patient.

3. Transparent dressings may be left in place for up to a week and changed with insertion of a new catheter or needle (CDC, in press).

4. Clients, families and significant others, and assistive personnel should be instructed to report any leakage, erythema, edema, or pain at injection site as soon as possible.

5. Infusion rates of 3–5 ml/hr are generally well tolerated.

I. Removal

1. Verify order or indication for removal.

2. Explain procedure to the patient.

3. Place the patient in a chair or bed for stabilization.

4. Discontinue all infusions.

5. Put on gloves, remove dressing, and observe site for edema, erythema, or discharge. Remove gloves and replace.

6. Pull catheter/needle out in the same angle as insertion while stabilizing the skin with sterile gauze.

7. Apply constant firm pressure to exit site if there is bleeding. Apply small bandage.

8. Instruct patient and caregiver to report any discomfort or signs of bleeding, bruising, erythema, edema, or drainage.

9. Document observations, patient tolerance, catheter integrity, and actions.

J. Administration of medications and fluids: No significant barriers to absorption of fluid or medications exist (Justad, 2009). Medications and fluid delivered SC easily enter the bloodstream by passing through the spaces between cells of the capillary. Blood flow and drug solubility are the major determinants of how fast absorption takes place.

1. Medications and fluids should be isotonic, nonirritating, nonviscous, and water soluble (Fonzo-Christe et al., 2005).

2. Medications (Fonzo-Christe et al., 2005)

  a) Any analgesic available for parenteral use is acceptable for SC infusion, except for meperidine hydrochloride, which causes tissue necrosis.

    (1) Morphine and hydromorphone are the preferred analgesics for home administration.

    (2) Hydromorphone is recommended as the most cost-effective analgesic because it is very potent and high doses can be delivered in small amounts. Stability has been found to be 28 days. Hydromorphone is at least as effec-

tive as morphine using the SC infusion route (Justad, 2009).

(3) Morphine was found to be equianalgesic for IV and SC routes when administered as a continuous infusion (Justad, 2009).

(4) Other commonly used opioids include methadone, fentanyl, and ketorolac.

(5) Methadone causes skin irritation with infusion (erythema and induration), but several authors have proposed successful interventions. These include the use of dexamethasone in the infusion, the use of hyaluronidase in the infusion, and site rotation every 24 hours.

(6) The IV opioid dose is considered clinically equivalent for SC use.

(7) The patient-controlled analgesia mode allows for rapid individual dose titration and provides sense of control for the patient. This can be done both in the hospital and in the home.

b) Other symptom management (Fonzo-Christe et al., 2005)

(1) Octreotide, scopolamine, and phenobarbital have been used for symptom management.

(2) Metoclopramide has been used for intractable nausea and vomiting in SC infusions.

(3) Hypercalcemia may be treated with SC infusion of clodronate.

3. Fluids

a) Solutions include 0.9% sodium chloride or a mixture of 0.9% sodium chloride and 5% dextrose; dextrose alone cannot be used because although it is isotonic, in the body it becomes hypotonic because of rapid metabolism (Lybarger, 2009). Potassium has been added without local irritation.

b) The addition of the enzyme hyaluronidase to SC fluid infusion acts as a physical adjunct to increase absorption and dispersion of fluid (Lybarger, 2009). It facilitates fluid absorption from the tissue, especially when the fluid is infused rapidly or in large quantities. The rate of perfusion is proportional to the amount of hyaluronidase present. The extent of diffusion is proportional to the volume of solution present. It may cause a systemic reaction; therefore, an intradermal test dose should be performed (0.02 of a 150 units/ml solution). Usual dose is 150 units in a liter or more of fluid. Availability includes

(1) Hylenex® (Baxter International Inc.) recombinant: Human source with less likelihood of local injection reaction

(2) Amphadase® (Amphastar Pharmaceuticals, Inc.): Bovine source

(3) Hydase™ (PrimaPharm, Inc.): Bovine source

(4) Vitrase® (ISTA Pharmaceuticals): Sheep derivative

c) Fluid replacement using SC infusion has been shown to be as effective as IV therapy with decreased cost and a trend toward fewer fluid therapy–related complications.

4. Rate of infusions

a) Recommended maximum infusion rate for medications is 3–5 ml/hr (Justad, 2009). Faster infusion rates result in tissue irritation and sloughing unless other measures are taken, such as using hyaluronidase in the infusate.

b) Concentrate the drug dose to ensure maximum flow rate of 3–5 ml/hr or less, taking bolus dosing into consideration.

c) Rates for fluid replacement depend on how quickly the replacement must be achieved but range from 20–80 ml/hr. Fluid replacement for some patients has been done at night only (Dasgupta, Binns, & Rochon, 2000).

d) An electronic infusion device should be used to deliver the infusion to lessen the likelihood of fluid overload or excess fluid into the SC tissue. Examples include an electronic syringe driver, elastomeric balloon pump, or peristaltic pump.

K. Complications (Fonzo-Christe et al., 2005; Hunter, 2008; Justad, 2009; Lybarger, 2009)

1. Adverse effects are minimal; they usually are local and are associated with the type of solution, infusion rate, and volume. Patients and caregivers should be taught to assess the SC site twice daily or every eight hours. Report any problems to the home health nurse or clinic.

2. Local reactions at the insertion site include erythema, edema, or induration.

a) Reactions may be caused by prolonged duration of catheter or needle placement, rapid infusion, or irritation from solution.

b) Remove needle and restart in another site.

3. Pain or discomfort at infusion site may develop.

a) Discomfort may be caused by needle migration, prolonged duration of needle placement, inadvertent placement in muscle tissues, or rapid infusion.

b) Assess for edema; if present, try slowing infusion, or restart in another site.

c) Warm compress at site may be used after needle removal for comfort.

4. Leakage or pooling of fluid at infusion site also may occur.

a) This may be caused by poor absorption or too-rapid infusion.

b) Stop infusion, remove catheter/needle, and restart in another site.

5. Edema

a) If it occurs in a small amount, slow infusion and monitor for absorption.

b) If it occurs in a large, generalized area, change site for SC infusion.

c) Gently massage the area, and monitor for underlying tissue damage. Excess or deep massage can cause tissue damage.

d) Reduce the rate of infusion.

e) Use hyaluronidase to aid in absorption.

6. Obstruction: If this occurs, restart in another site.

7. Sloughing of tissue, infection, and puncture of vessels with bleeding and bruising are rare complications. Frequently assess the site and avoid using SC infusion in patients with co-agulation or bleeding disorders to minimize the possibility of these occurring.

8. Fluid overload is possible even with SC infusion. Careful patient selection, frequent assessment, and the use of an infusion device will minimize this risk.

9. Sensitivity reaction to the absorption of adjunct hyaluronidase if used: Intradermal test dose of hyaluronidase is recommended prior to using in SC therapy.

L. Education and documentation (see Section X)

M. For a practicum on SC infusion, see Appendix 6.

IV. ARTERIAL ACCESS DEVICES

A. History

1. Arterial therapy with chemotherapy, especially to the liver, has been used for many years. Implantable pumps were introduced in the 1980s for long-term hepatic artery infusions (HAIs) (Bertino, 2008).

   a) Percutaneous short-term catheters also have been used to arterially administer chemotherapy to tumors in specific locations such as with osteosarcoma, where the arterial chemotherapy is directed to the involved bone, such as the femur, in combination with systemic IV therapy.

   b) In recent years, intra-arterial delivery of chemotherapy to head and neck cancers has been reinitiated.

   c) As improved techniques and newer cancer treatments are developed, the use of arterial access devices will increase.

2. Novel therapies such as replicating viruses and combination drug therapies are being examined using HAI to deliver treatment to tumors (Bertino, 2008).

B. Description and types of arterial access

1. Catheters for arterial use have smaller internal diameters; the catheter wall is thicker because of higher vascular arterial pressures. Catheter sizes range from 2–5 Fr with the most frequent size for HAI being 2.6–2.8 Fr.

2. Catheters on ports/pumps may have an opening at the end or have a side hole with a closed end.

3. Some catheters have one-way valves to prevent retrograde blood flow.

4. Nontunneled percutaneous arterial catheter: Short-term access. This type of approach is used in clinical trials, and the catheter is connected to an external pump for infusing the chemotherapy agent. The catheter is removed immediately after chemotherapy has finished infusing (Barber, Mavligit, & Kurzrock, 2004; Ensminger, 2008).

5. Implanted arterial port

   a) Consists of a portal body with a self-sealing silicone septum. Accessed by using a noncoring needle similar to a venous port. Catheter is a single-lumen silicone radiopaque beaded/branded catheter placed into the appropriate artery to be infused.

   b) Several companies manufacture these ports; it is important to know the type used at one's institution.

6. Implanted arterial pump

   a) A flexible medication delivery pump is the SynchroMed® (Medtronic Inc.) electronic pump. Pump contains a collapsible reservoir that can be filled with medication. A peristaltic mechanism pushes the medication through a bacteriostatic filter into the catheter to infuse.

   b) Fixed rate pumps are the Codman® Implantable Infusion Pump (Codman and Shurtleff, Inc.) and the Medtronic IsoMed® Constant-Flow Infusion System. One chamber holds the medication, and the other holds a charging fluid. Once inserted into the abdomen or infraclavicular fossa, the pump is regulated to the temperature of the body, leading to the expansion of the charging fluid, which pressurizes the medication chamber to push the drug through the catheter.

   (1) Constant or variable-rate infusions provide infusion over long periods of time, which may be several weeks to years with minimal human intervention (refilling or reprogramming). External control of rate and volume of primary and/or supplemental drug delivery is maintained.

   (2) The FDA has approved two types of implantable pumps for marketing at this time: a nonprogrammable vapor-pressured powered (fluorocarbon propellant) pump and a programmable peristaltic pump (direct electromechanical action powered by a battery).

   (3) Programmable pumps have the advantage of variable delivery rates that are set and adjusted through radiofrequency control.

   (4) Nonprogrammable pumps have predetermined constant rates of infusion and thus are limited in their ability to modify any pattern of delivery.

   (5) The pumps are labeled for specific drugs and routes of administration (i.e., intra-arterial floxuridine).

(6) When pumps are not infusing chemotherapy, they are infusing heparinized saline.

7. Costs: The arterial pump and catheter cost approximately $6,000. Implantation including hospitalization and physician fees can range from $20,000–$30,000.

8. Usage

   a) Arterial chemotherapy delivery has lower systemic toxicities and higher tumor response rates (Damascelli et al., 2007).

   b) Properties of drug suitability for intra-arterial therapy include (Ensminger, 2008)

     (1) Efficacy in tumor type

     (2) Ability to have high regional exposure but low systemic exposure with high total body clearance and regional extraction of drug.

   c) When using regional perfusion, the entire tumor must be able to be perfused; however, perfusion needs to be limited to the specific area of the tumor. Thus, some areas must have extra blood supply vessels eliminated with ligation or mechanical/chemical embolization.

   d) For hepatic infusion, infusing the drug into the hepatic artery that mainly supplies blood to hepatic metastases is preferred because the portal vein mainly supplies normal liver cells (Homsi & Garrett, 2006).

   e) Chemoembolization is a process in which large-diameter particles called microspheres and some drugs can be given together. It is a standard of care in hepatic cellular carcinoma and liver metastases from neuroendocrine tumors. The drugs usually used are a solution of doxorubicin or cisplatin. Small particles, usually Gelfoam® (Pfizer, Inc.) and Ivalon® (Fabco), are used until blood flow to the tumor stops (Ensminger, 2008).

     (1) In 2002 the FDA approved SIR-Spheres® (Sirtex Medical Inc.), a resin microsphere containing Y^{90} for use in chemoembolization (Ensminger, 2008).

     (2) Chemoembolization of hepatic malignancy represents an important therapeutic procedure in individuals with liver-dominant neoplasms (Brown et al., 2006; Dayani et al., 2009).

C. Advantages and disadvantages of arterial therapy (see Table 7)

  1. Advantages

   a) Intra-arterial chemotherapy has the potential to deliver higher doses of drug to the tumors with less systemic toxicity compared to systemic treatment. Studies have demonstrated increased response rate and overall survival with HAI compared to systemic treatment (Bertino, 2008).

   b) HAI demonstrated improvement in response and time to progression in patients with colorectal cancer with liver metastasis when compared to IV chemotherapy. HAI FUDR (floxuridine) meta-analysis showed increased survival at one year (10% or p = 0.041) and two years (6% or p = 0.124) over IV therapy (Homsi & Garrett, 2006).

   c) In the adjuvant setting, HAI showed a decrease in recurrence and improvement in survival (Homsi & Garrett, 2006).

   d) In the neoadjuvant setting, HAI has enabled some patients who had been deemed unresectable before receiving HAI to undergo surgical resection of liver metastasis (Homsi & Garrett, 2006).

  2. Disadvantages

   a) Regional perfusion chemotherapy can be logistically and technically complicated to deliver (Homsi & Garrett, 2006).

   b) HAI should be done only in centers with expertise and trained personnel (Bertino, 2008). Thus, availability is limited outside of large medical centers.

   c) Because arterial therapy is only for local control, the potential for development of distant metastasis is present. If distant metastasis is already present, IV chemotherapy is done in combination.

D. Patient selection criteria

  1. Suitable patients for HAI

   a) Disease confined to liver

   b) Individual hepatic arterial anatomy mapped with hepatic angiography

   c) Deemed an appropriate surgical candidate for a pump placement (Homsi & Garrett, 2006)

   d) If not appropriate for pump placement, patient needs to be assessed for nonsurgical port placement or temporary percutaneous catheter.

  2. Suitable patients for arterial perfusion (Matthews, Snell, & Coats, 2006)

   a) Those who have arterial access that will give total perfusion to the tumor

   b) Tumor location is such that systemic exposure to chemotherapy will be limited

   c) Patients with less than or equal to 30% of hepatic tumor involvement, limited weight loss, no severe ascites, and no hyperbilirubinemia (Barber et al., 2004)

Table 7. Advantages and Disadvantages of Arterial Catheters/Ports/Pumps

Device	Advantages	Disadvantages
Percutaneous short-term arterial catheters (those removed at the end of each infusion cycle)	Used in phase I trials of new agents until efficacy decided Can be used for multiple drug infusions at one setting Can be used with abnormal liver anatomy Can be used in palliative or neoadjuvant setting No device in place after the procedure	Bed rest required until catheter removed (if femoral access is used) Hospitalization required (although short-term infusions of 8 hours or less can be done during a 23-hour observation instead of full hospitalization admission) Insertion of catheter is done in interventional radiology department by trained personnel, so not available at every institution Tip of catheter stability less than with implanted devices Complications secondary to repeated insertions into artery Monitoring of site during infusion required Cost of initial insertion (can be done in interventional radiology department as an outpatient in centers with trained personnel)
Arterial ports	Allow repeated access to arterial system Allow for long-term use Can be used for multiple drug infusions at one setting (combination therapy has begun in clinical trials) Tip of catheter stability increased compared to with percutaneous temporary catheter Depending on insertion site, patient may be able to ambulate during infusion More cost-effective if long-term use is planned Can be used in an outpatient or inpatient setting if properly trained personnel are available	Patient discomfort with needlesticks Special noncoring, single-use needle required Monitoring of site during infusion required Cost of initial insertion (can be done in interventional radiology department as an outpatient in centers with trained personnel) High rate of device malfunction compared to implanted pumps or temporary percutaneous catheters
Arterial implanted pumps	Allow prolonged access to arterial system Allow repeated access to arterial system No immobility required Tip of catheter stability increased compared to percutaneous temporary catheter Has lower rate of malfunction than arterial ports	Need a flexible medication pump, not drug-specific pump; so not the device for clinical trials Cost of initial insertion Trained personnel needed to refill implanted pump with chemotherapy

3. Contraindications for placement of implantable port/pump for HAI
   a) Portal vein thrombosis
   b) More than 70% of liver replaced by tumor
   c) Significant impairment of liver function
   d) Hepatic artery anatomy that precludes perfusion of the entire liver (Homsi & Garrett, 2006). "Standard" hepatic anatomy is seen in only 55% of patients (Ganeshan, Upponi, Hon, Warakaulle, & Uberoi, 2008).
4. Contraindications for using arterial access include active infection, inadequate neutrophil count, or severe coagulopathy.
5. Treatment-related toxicities contraindicated in arterial therapy
   a) Chemical hepatitis: Most commonly (42%) presents with elevated liver enzymes or bilirubin

   b) Biliary sclerosis
   c) Peptic ulceration (Homsi & Garrett, 2006)
6. Implanted devices are available for children as well as adults, although temporary percutaneous catheters may be used depending on the length of therapy.
7. Consideration of any comorbidities that would preclude the patient from undergoing procedural or surgical placement of access
E. Insertion procedures
   1. Prior to placement of any catheter, obtain an accurate assessment of arterial anatomy with noninvasive computed tomography (CT) angiography or magnetic resonance angiogram techniques (Ganeshan et al., 2008).
   2. Implantation of ports/pumps for HAI usually is performed in the operating room at the

time of any tumor resection (Ganeshan et al., 2008). Advantages include

a) One procedure instead of multiple

b) Direct visualization of anatomy

c) Accessory vessels easily ligated

d) Gallbladder removal (if present) may be done to prevent biliary sclerosis and cholangitis from hepatic artery perfusion.

3. More recently, percutaneous implanted catheters have been inserted into the hepatic circulation in interventional radiology (Arai et al., 2007).

a) Limited invasiveness compared to surgery or laparotomy

b) Fewer problems with hepatic arterial occlusion

c) Fewer problems with catheter dislocation and kinking

d) A "tip-fixation method" is used and a catheter with a side hole is inserted into the gastroduodenal artery, adjusting the side hole to infuse the common hepatic artery. The catheter is fixed using coils and/or liquid embolic material, such as n-butyl-2-cyanoacrylate (NBCA) mixed with iodized oil (Arai et al., 2007).

4. Laparoscopic approach for HAI catheter placement

a) Resection of primary tumor and/or liver metastases can be done at the same time.

b) Arteriograms are obtained, and if multiple arteries are found to supply the liver, they are united into a single artery by using coils and/or surgical ligation. A side-hole catheter is inserted into the gastroepiploic artery via the gastroduodenal artery, and the side hole is placed at the orifice of the common hepatic artery. The right gastric artery is then ligated, and the gastroduodenal artery is clipped (Watanabe et al., 2004).

5. When the hepatic artery is not the artery to be infused, then the artery used will be based on

arteriogram data, tumor location, and risk/benefit of a temporary access versus a more permanent access, which depends on patient selection and medical team expertise.

6. After catheter placement, the catheter is connected to port/pump if not already attached.

7. The port/pump is placed in an SC pocket.

8. Usually SC pocket placement for port/pump is in the upper chest wall over a bony prominence under the infraclavicular fossa or in the lower abdomen (but may be placed anywhere on the trunk of the body).

a) It is important that the incision does not transverse the septum of the port/pump device, which will cause problems with access.

b) Temporary insertion of a percutaneous catheter is done in interventional radiology.

c) The subclavian, hypogastric, femoral, and brachial arteries have all been used in the placement of HAI catheter, with the left subclavian and femoral artery being the most common (Ganeshan et al., 2008).

d) Precise placement of the catheter tip position is pivotal to minimize extrahepatic cytotoxic side effects and optimize the hepatic chemotherapy infusion treatment (Ganeshan et al., 2008).

9. Postprocedure care

a) Surgically placed internal catheter connected to a port or implant pump

(1) Provide routine postoperative care, including pain control and incisional care.

(2) Observe site of port/pump insertion for drainage, bleeding, edema, erythema, or tenderness.

b) Percutaneously placed internal catheter connected to a port or implanted pump: Observe puncture site and site of port/pump insertion for drainage, bleeding, edema, erythema, or tenderness.

c) Percutaneously placed temporary catheter connected to an external pump

(1) Observe dressing for drainage or bleeding.

(2) Ensure that all connections have been Luer-locked or capped securely to prevent any type of leakage.

(3) Secure catheter so as not to kink to ensure good flow of infusate.

(4) Unless chemotherapy is infusing, the catheter should have heparin infusing to maintain patency. Whether coagulation studies need to be done before discontinuation of catheter will depend

on length and amount of heparin infused. Short-term infusions of chemotherapy of fewer than six hours with immediate discontinuation of arterial line after chemotherapy is flushed through do not usually need coagulation studies. However, always follow institutional policies.

(5) Assess the involved limb for peripheral pulses, color, temperature, capillary refill, numbness or tingling, swelling, or signs of bleeding or hematoma formation. This assessment should be done with each set of vital signs.

(6) Patients should be monitored following the procedure with vital signs every 15 minutes for at least 2 hours (Ganeshan et al., 2008). Monitoring varies among institutions with most requesting vital signs every 15 minutes times 4; then 30 minutes times 2; then every hour times 2–4; then every 4 hours.

(7) No venous punctures or blood pressures should be done on the extremity being used for access.

(8) If femoral access is used, patient should be on bedrest to keep catheter from becoming disconnected or dislodged (Ensminger, 2008).

   (a) If a restraint is used on the lower extremity, follow institutional guidelines on use of restraints.

   (b) Deep vein thrombosis prophylaxis should be used, such as antiembolic stockings or sequential compression devices. Follow institutional guidelines regarding deep vein thrombosis prophylaxis.

   (c) Rarely should any type of ambulation occur during infusion. It must have health provider order and must be done under supervision so that prompt intervention can be implemented in case problems with the catheter or pump occur.

(9) If brachial or subclavian access is used, secure the arm in a sling or some type of immobilization device. An advantage of these approaches for percutaneous insertion is that the patient can be ambulatory (Ensminger, 2008; Ganeshan et al., 2008).

F. Maintenance procedures (see Table 8)

1. If the patient has an implanted port/pump, chemotherapy usually is given in the outpatient setting (unless the infusion time with a port is prohibitive, such as when the port is connected to an external pump).

2. It may be possible to find a home health agency to assist in administration. However, they must

   a) Have knowledge regarding arterial infusion and clinical competence in administration of chemotherapy via arterial route

   b) Know the chemotherapy being administered and all the side effects

   c) Be knowledgeable in the safe handling of chemotherapy agents and know how to use personnel protective equipment

   d) Be on 24-hour call for any problems or complications that may arise with infusion.

3. Patients with temporary percutaneous catheters are either inpatients or under 23-hour observation (considered outpatient) depending on length of infusion.

   a) During the procedure for placement of catheter, the patient is monitored with heart rate, oxygen saturation, and electrocardiogram recordings by a trained nurse.

   b) Neither conscious sedation nor antibiotic prophylaxis is routinely used (Ganeshan et al., 2008).

4. Drug delivery with arterial access

   a) For HAI, several hours of hydration is recommended prior to chemotherapy infusion (Brown et al., 2006; Ganeshan et al., 2008).

   b) Perfusion scan can be used to document catheter position/function prior to use (Compton & Raaf, 2006).

   c) With a temporary catheter, document position with each insertion. For port/pumps, follow institutional guidelines.

   d) Any signs that suggest catheter migration (e.g., regional side effects, edema, leakage, inability to infuse) of an implanted port where the catheter had been secured and confirmed in place when implanted require a position check prior to administering chemotherapy to verify position of catheter tip.

   e) Review any laboratory tests ordered before chemotherapy to ensure that patient is within the limits for both the type of chemotherapy to be infused and the procedure (for temporary catheter placement, coagulation profile is needed). These include complete blood count, kidney function, electrolytes, and liver function tests if HAI is being done.

   f) If a port or temporary catheter is used, connect to an external pump for infusion. Label all tubing as arterial access.

Table 8. Maintenance and Care of Arterial Access Devices		
Type of Device	**Flushing**	**Exit-Site Care and Dressing**
Catheter	Flush before and at the end with 10 ml of normal saline (NS). (Note: If chemotherapy is not compatible with NS, flushing with dextrose 5% in water (D5W) may be needed between the NS flushes and the chemotherapy.) If capping is needed (extremely rare), catheter should be flushed prior to capping. After NS flush, flush with heparin 1,000–5,000 IU/ml 3–5 ml every day or follow your institutional guidelines.	Perform incision care as indicated. Maintain sterile occlusive dressing. Change dressing every two days for gauze and weekly for transparent semipermeable dressing.
Port	Flush before and at the end of infusion with 20 ml NS for each chemotherapy drug. (Note: If chemotherapy is not compatible with NS, flushing with D5W may be needed between the NS flushes and the chemotherapy.) Final flush: Flush with additional 5–10 ml of saline followed by 2,000–5,000 IU heparin/ml 5 ml every week.	Change port needle every seven days. Use 2% chlorhexidine/70% alcohol–based skin preparation prior to needle insertion. Make sure that the skin preparation solution has time to dry prior to needle insertion. Do not use topical antibiotic ointment or creams at the insertion site, as potential exists to promote fungal infections and antimicrobial resistance. Some type of wrap may be used to protect the catheter and keep the patient from pulling or dislodging the catheter while in use (e.g., gauze, netting).

Note. It is assumed that personal protective equipment is used when dealing with these arterial access devices and that the nurse will maintain good aseptic technique.

g) Refilling and accessing pumps is done via a Huber needle, which is inserted into the pump reservoir septum. The location of the septum is determined by palpation or by a template/tattoo-like mark placed on the skin (Compton & Raaf, 2006). Accessing needs to be done by a nurse who has shown competency in the procedure and in some states must be performed by an advanced practice nurse (APN).

h) The number of cycles may be specific based on the drug or may continue until disease responds and can be resected or disease progression.

i) The following drugs have been delivered via arterial route: cisplatin, 5-fluorouracil, floxuridine, irinotecan, mitomycin, oxaliplatin, paclitaxel, protein-bound paclitaxel (Abraxane®, Abraxis BioScience, LLC), vinblastine, doxorubicin, and tumor necrosis factor.

j) Two of the drugs listed are lipid/protein bound (doxorubicin and Abraxane). This is important because usually all temporary catheters have in-line filters, and these two drugs cannot be given through a filter. To date, these drugs have been given HAI in clinical trials only. There is no literature on the monitoring of infusions without a filter. Institutions that administer these drugs have developed an in-house standard. Close monitoring is mandated, and the nurse must be within hearing distance of the pump alarm and should check on the infusion every 10–15 minutes.

k) At present, FUDR is the only noninvestigational anticancer drug approved for intra-arterial use by the FDA (Ensminger, 2008).

l) Arterial access devices are not to be used for infusion of TPN or lipid administration.

5. Access, flushing, and dressings (see Table 8)
   a) Nurses should know the devices used within the institution in which they are employed, including the care, recommendations, and precautions of the manufacturer.
   b) Nurses should know their institution's standard of care for accessing, flushing, site care, and dressing for the different devices.
   c) Aseptic technique should be used during all catheter care.
   d) Catheter access at the hub
      (1) Clean catheter connection with CHG plus isopropyl alcohol (allowing time for solution to dry) (CDC, in press).
      (2) Always clamp catheter during tubing or cap changes.
      (3) Some institutions that insert temporary catheters connect the heparinized so-

lution with the pump at the time of insertion in interventional radiology after confirmation of tip placement under fluoroscopy (see Figure 14).

e) Dressing changes depend on the type of dressing, with gauze changed every two days, or if transparent semipermeable dressing is used, at least weekly (CDC, in press). Always change a soiled dressing immediately.

f) Flush a port to verify patency; port should allow easy flow and cause no discomfort.

g) Blood return should be brisk unless the catheter has a one-way valve, which will prevent any blood return.

h) Flushing to maintain patency varies among institutions; however, most will follow manufacturer's recommendations (Watanabe et al., 2004).

   (1) Typically catheters are flushed with 3–5 ml of heparin every day with 1,000–5,000 IU/ml.

   (2) Ports are flushed with 2,000–5,000 IU/ml of 5 ml heparin weekly.

i) When ports or external catheters require a "keep-open" flow rate, usually a heparin solution is infused to maintain patency, with the medical team determining the concentration.

G. Removal of catheter/port/implanted device

  1. Whether a trained RN or APN can remove arterial short-term catheters (not arterial lines for intensive care unit monitoring) depends on the individual state board of nursing. For states that do permit RNs to remove arterial catheters, training and competency records must be maintained.

  2. Removal of a percutaneous temporary catheter

Figure 14. Arterial Line

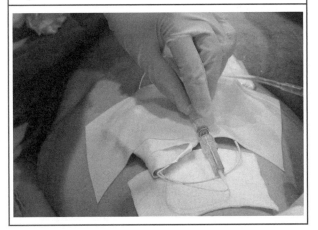

a) After the catheter is removed from the artery, manual compression may be done or, if femoral access was used, a vascular closure device may be used (Dauerman, Applegate, & Cohen, 2007).

b) Manual compression has remained the gold standard since first introduced for closure of a percutaneous arterial vascular access. Procedures for manual compression in regard to exact method and hand position hold time vary widely across institutions (Tu & Tremmel, 2007).

c) Place an occlusive pressure dressing over the site. Use of any type of antibiotic ointment at the site is controversial.

d) There is no evidence for the use of a sandbag over the site to reduce bleeding. However, it will help to keep the extremity immobile.

e) After the catheter is pulled, monitor extremity pulse, skin color, and skin temperature per institutional guidelines. This includes monitoring the site for any bleeding or swelling. Usually these checks are every 10–15 minutes for four to six times then hourly for four to six hours.

f) After at least eight hours, the pressure dressing may be removed and a small dressing or adhesive bandage applied.

g) If infusion is done as an outpatient procedure, the patient should not shower or submerge extremity until the pressure dressing is removed. It is preferred that the patient not take a tub bath for at least 48 hours to give time for arterial site to heal, but the patient may shower the day after the procedure.

  3. Repair or replacement of malfunctioning port systems requires additional surgery. Advancements in interventional radiology have made it possible for some repairs to be performed percutaneously under local anesthesia (Ganeshan et al., 2008).

  4. Surgery may still be needed for port/pump removal if repair or removal cannot be done percutaneously.

H. Complications (see Table 9)

  1. Most common complications seen with arterial access include catheter dislodgement, hepatic artery occlusion, thrombotic occlusion of the catheter, and infection of catheter insertion site (Ganeshan et al., 2008).

  2. Complications of implantable pumps/ports include infection, hematoma or seroma formation of pump pocket; catheter occlusion, pump malfunction, difficulty assessing port, overinfusion, extrahepatic perfusion, and wound de-

hiscence (Barber et al., 2004; Lorente, Santa-creu, Martin, Jimenez, & Mora, 2006).

3. Catheter migration in temporary percutaneous catheters occurs less than with port catheters, and rate increases if axillary or brachial artery access is used (Ganeshan et al., 2008).

4. Cerebral infarction has been described as a serious complication in patients with HAI catheters inserted via subclavian and brachial routes (Ganeshan et al., 2008). Prophylactic use of anticoagulation is not generally considered to reduce these complications significantly (Ganeshan et al., 2008).

5. Fibrinolytic therapy with tPA can be useful in cases of acute arterial or catheter thrombosis (Ganeshan et al., 2008).

6. High-pressure irrigation should be avoided but may be done by an experienced clinician if chemical lysis is not effective. An arteriogram is necessary after this maneuver because catheter displacement or rupture is possible (Crompton & Raaf, 2006).

   a) This is used to relieve an obstruction from a kink in catheter or migration.

   b) Technique is never used for thrombosis because of the risks of catheter rupture and fracture.

7. Tumor that becomes necrotic from treatment is susceptible to bacterial growth and the risk of infection increases, especially with tumors in the liver, which causes abscesses (Ensminger, 2008).

I. General practice issues for arterial access devices

1. Use positive pressure pumps.

2. Maintain positive pressure or clamp when withdrawing needle from port.

3. Use Luer-lock connections.

4. Never leave system open to air. Maintain a closed system.

5. Make sure tubing is secure without kinks to prevent accidental disconnection.

6. DO NOT USE arterial access devices for routine blood sampling.

J. Education and documentation: See Section X.

K. For a practicum on arterial catheter care, see Appendix 7.

Table 9. Major Complications Associated With Arterial Access Devices

Complication	Incidence	Prevention	Signs and Symptoms	Intervention
Infection	Varies in literature but up to 25% with implanted systems; however, ports have higher rate than implanted pumps Removal of implanted systems for infection average about 2%–3% of those infected	Good aseptic techniques Sterile, occlusive dressings over ports when accessed and over percutaneous catheters until removed Remove percutaneous catheters as soon as possible (within four days is optimal, after which the risk of infection increases)	Tenderness, erythema, or drainage at site Fever	If chemotherapy is infusing, notify MD, as infusion may need to be stopped. Culture site and catheter exit tip. Administer antibiotics as ordered. Have interventional radiology or trained provider assess if device needs to be removed. If removed, send catheter for culture. Need provider order for culture.
Catheter migration/ dislodgment	Percutaneous placed catheters: 6%–18% Catheter port systems: 2%–44% (higher if axillary or brachial access used)	Surgical or interventional placement of catheter that is sutured in place Use of braided or beaded catheter to secure in place Routine check of placement with flow study	If hepatic artery infusion (HAI), epigastric pain, nausea, vomiting, or diarrhea may occur. Pain over site or in surrounding area of infusion site when infusion is not to the liver Edema or erythema over site being infused if not HAI For any arterial infusion, weak or absent peripheral pulse Inability to infuse Patient discomfort during infusion	Stop infusion and notify MD or interventional radiologist. Flush catheter (after talking to attending physician and getting order) with normal saline or compatible solution for the chemotherapy that was infusing (do not discard the chemotherapy until ordered). Trained personnel will differentiate between chemotherapy-related problems versus perfusion of ancillary organs. Obtain perfusion study as ordered. Results of this evaluation will determine whether device needs to be removed.

(Continued on next page)

Table 9. Major Complications Associated With Arterial Access Devices *(Continued)*

Complication	Incidence	Prevention	Signs and Symptoms	Intervention
Occlusion/ thrombosis	Implanted ports: approximately 9%–15% Implanted pumps: 10%–15%, average of 6% Percutaneous placed catheters: average 11%	Applying positive pressure when deaccessing a catheter or port Flushing with saline or compatible solution between drugs Using heparinized solution for flushing catheter between use: addition of heparin to infusate or 1,000–5,000 IU per day can be used. With implanted ports, the dose is usually 400 IU per day (may be increased based on clinical situation).	Unable to flush or withdraw fluid (if catheter has a one-way valve, withdrawal of fluid is not possible) If temporary percutaneous catheter is in place, a change in color, pulse, and temperature of involved extremity If catheter tip is in hepatic artery—any abdominal pain needs to be assessed immediately.	DO NOT force flush (could cause rupture of catheter or diaphragm). After assessment by trained personnel, may use tissue plasminogen activator. Evaluate need to remove device (replacement will be based on clinical situation, as replacement may not be able to be done at same time as removal). Notify MD-mid-level provider.
Bleeding at exit site	Less than 1%	Baseline and frequent observation of exit site	For temporary percutaneous catheter placement, more drainage than what would be expected for accessing the artery should be considered a problem.	Apply a pressure dressing. Notify MD-mid-level provider. May use sandbag at site (literature on this is controversial on whether it provides any benefit to reduce bleeding). Educate patient to report any swelling, erythema, or pain over pump site immediately.
Device failure	Implanted ports: as high as 90% over first year Implanted pumps: 32% over first year	See Catheter migration/ dislodgment and Occlusion/thrombosis.		

Note. Skin necrosis over implanted devices has been seen but is rare (less than 1%).

Note. Based on information from Bacchetti et al., 2009; Barber et al., 2004; Compton & Raaf, 2006; Conly, 2005; Dumont et al., 2006; Ensminger, 2008; Ganeshan et al., 2008.

V. INTRAVENTRICULAR ACCESS DEVICES

A. History: Dr. Ayub Ommaya (1963) created Ommaya SC reservoirs for sterile access to the ventricular system as an alternative to repeated lumbar punctures in managing cryptococcal meningitis.

B. Description of the device
1. The device is a dome-shaped, self-sealing silicone reservoir attached to a catheter.
2. Reservoir volume is 1.5–2.5 ml.
3. Dome size is 1.5–3.5 cm in diameter.
4. Catheter length is measured and cut intraoperatively to fit within the frontal horn of the ipsilateral lateral ventricle (Dickerman & Eisenberg, 2005).
5. Reservoir is radiopaque and will not interfere with imaging studies (see Figure 15).
6. May be revised to include a ventriculoperitoneal shunt with on/off valve.
7. Global cost of Ommaya reservoirs, including surgical placement, is approximately $15,132.

C. Advantages and disadvantages: See Table 10.

D. Patient selection criteria
1. Patients with malignant cerebrospinal fluid (CSF) leukemias or lymphomas, meningeal carcinomatosis, or CSF infections
2. Patients who require intermittent administration of chemotherapy, antibiotics, or antifungals into the CSF
3. Patients who do not wish to undergo repeated spinal tap for CSF access
4. Patients receiving treatment for leptomeningeal carcinomatosis in primary breast cancer with good performance status (Waki et al., 2008)

E. Insertion procedures (Dickerman & Eisenberg, 2005)

Table 10. Advantages and Disadvantages of Intraventricular Reservoirs

Type of Catheter	Advantages	Disadvantages
Intraventricular reservoir	• Provides relatively painless access to the cerebrospinal fluid (CSF) • Obviates the need for repeated spinal taps • Permits consistent and predictable drug delivery through the CSF • Allows for measurement of intracranial pressure • Can be used for multiple therapies, such as chemotherapy, antibiotics, antifungals, and pain medication • Allows for sampling of CSF	• Requires surgical insertion • Catheter may migrate. • Expensive to implant • May become infected

1. Discuss the procedure, including rationale and risks, with the patient and significant others, and obtain informed consent.
2. The device is inserted in the operating room while the patient is under local or general anesthesia.
   a) The patient is placed in a supine position, and the area is cleaned and draped.
   b) A flap is created by cutting a U-shaped incision in the scalp, and a burr hole is made through the cranial bone.
   c) The reservoir then is surgically implanted subcutaneously under the scalp above the frontal lobe and secured to the pericranium while the catheter is threaded through the burr hole into the ipsilateral frontal horn of the lateral ventricle.
   d) The reservoir is covered by the flap of scalp tissue, which is then sutured closed. The patency of the catheter is verified by withdrawal of CSF through the reservoir, and sterile dressing is applied.
3. Postoperative CT scan is done to confirm placement within the ipsilateral frontal horn of the lateral ventricle.

F. Postoperative care
1. The original sterile dressing should remain in place for at least 24 hours; afterward, a gauze and tape dressing is applied for several days, and then the area is left open to the air.

Figure 15. Magnetic Resonance Imaging of Brain Showing Placement of Ommaya Reservoir

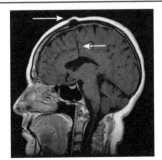

The top arrow points to the Ommaya reservoir port. The bottom arrow points to the catheter, which descends to the lateral ventricle.

Note. Photo courtesy of the University of Texas M.D. Anderson Cancer Center. Used with permission.

_____

_____

_____

_____

_____

_____

_____

2. Monitor the site for bleeding, leakage of CSF, and excessive edema.
3. Monitor and notify the physician for neurologic changes, such as headache, vomiting, cognitive changes, vision changes, progressive lethargy, dysarthria, or seizures.
4. Monitor and notify the physician for signs of infection, including fever, stiff neck, headache, or other neurologic changes (Halaby, Leyssius, & Veneman, 2007).
5. Cisternogram should be done to verify patency of Ommaya catheter and CSF flow tracts prior to administering medication into the Ommaya reservoir.
6. Sutures will need to be removed in 7–10 days and should be kept dry until then.
7. Advise the patient to avoid trauma to the area in order to prevent damage to the reservoir or dehiscence of the surgical wound.

G. Removal of device
1. An intraventricular reservoir is rarely removed once implanted, unless the device malfunctions or the body develops an infection that cannot be resolved with the device in place.
2. Intraventricular reservoirs must be surgically removed.
3. Intraventricular reservoirs may be removed if implanted for the purpose of delivering prophylactic therapy only.

H. Maintenance and care: Access, dressing, and flushing procedures
1. Controversy exists as to when an Ommaya can be accessed after placement. Opinions differ from waiting 24 hours after placement to accessing the same day as surgery.
2. Before accessing Ommaya reservoirs, check with one's state nursing board and institution for restrictions.
3. Observe strict aseptic technique at all times when accessing an Ommaya reservoir (Holmfred, Vikerfors, Berggren, & Gupta, 2006). Use of sterile gloves, face mask, and sterile field is important to prevent iatrogenic meningitis.

4. Preservative-free drugs and diluent must be used at all times to prevent meningeal irritation (Aiello-Laws & Rutledge, 2008).
5. Use of a 25-gauge or smaller needle will preserve the integrity of the dome.
6. Review institutional policies regarding procedure with and without administration of chemotherapy.
   a) Discuss the procedure, including risks and rationale, with the patient, and obtain informed consent.
   b) Perform time-out procedure to verify right patient, right procedure, and right procedure site.
   c) Intraventricular medications should be checked against the original order and verified by two licensed personnel. This should be reflected in the procedure note and on the medication administration record (Joint Commission, 2005).
   d) Assess the patient's vital signs and neurologic status.
   e) Wash hands and assemble all equipment for drug injection or CSF sampling.
      (1) Sterile field
      (2) 25-gauge butterfly needle with attached extension tubing
      (3) Sterile 2 × 2 gauze
      (4) Syringe with medication to be infused should be labeled individually and is not considered sterile. Therefore, the hand that retrieves it is no longer sterile and should touch only the nonsterile syringe throughout remainder of procedure.
      (5) Three alcohol swabsticks
      (6) Three povidone-iodine swabsticks. Chlorhexidine use is controversial as a skin preparation prior to Ommaya access. The FDA requires a label warning regarding possible contact with meninges; therefore, it is advisable to avoid the use of chlorhexidine for site preparation prior to Ommaya access.
      (7) Sterile gloves
      (8) CSF sample containers
      (9) Two or more 10 ml syringes for withdrawing CSF
      (10) Electric razor to shave area, if necessary. Standard blades may damage skin integrity, which puts the patient at increased risk for iatrogenic meningitis.
   f) Ensure that the patient is comfortable.
      (1) Assist the patient to a comfortable supine or semi-reclining position.

(2) Place plastic-backed absorbent material beneath site if giving chemotherapy. The patient's head may be supported with a pillow.

g) May lightly shave site with electric razor or clip hair if necessary.

h) Prepare a sterile field, and open equipment.

i) Examine area over the reservoir for signs of infection or trauma.

j) Gently palpate the reservoir. May pump reservoir three to four times to fill with CSF from ventricle. If giving chemotherapy, don long-sleeve, low permeability gown and double gloves. Top pair of gloves should be sterile. Maintain sterile technique throughout procedure.

k) Using three alcohol swabs, cleanse the area over the site in a circular motion, beginning with the center and moving outward, and avoid covering the same area twice with the same swab.

l) Repeat with the three povidone-iodine swabsticks.

m) Allow povidone-iodine to air-dry for one to two minutes.

n) Insert the butterfly needle with extension tubing at a 45°–90° angle into the reservoir (see Figure 16). A release of resistance

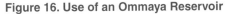

Figure 16. Use of an Ommaya Reservoir

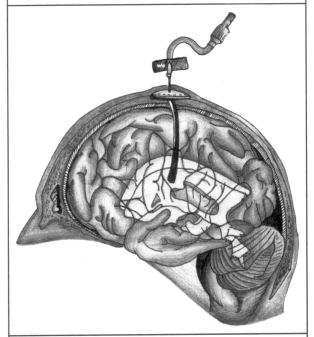

Note. From "Vascular Access Devices" (p. 64), by J.S. Webster in M.M. Gullatte (Ed.), *Clinical Guide to Antineoplastic Therapy: A Chemotherapy Handbook,* 2001, Pittsburgh, PA: Oncology Nursing Society. Copyright 2001 by the Oncology Nursing Society. Reprinted with permission.

---

will be felt when reservoir is punctured. If blood appears in tubing, withdraw and reinsert at a 90° angle to avoid tunneling between scalp and dome of reservoir. May attach a sterile three-way stopcock if administering medication.

o) Gently withdraw CSF into the syringe. CSF should flow freely into the syringe. If resistance is noted, remove butterfly and attempt again with new butterfly. If resistance is still noted, or if the patient complains of discomfort, stop the procedure and notify the physician. Withdraw CSF equal to the amount of drug to be infused, plus an additional 3 ml to use as flush following the procedure, and set aside on a sterile field, maintaining the sterility of the syringe. May use a three-way stopcock to maintain closed system.

(1) If CSF is bloody or cloudy: Preserve the specimen, notify the doctor, and stop the procedure. May send sample for culture, sensitivity, gram stain, protein, glucose, and cell count with differential.

(2) Little information is available on how rapidly to inject intraventricular medications, but some consensus exists on the need to premix the drug with CSF to enhance equilibrium of drug concentration in CSF. This may be accomplished by using a barbotage technique (Bering, Rall, Walker, Leventhal, & Ommaya, 1969). Barbotage may be done safely by withdrawing about 1 ml of CSF into the syringe prior to injection, thus allowing CSF to mix with medication in the syringe. This process can be continued until the syringe is empty.

(3) Following medication, flush with reserved CSF or preservative-free normal saline. Controversy exists over whether to use preservative-free normal saline or reserved CSF to flush following medication administration. The recent literature contains a paucity of information. A three-way stopcock can be used during intraventricular administration to retain a closed sterile system throughout the procedure. One syringe contains chemotherapy (or medication) and the other CSF. This eliminates the need to change syringes during the procedure and reduces the risk of infection.

(4) If the patient is receiving liposomal cytarabine, 4 mg of dexamethasone must be taken two times per day beginning the day of administration and continued for four additional days to limit arachnoiditis (Enzon Pharmaceuticals, Inc., 2007).

p) Remove needle, and apply gentle pressure with a sterile 2 × 2 gauze.

q) Gently pump the reservoir three to five times to help distribute the drug; this is particularly important if barbotage was not done during administration.

r) Instruct the patient to report headache, nausea, dizziness, neck or back pain or stiffness, or other neurologic symptoms.

s) Obtain vital signs, and assess neurologic status following the procedure. The patient may ambulate immediately following the procedure if stable. The patient may be released from outpatient facility immediately following procedure if vital signs are stable and the patient is clinically stable.

I. Complications
   1. Infection
      a) Etiology
         (1) Improper technique when accessing the system
         (2) Surgical contamination
         (3) Systemic complication of immunosuppressed patient
         (4) Non-iatrogenic trauma to site
      b) Signs and symptoms (Halaby et al., 2007)
         (1) Site tenderness, warmth, erythema, or drainage
         (2) Fever
         (3) Headache with or without vomiting, neck stiffness
         (4) Bloody or purulent CSF from reservoir
      c) Laboratory: Elevated white blood cell count, elevated protein, and microbial growth in CSF specimen
      d) Prevention
         (1) Maintain strict sterile technique when accessing the system.
         (2) Ensure that only specially trained personnel access the device.
         (3) Protect the device from trauma and damage.
      e) Interventions
         (1) Obtain a sample from the reservoir for culture and sensitivity, gram stain, protein, glucose, and cell count with differential.
         (2) Infection frequently can be treated by instillation of antibiotics or antifungals into the reservoir or by IV antibiotic therapy (Elvy, Porter, & Brown, 2008; James & Bradley, 2008).
         (3) Persistent infection requires device removal.
   2. Malposition or migration of catheter
      a) Etiology
         (1) Kinking of catheter
         (2) Migration of catheter out of ventricle
      b) Signs and symptoms
         (1) Poor or absent refilling of the reservoir when depressed
         (2) Inability to gently aspirate CSF
         (3) Inability to instill fluid into the reservoir
         (4) CSF leakage around the reservoir
         (5) Change in neurologic status: Dizziness, headache, lethargy
      c) Interventions
         (1) Notify physician.
         (2) Verify placement by radiologic imaging (CT or magnetic resonance imaging [MRI] of brain)
         (3) Attempt to gently irrigate catheter.
         (4) Refer to neurosurgeon to evaluate need for revision of or removal of device.
   3. Blood in CSF
      a) Etiology
         (1) Intraventricular hemorrhage
         (2) Subdural hematoma
         (3) Subarachnoid hematoma
         (4) Improper positioning of butterfly needle during access (actually SC bleeding)
      b) Assessment
         (1) Change in neurologic status
         (2) Sensory or motor deficits
      c) Interventions
         (1) Notify physician.
         (2) Condition may require surgical intervention (craniotomy).
         (3) Order radiographic studies to verify placement.
J. Patient education
   1. Care of device
      a) Avoid getting incision wet while sutures are present.
      b) No special care is required once sutures are removed.
      c) Hair is allowed to grow back, except for a small 2–3 cm area over the device.
      d) Avoid trauma to the site to prevent wound dehiscence or damage to the reservoir.

2. Signs and symptoms of infection or device malfunction
    a) Site tenderness, warmth, erythema, or drainage
    b) Fever
    c) Headache with or without vomiting, neck stiffness
    d) Bloody or purulent CSF from reservoir
    e) Vision changes
    f) Nausea and vomiting
    g) Ataxia or slurred speech
    h) Change in mentation or level of consciousness
K. Special considerations (Jansen et al., 2008; Kolaski & Logan, 2007; LaFay-Cousin & Strother, 2009)
    1. Pediatric
        a) Cognitive development may be affected by treatments.
        b) Intrathecal chemotherapy may have less effect on cognitive function than radiation therapy.
        c) Studies are limited by size and wide variations in age of patients.
        d) Nursing care should be developmentally appropriate.
    2. Older adults: Underlying dementia may complicate assessment and diagnosis of medication-induced mental status changes in patients receiving intrathecal chemotherapy.
L. Education and documentation: See Section X.
M. For a practicum on intraventricular reservoirs, see Appendix 8.

VI. EPIDURAL AND INTRATHECAL ACCESS DEVICES

A. History (Brill, Gurman, & Fisher, 2003; Frolich & Caton, 2001)
   1. Description of infiltrating morphine around a peripheral nerve was first published by Francis Rynd in 1845.
   2. First epidural analgesia was discovered accidentally by Leonard J. Corning in 1885 when he introduced cocaine between the lumbar vertebral processes in a patient whom he was treating for habitual masturbation.
   3. In 1898 in England, August Bier and his assistant experimented with intrathecal anesthesia by administering cocaine intrathecally to each other.
   4. Rudolph Matas of the United States first performed intrathecal anesthesia using morphine in 1899.
   5. Reports of lumbar epidural anesthesia were published in 1921.
   6. Spinal catheters were described in 1944 when Edward Tuohy threaded a No. 4 silk catheter through a Barker needle for continuous spinal anesthesia. Because silk was difficult to sterilize, the development of plastic catheters, which could withstand the heat of autoclaving, began to surface around 1949.
B. Description and types of access devices
   1. Definitions
      a) Epidural: Dura mater is the most exterior membrane covering the spinal cord. This area forms the inner border of the epidural space.
      b) Intrathecal: The area below the dura where CSF circulates
   2. Epidural and intrathecal implantable systems
      a) Similar to venous, arterial, and peritoneal ports (all have a portal body, reservoir, septum, and catheter), except epidural and intrathecal ports have a 60 micron filter within the reservoir, and the low-profile systems have a 20 micron filter that prevents large particulate matter from entering the catheter (see Section II.G for information on implanted ports)
      b) Volume of reservoir in portal body: Approximately 0.5 ml
      c) Radiopaque polyurethane, nylon, Teflon, and wire-reinforced catheter
         (1) Epidural: Outer diameter of 1.2 mm and internal diameter of 0.5 mm is attached or unattached to portal body.
         (2) Intraspinal: Outer diameter of 0.9 mm and internal diameter of 0.5 mm is attached or unattached to portal body.
      d) Portal body designed with polysulfone on the outside and titanium on the inside
   3. Catheters
      a) Temporary: Epidural and intrathecal
         (1) Radiopaque polyamide, polyurethane, Teflon, or nylon catheters are available with open- or closed-end tips with three-eyed multiport configuration.
         (2) Outer diameter of 0.85 mm. Catheter can be inserted through an 18-gauge or 20-gauge epidural or spinal needle.
         (3) Catheter can produce skin irritation at the site of insertion; therefore, these catheters are not suitable for long-term therapy.
      b) Tunneled catheter: Epidural and intrathecal (see section II.F)
         (1) Outer diameter of 1.3 mm and includes an attached Dacron® (Invista, Inc.) cuff and/or VitaCuff® (C.R. Bard, Inc.)
         (2) Silicone polyurethane material with radiopaque material
   4. Implantable pump with catheter attached (see Section VIII for pump description)
   5. Costs: Global cost, including surgical placement and catheter, is approximately $5,481.
   6. Purpose of epidural and intrathecal access
      a) Administration of opioid analgesics and anesthetic medications for chronic intractable pain that is inadequately controlled by aggressive pharmacologic interventions with oral, rectal, IV, or transdermal methods (Ghafoor et al., 2007; Heran, Smith, & Legiehn, 2008)
      b) Administration of chemotherapy agents intrathecally
      c) Administration of antispasmodic agents intrathecally (Brashear & Lambeth, 2009; Kolaski & Logan, 2007)
C. Advantages and disadvantages: See Table 11.
D. Patient selection for epidural and intrathecal access devices (Brashear & Lambeth, 2009; Clayton et al., 2008; Ghafoor et al., 2007; Heran et al., 2008)
   1. Patient with chronic intractable cancer pain
   2. Patient with chronic intractable back or pelvic pain
   3. Patient with postsurgical pain and needs temporary epidural anesthesia or patient-controlled anesthesia
   4. Placement of intrathecal baclofen pumps for patients with spasticity
   5. Frequent administration of intrathecal chemotherapy for patients with primary neurologic cancers or neoplastic meningitis

Table 11. Advantages and Disadvantages of Epidural or Intrathecal Access Devices

Type	Advantages	Disadvantages
Overall (compared to other routes)	• Less sedation with narcotics than with other routes, such as IV • Less effect on cardiovascular or respiratory status	• Requires skilled personnel to manage catheter, which may be problematic in some rural areas • Medications used with epidural and intraspinal may be difficult to obtain in rural areas.
Temporary catheter	• Indicated postoperatively for short-term pain control (e.g., trauma pain, postoperative pain) • Indicated for infrequent access for medications • Ease and speed of insertion • Used for pain control when life expectancy is weeks	• Cannot be easily secured, thus falls out readily or leaks around insertion site • Requires frequent, meticulous site care • Maintenance supplies add to cost.
Permanent catheter	• Facilitates ambulation and activities of daily living with adequate pain control • Less risk of catheter dislodgment • Can be used for more than a year	• Requires surgical placement and removal • Placement costs are expensive when compared to temporary catheters. • Cost of maintenance supplies • Greater risk of infection
Implantable port	• Less chance of infection • Facilitates ambulation and activities of daily living with adequate pain control • Less risk of catheter dislodgment • Can be used for months or years	• Requires surgical procedure for placement and removal • Involves expensive placement costs compared to temporary catheters • Requires access with a noncoring needle
Implantable pump	• Less chance of infection • Infusion rates can be changed by a computer. • Less risk of catheter dislodgment • Catheter can be placed epidurally or intrathecally. • Because of the pump reservoir's capacity, refills are required only every one to three months.	• The complexity of the technology requires healthcare professionals who are trained in computer technology and internal pump access. • Initial cost of equipment and implantation is high. • Requires needlestick for access • Because the life of the pump may be shorter than the patient's life expectancy, it may have to be surgically replaced. • Patient can form granulomas on catheter tip and may require catheter removal.

E. Insertion procedure and postoperative care
  1. Patient preparation
    a) Review recent imaging studies, laboratory studies, medications, and clinical notes.
      (1) Notify physician of neutropenia, thrombocytopenia, current anticoagulation therapy, and abnormal imaging results.
      (2) If the patient is on low-molecular-weight heparin, physician may instruct to hold medication for 24 hours prior to procedure to reduce risk of epidural or intrathecal hematoma (Pian-Smith & Nishida, 2007).
      (3) If the patient is taking warfarin, physician may instruct to hold dose for three to five days prior to procedure to reduce risk of epidural or intrathecal hematoma (Pian-Smith & Nishida, 2007).
    b) Discuss the procedure, risks, and rationale with the patient and obtain informed consent.
    c) Observe strict aseptic technique to avoid iatrogenic meningitis or sepsis.
      (1) Wear sterile gloves and mask (Halaby et al., 2007).
      (2) Use sterile barriers.
    d) Clean the area of insertion.
      (1) Ten percent povidone-iodine and 0.5% chlorhexidine have been shown to be effective as cleansing agents.
      (2) Ten percent povidone-iodine, chlorhexidine, and alcohol all have the potential to be toxic to the central nervous system (CNS) if introduced during access.
      (3) The American Society of Regional Anesthesia and Pain Medicine recommends use of chlorhexidine for skin preparation prior to regional anesthesia (Hebl, 2006).
  2. Epidural and intrathecal port placement (Pian-Smith & Nishida, 2007)

a) Placement is performed in the operating room with the patient under local anesthesia.

b) Patient is placed in a lateral decubitus or sitting position.

c) Catheter is inserted percutaneously into the epidural space approximately 4 cm, usually at L2–3, L3–4, or L4–5.

   (1) Dura mater is the most exterior membrane covering the spinal cord, which forms the inner border of the epidural space. The ligamentum flavum and periosteum of the vertebral column form the outer border. The epidural space is a potential space between these boundaries.

   (2) Epidural space extends from the foramen magnum to the sacral hiatus.

   (3) Contents of the epidural space are composed of adipose and connective tissue as well as blood vessels.

   (4) For intrathecal administration, the catheter is advanced below the dura where CSF circulates. Presence of CSF within the spinal needle hub verifies correct placement.

d) The proximal end of the catheter is subcutaneously tunneled around the flank to the abdomen or anterior chest wall and connected to the portal body.

e) The portal body is sutured to the fascia over a bony prominence, such as the lower rib.

3. A temporary catheter may be placed for up to seven days.

   a) It may be inserted at the bedside or in the operating room using local anesthesia and placed into the epidural space or intrathecal space of the spine.

   b) External portion is taped up the patient's back to the anterior chest wall or around the flank and taped to the abdomen.

   c) Assess site for CSF drainage, which could indicate a disconnected temporary catheter.

4. Tunneled catheter

   a) Catheter is inserted in the operating room using local anesthesia, with the distal tip of the catheter inserted into the epidural or intrathecal space.

   b) Proximal tip is tunneled under the SC tissue, exiting at the waist or side of the abdomen.

5. SC implantable pump

   a) Pump is inserted in the operating room while the patient is under local anesthesia.

b) Pump is implanted into a created SC pocket, and the catheter is tunneled and threaded into the intrathecal space.

6. Immediate postoperative care

   a) Check dressing for bleeding or drainage.

   b) Assess site for hematoma or excessive postoperative edema.

   c) Change dressing daily until site is healed.

   d) Perform frequent neurologic assessments.

   e) Monitor vital signs per postoperative routine and then every four hours until they are stable.

   f) Assess for pain.

F. Maintenance and care procedures

1. Before accessing epidural or intrathecal device, check with the state nursing board and institution for restrictions.

2. Nurses must be knowledgeable of the principles of epidural drug administration.

   a) The patient will be monitored and managed with the initial dose of opiate and with each subsequent increase in dose.

   b) The patient needs to be weaned off other opioids while receiving epidural analgesia.

   c) Monitor the patient for signs of infection (Halaby et al., 2007; Holmfred et al., 2006; Rhinehart & McGoldrick, 2005).

      (1) Systemic signs: Fever, headache, nausea or vomiting, neck or back pain or stiffness, seizure, altered mental status, or sepsis

      (2) Local signs: Tenderness, erythema, edema, CSF leakage, bleeding, purulent drainage at the insertion site, or wound dehiscence

   d) Monitor for signs of device failure, catheter migration, or mass at catheter tip (Deer, Raso, & Garten, 2007; Gibbins et al., 2008; Harney & Victor, 2004; Jhas & Tuli, 2008): Resistance upon infusion of fluids, alteration of circulation, CSF leakage, sensory changes, inability to aspirate CSF from intrathecal catheter, weakness or decreased mobility in lower extremities, bowel or bladder incontinence or retention, cranial nerve deficits if CSF leak is present (particularly sixth nerve palsy), or pain

   e) Always use Luer-lock connections. Avoid tubing with injection ports, or place tape over any injection ports to prevent inadvertent administration of other drugs into the epidural or intrathecal catheter.

   f) Epidural and intrathecal catheters should be clearly labeled to avoid being confused with venous catheters (Arrow International, Inc., 2007).

g) With continuous infusion administration of medication, tape a tension loop of tubing to the patient's body to prevent accidental dislodgment.

h) Only preservative-free normal saline or Elliotts B® solution (QOL Medical) may be administered or used as a diluent in intrathecal medications. Elliotts B solution is an artificial fluid that approximates the normal ionic composition of CSF.

i) Check placement prior to drug administration by gently aspirating. If clear fluid volume is greater than 0.5 ml or if blood is obtained, notify physician and do not administer drug. The presence of CSF indicates that the catheter has punctured the dura, and the presence of blood may indicate that the catheter has punctured the vasculature.

j) Assess the patient for symptoms of respiratory and CNS depression by monitoring the following.
   (1) Quality and rate of respirations
   (2) Breath sounds
   (3) Color of lips and nail beds
   (4) Level of consciousness, sensorium, and arousability

k) Use of an apnea monitor or pulse oximetry is recommended for the first 24 hours of intrathecal or opioid administration because the risk of respiratory depression is highest during this period. Respiratory depression may not occur in patients who have been taking an opiate on a long-term basis.
   (1) Delayed respiratory depression usually occurs 3–12 hours after administration, but it can occur as long as 24 hours after.
   (2) Have an oral airway, Ambu® bag (Ambu Inc.), and naloxone hydrochloride at the bedside for management of respiratory depression.

l) All patients must have an IV line or intermittent locking device in place for at least 24 hours for administration of naloxone, as needed.

m) Keep head of bed elevated 30°.

n) Assess for signs and symptoms of urinary retention, pruritus, nausea, vomiting, and loss of sensation in lower extremities as indications of opioid toxicity or catheter migration.

o) Intensive homecare teaching is imperative to the patient and caregiver.

   (1) Explain injection of medication technique, catheter care, dressing changes, infection precautions, and signs to report to the physician.
   (2) Maintain frequent telephone contact or home visits.

3. Maintain strict aseptic technique with mask and sterile gloves with any access or maintenance procedures (Rhinehart & McGoldrick, 2005).
   a) Strict aseptic technique
      (1) Wear mask and sterile gloves.
      (2) Use povidone-iodine or chlorhexidine to clean, as alcohol is contraindicated (Arrow International, Inc., 2007).
   b) Dressing changes: Clear dressing should be applied to allow for visualization of the site.
   c) Flushing
      (1) Catheter (temporary and permanent): 1–2 ml of preservative-free normal saline after use
      (2) Port: 3 ml of preservative-free normal saline after use
      (3) Pump: No flushing required
      (4) Routine flushing not necessary because tip is in CSF
   d) Daily site inspection for drainage, erythema, and edema

4. Administering analgesics through catheter or port (see Section II.G for information on port access)
   a) Follow strict aseptic technique using mask and sterile gloves (Rhinehart & McGoldrick, 2005).
   b) Check label on catheter to verify epidural or intrathecal placement.
   c) Gently aspirate 1 ml of fluid. If blood or greater than 0.5 ml of serous fluid is aspirated from epidural catheter, notify the physician and do not administer drug.
   d) Blood should not be aspirated from intrathecal catheter. CSF should be present if intrathecal catheter is properly positioned.
   e) Slowly and steadily inject the medication through a 0.2 micron filter without surfactant.
   f) Flush the catheter with 1–2 ml of preservative-free normal saline. The port may be flushed with up to 3 ml of preservative-free normal saline to ensure that medication has reached epidural or intrathecal space.

5. Filter and injection cap change: A filter may not be required if the drug is filtered prior to drug administration or if the portal body contains a filter.

a) Change filter and injection cap every week or more frequently if damage or leaks occur.

b) Wash hands.

c) Prepare appropriate equipment for the procedure.

d) Apply mask and sterile gloves.

e) Attach the new injection cap to the new filter, and flush the system with preservative-free normal saline.

f) Clean the connection between the catheter and the filter with a povidone-iodine swab, allowing it to dry completely.

g) If any excess povidone-iodine remains, remove with sterile gauze.

h) Remove old filter and injection cap.

i) Screw on the new filter and injection cap securely.

j) Place a label saying "epidural" or "intrathecal" around the tubing near the hub.

6. Contact homecare agency for follow-up and patient support, if appropriate.

G. Removal of device

1. Temporary catheters can be pulled directly out of epidural and intraventricular systems after applying sterile gloves at the bedside. Catheter is assessed for integrity. Whether a trained RN or APN can remove temporary catheters depends on the individual state board of nursing. Training and competency records must be maintained.

2. Pumps and ports are removed in the operating room under sterile technique. Often these devices are left in place and not removed except in the occurrence of catheter migration, infection, CSF leak, hematoma, meningitis, catheter occlusion, or severe spinal headaches.

H. Complications of epidural and intrathecal access devices

1. Infection (Halaby et al., 2007; Holmfred et al., 2006; Rhinehart & McGoldrick, 2005)

a) Sites of possible infection: Exit site, tunnel, port pocket, pump pocket, epidural space, CSF, and surgical wound

(1) Bacteria from the patient's skin have direct access to the CNS via an epidural or intrathecal catheter and are responsible for a significant number of wound infections.

(2) The patient and caregivers returning home with a catheter must be educated on aseptic technique and its importance.

b) Assessment: Edema, tenderness, local warmth, drainage, headache, pain during injection, decreased analgesic effects after pain medications are administered, fever, change in sensory or motor function, nuchal rigidity, mental status changes, port or pump pocket erythema, seizure, and photophobia

c) Prevention

(1) Strict sterile technique during insertion of device, as well as during routine maintenance and medication administration, is vital in preventing meningitis.

(2) Protect the exit site from injury and the device from damage.

(3) Use a microporous filter to decrease introduction of pathogens.

(4) Use of a face mask by healthcare provider can significantly reduce the risk of iatrogenic meningitis caused by *Streptococcus salivarius*.

d) Intervention and treatment

(1) Obtain CSF culture, gram stain, cell count with differential, and protein and glucose levels.

(2) Administer antibiotics either IV or through the device.

(3) Remove device if persistent infection is present. Culture tip of catheter.

2. Displacement or migration of catheter (Gibbins et al., 2008; Harney & Victor, 2004; Narouze, Yonan, Kapural, & Malak, 2007)

a) Etiology: Kinking or blockage of catheter, catheter migration out of epidural space, catheter compression, inadvertent dural puncture during epidural placement, or spinal cord puncture either by migration of intrathecal catheter or during insertion

b) Associated with a variety of mal effects including ineffective pain control, traumatic syrinx, epigastric arterial erosion, and cerebral hypotension and herniation because of excessive CSF leakage

c) Assessment parameters

(1) Change in neurologic status

(2) Spinal headache

(3) CSF leakage around the exit site, port, or pump pocket

(4) Slow or resistant filling of pump reservoir or port

(5) Easy mobility of port under the skin

(6) Increase in pain

(7) Outward migration of catheter judged by catheter marks outside the patient's body

c) Prevention: Avoid trauma to the implant site or device.

d) Intervention and treatment (Harney & Victor, 2004)

(1) Attempt to gently irrigate with preservative-free normal saline.

(2) Notify physician if blood or greater than 0.5 ml of CSF is aspirated from epidural catheter, and do not administer drug.

(3) Perform a neurologic assessment.

(4) Conduct a CT or MRI to assess placement of catheter. (NOTE: intrathecal/epidural pumps must be turned off prior to MRI.)

(5) Consider the use of radiation therapy to decrease size of tumor if tumor growth blocks the catheter.

(6) If a dural puncture inadvertently occurs, increase fluid and caffeine intake, and keep the patient flat in bed for 12–24 hours.

(7) Administer pain medications as needed for dural headache.

(8) Remove device.

3. Bleeding

a) Epidural or subarachnoid bleeding

b) Assessment parameters

(1) Change in neurologic status

(2) Severe back pain

(3) Sensory or motor deficits

c) Intervention and treatment

(1) Notify physician, and order CT or MRI.

(2) Establish IV access.

(3) Elevate head of bed 30°.

(4) Monitor neurologic status and vital signs.

(5) Obtain neurosurgery consult if neurologic status is deteriorating.

(6) Physician may need to remove device if bleeding persists.

4. Stroke (Heran et al., 2008)

a) Etiology is unclear. May be related to inadvertent trauma to artery upon puncture.

b) May occur in either the brain or the spinal cord. Most common with cervical spine injections.

5. Fibrin formation at catheter tip (Deer et al., 2007; Jhas & Tuli, 2008)

a) Etiology: May result from fibrin sheath formation around catheter distal tip applying pressure to the dorsal nerve, nerve roots, and spinal cord

b) Symptoms: Inadequate pain management, neurologic deficits, paralysis, and bowel or bladder retention or incontinence

c) Pain occurs with injection; radicular pain is more frequent with intrathecal catheters.

d) Backtracking of drug can occur outside the catheter, with deposition of drug into the SC tissue.

e) Intervention and treatment: Inject drug slowly. If pain persists, evaluate location of catheter tip by x-ray. Removal of device may be necessary.

6. Dislodgment of needle from port

a) Assessment: Edema at port or reservoir site, uncontrolled pain, erythema at port site

b) Prevention: Secure needle using Steri-Strips securement device or tape across the needle hub with occlusive dressing. Tape a tension loop of tubing to skin.

c) Intervention/treatment: Reaccess device.

I. Pediatric considerations (Jansen et al., 2008; Kolaski & Logan, 2007; Lafay-Cousin & Strother, 2009)

1. Cognitive development may be affected by treatments.

2. Intrathecal chemotherapy may have less effect on cognitive function than radiation therapy.

3. Complications related to intrathecal baclofen are more likely in children.

4. Studies are limited by size and wide variations in age of patients.

5. Nursing care should be developmentally appropriate.

J. Geriatric considerations (Chau, Walker, Pai, & Cho, 2008)

1. Older adult patients may metabolize opiates differently.

2. Polypharmacy frequently complicates management of pain.

3. If dementia is present, the patient may be unable to report either pain or relief of pain. Thus, the potential for undertreated pain is high in this group.

K. Education and documentation: See Section X.

L. For a practicum on epidural and intrathecal device care, see Appendix 9.

VII. INTRAPERITONEAL (IP) CATHETERS

A. History (Twardowski, 2004)

1. Began with the need to access the peritoneal cavity for drainage of ascites fluid and for peritoneal dialysis

2. As early as 1923, available equipment that was used for other purposes, such as metal trocars and glass cannulas used for surgical drains, were adapted to access the peritoneal cavity. The rigidity of the materials led to problems of leakage, infection, and catheter occlusion.

3. In the 1940s and 1950s, discovery of less rigid materials, such as nylon and polyvinyl, improved the drainage of peritoneal fluid, yet infection and leakage remained a problem.

4. In the 1960s, a silicone rubber model with the coiled IP end with multiple perforations extending 23 cm from the tip with a long SC tunnel became the prototype of the current peritoneal catheters.

5. Henry Tenckhoff, in 1965, improved the peritoneal catheter for peritoneal dialysis. The intra-abdominal flange was replaced by a Dacron cuff, the SC tunnel was shortened, and a second, external cuff was used to decrease the length of the catheter.

6. Research continues with catheter modifications in an effort to decrease infection, leakage, and obstructive complications.

7. Implanted ports were first used for peritoneal access in the early 1980s.

B. Description of devices

1. Catheters are temporarily or permanently implanted into the peritoneal cavity.

2. They provide repeated access to the peritoneal cavity for the administration of IP therapies (e.g., chemotherapy, biologic response modifiers, dialysis), as well as the removal of peritoneal fluid for diagnosis, analysis, and palliation of ascites.

3. Catheter may contain a single lumen or have multiple holes (fenestrated) that permit increased distribution of solutions.

4. Cost: See Table 12.

5. External tunneled catheters (see Figure 17)

   a) May be temporary catheters used for one-time access, either for paracentesis or delivery of medications into the peritoneum, or semipermanent catheters, such as the Tenckhoff, used for repeated access into the peritoneum (Covidien, n.d.)

   b) Materials: Silicone or polyurethane with radiopaque stripe for identification on radiologic studies

   c) Size: Consists of three parts

      (1) External segment is 20 cm.

      (2) SC segment is 2–10 cm long.

      (3) Intra-abdominal segment is 31–48 cm long.

   d) Catheters are available in multiple styles, sizes, and configurations for infant (31 cm), child (35 cm), and adult (42 cm) lengths.

   e) Internal portion of the catheter may be coiled or straight with outer diameters ranging from 8–15 Fr. Coiled catheters decrease the incidence of catheter migration (Covidien, n.d.).

   f) May have single or double Dacron cuffs on the catheter to secure its position and prevent infection within the IP cavity

      (1) One cuff: Located between the external exit site and SC segments, placed 2–3 cm from the catheter exit site, deep subcutaneously to prevent cuff infection and extrusion (Covidien, n.d.)

      (2) Two cuffs: One located between the external exit site and SC segments and one between the SC and intra-abdominal segments, anchored to the rectus sheath, making a watertight seal to prevent leakage and infection (Covidien, n.d.; Rosot Enterprises, Inc., n.d.)

   g) VitaCuff also is available. The VitaCuff is a short-term antimicrobial barrier cuff that protects against infection (Bard Access Systems, Inc., 2007a).

   h) External catheters for IP use also may have an optional BD™ (Becton, Dickinson and Co.) clamp placed on the tubing to prevent backflow of fluid from the peritoneal cavity. This optional clamp can be used on either a permanent or temporary catheter.

6. Implanted SC ports (see Figure 18)

   a) Materials: Titanium or plastic portal body has a self-sealing silicone septum and may have a preattached or attachable radiopaque polyurethane or silicone single-lumen or

Table 12. Approximate Costs of Intraperitoneal Catheters

Catheter	Cost of the Device	Physician Fee	Radiology Fee	Facilities Fee (National Charge Percentile)
Implanted port with no Dacron® (DuPont) cuff, fenestrated tubing	$595	Insertion $950–$1,500 Removal $950–$1,200	Insertion $1,500 Removal $1,000	$3,200 $2,348
Implanted port with one Dacron cuff, fenestrated tubing	$642	Insertion $950–1,500 Removal $950–$1,200	Insertion $1,500 Removal $1,000	$3,200 $2,348
Venous access device for IP use, single-lumen opening	$665	Insertion $950–$1,500 Removal $950–$1,200	Insertion $1,500 Removal $1,000	$3,200 $2,348
External IP catheter with one Dacron cuff	$75	Insertion $950–$1,500 Removal $950–$1,200	Insertion $1,500 Removal $1,000	$3,200 $2,348
External IP catheter with two Dacron cuffs	$85	Insertion $950–$1,500 Removal $900–$1,200	Insertion $1,500 Removal $1,000	$3,200 $2,348

Note. Information was obtained from catheter companies Covidien and Bard Access Device Systems and was accurate at the time of publication. Physician, radiology, and facilities fees obtained from local hospital and based on CPT (procedural) codes for 2009 and the allowable fee that is charged to patients for this service.

fenestrated catheter (Bard Access Systems, Inc., 2007a).

b) Size: Septum diameter is 11.4 mm, and catheter length is 31–48 cm.

c) Diameter: Attached catheter has an outer diameter ranging from 6.6–9.6 Fr. This system can only be accessed with a noncoring needle (19–22 gauge).

d) The cuff, if one is used, is located between the IP and the SC sections of the catheter.

e) Ports are available in adult and child sizes.

C. Advantages and disadvantages of peritoneal devices: See Table 13.

D. Patient selection criteria

1. Patients receive IP therapy for the following malignancies.

a) Ovarian cancer: In 2006, the National Cancer Institute (NCI) announced the use of IP chemotherapy as an option for first-line therapy for patients with stage III optimally debulked ovarian cancer. For this patient population, IP chemotherapy was shown to increase the tumor-free interval and overall survival over IV chemotherapy alone (Armstrong et al., 2006; Markman, 2007).

(1) Microscopic residual disease (less than or equal to 1 cm) after initial surgical debulking

(2) Consolidation therapy after conventional IV therapy or after negative second-look surgery

(3) Extended therapy after second-look exploration for patients with small-volume residual disease (less than or equal to 1 cm)

b) Gastrointestinal malignancies

(1) Initial treatment in patients with small-volume IP disease of low-grade gastrointestinal and appendiceal carcinoma (Marin, Oleszewski, & Muehlbauer, 2007; National Institutes of Health, 2007a)

(2) Adjuvant therapy for patients with a high risk of relapse

c) Pseudomyxoma peritonei syndrome, an uncommon, slowly progressive condition that usually arises from perforation of a histologically benign adenoma in the appendix, characterized by mucin accumulation in the peritoneal cavity (Sugarbaker, 2006)

Figure 17. External Peritoneal Catheter

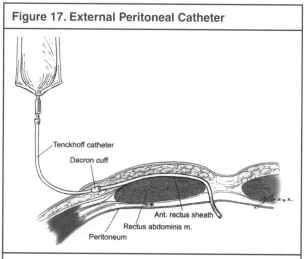

Tenckhoff catheter
Dacron cuff
Ant. rectus sheath
Rectus abdominis m.
Peritoneum

Note. From "Surgical Techniques" (p. 746), by J.S. Berek in J.S. Berek and N.F. Hacker (Eds.), *Practical Gynecologic Oncology* (4th ed.), 2004, Philadelphia, PA: Lippincott Williams & Wilkins. Copyright 2004 by Lippincott Williams & Wilkins. Reprinted with permission.

Figure 18. Implanted Peritoneal Port

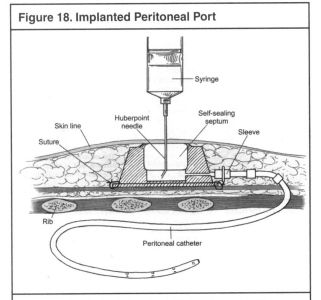

Note. From "Surgical Techniques" (p. 747), by J.S. Berek in J.S. Berek and N.F. Hacker (Eds.), *Practical Gynecologic Oncology* (4th ed.), 2004, Philadelphia, PA: Lippincott Williams & Wilkins. Copyright 2004 by Lippincott Williams & Wilkins. Reprinted with permission.

d) Used in clinical trials for patients with peritoneal carcinomatosis secondary to abdominal and pelvic malignancies (Yung et al., 2009)

e) Malignant peritoneal mesothelioma that is limited to the peritoneum (Hesdorffer, Chabot, DeRosa, & Taub, 2008)

f) Palliative treatment for ascites in lymphoma and gynecologic, gastrointestinal, lung, and breast cancers (Inan et al., 2008)

2. Patient characteristics

a) Peritoneal disease should be maximally cytoreduced or debulked to improve response to the IP treatment (Bryant et al., 2004; Trope & Kaern, 2006).

b) Tumor is confined to the peritoneal cavity.

c) The patient should be free of abdominal adhesions, which would limit even distribution of IP therapy (Berek, 2004). Peritoneal distribution can be checked in the radiology department by inserting radiopaque dye diluted in 2 liters of fluid, followed by CT scan of the abdomen (Berek, 2004).

d) If inserted during initial surgical exploration, therapy should begin after seven days (Berek, 2004).

e) If bowel resection or vaginal entry has occurred, the patient may need additional healing time before initiation of IP chemotherapy treatment (Walker et al., 2006).

f) The patient or caregiver must have the physical and cognitive ability to care for a catheter.

g) The patient must have a good performance status to be able to tolerate an aggressive treatment schedule and side effects.

h) The patient should be able to tolerate large volumes of IP fluid.

i) With pediatric and older adult patients, the volume of fluid for IP treatment can be adjusted to the size of the patient, using the reference of 1 liter of fluid per body surface area (BSA) (i.e., for BSA 1.5, volume can be 1.5 liters).

j) IP chemotherapy is rarely used in the pediatric population, as this cohort of patients typically is diagnosed with nonepithelial gynecologic cancers that are best treated with IV chemotherapy. If a pediatric patient requires an IP catheter, it is mostly likely being used for peritoneal dialysis.

3. The type of IP therapy will determine what type of catheter will be used.

a) Infusion of chemotherapeutic agents perioperatively, postoperatively, and as consolidation therapy for first-line and recurrent disease

b) May be administered during initial cytoreductive surgery as hyperthermic intraperitoneal chemotherapy (HIPEC), postoperatively, or as a combination of both. During cytoreductive surgery, the patient is cooled to 34°–35°C, and IP fluid is warmed to 40°–43°C. The rationale is that the increased temperature of the drug will increase tumor cell kill. HIPEC is being studied in pseudomyxoma peritonei, malignant peritoneal mesothelioma, and gynecologic and gastrointestinal malignancies (Murphy, Sexton, & Moran, 2007; Sugarbaker, 2009).

c) Infusion of chemotherapy for palliative treatment of carcinomatosis or ascites

d) Drainage of chronic ascites accumulation in the palliative setting for lymphoma and gynecologic, gastrointestinal, and other cancers. Patients experience severe discomfort from fluid accumulation, as evidenced by shortness of breath, inability to eat, decreased mobility, abdominal pain, and fatigue (Winkelman, 2004).

   (1) The patient has intractable ascites that requires multiple paracentesis.

   (2) Ascites fluid must be clear and nonmucinous.

   (3) Prognosis must be greater than one month.

Table 13. Advantages and Disadvantages of Intraperitoneal Devices

Type	Advantages	Disadvantages
External Tenckhoff peritoneal catheter	• Serves as a semipermanent access device that allows cyclic treatments over a long period of time • Decreases risk of visceral or bowel perforation when compared to temporarily placed intraperitoneal catheters for peritoneal access • Permits faster fluid infusion rate: 2 liters in 10–15 minutes • Permits rapid drainage of fluid • Allows for collection of fluid samples • Allows for high-pressure forced irrigation or manipulation to loosen fibrin clots • Access is less painful to the patient. • Can be removed at the bedside or as outpatient if a Dacron® (DuPont) cuff is used • Repair kits are available for external portion of the catheter. • Catheter is inexpensive. • Patient and caregivers can learn how to care for the catheter and how to drain fluid for palliation of ascites.	• Increased risk of infection because of an external portion; exposed tubing provides direct access to peritoneal cavity. • Increased risk of leakage around the exit site • Insertion must be performed in the operating room. • Increased risk of dislodgment • Requires maintenance by patient and others: Dressing changes, exit-site and catheter care • Increased cost because of necessary maintenance supplies • May require more office visits or use of home health agency, adding to cost • Inconvenient to patient: Limits ability to swim, bathe, and wear certain clothing • Can have a negative impact on patient's body image: Reminder of disease, may affect sexuality, increased anxiety about risks described earlier
Implanted peritoneal port	• Serves as a semipermanent access device that allows cyclic treatments over a long period of time • Potentially decreased risk of infection because of a lack of external portion • No risk of accidental removal • Does not require dressing or flushing between treatments • Does not affect body image; no restrictions on activity, bathing, or swimming • Increased patient acceptance because of lack of external component • Potential decreased patient anxiety	• Must be surgically placed and removed in the operating room • Requires a needlestick to access device, which may cause discomfort to patient • Does not allow for high-pressure forced irrigation or manipulation to dislodge fibrin • Slower infusion rate: 2 liters in 30–45 minutes because of needle size limitations • Decreased rate of fluid return: 2 liters in 1–2 hours • Inability to drain off or aspirate fluid because of needle size limitations • Device is more expensive and has increased cost with insertion.

(4) Benefits of IP catheter must outweigh risks.

(5) The patient and family must be able to care for the external catheter.

4. Rationale for IP chemotherapy treatment (Markman & Walker, 2006).

  a) IP chemotherapy delivers a high concentration of drug directly to the peritoneal space. Drugs that achieve the best peritoneal/plasma concentration ratio are those that have a high molecular weight, extensive first pass hepatic inactivation, and rapid plasma clearance.

  b) Chemotherapy can directly penetrate into the tumor by means of free surface diffusion and through the blood vessels that nourish the tumor.

  c) Drugs can be given in higher doses than with the IV route, providing prolonged tumor exposure with decreased systemic effect (as the majority of drug is detoxified by the liver) to minimize drug resistance and to obtain higher clinical response.

  d) Drug remains in the peritoneal cavity according to the drug clearance properties.

    (1) Drugs used are specific to the disease being treated.

    (2) Drugs considered venous irritants and vesicants have a similar effect on the peritoneum, causing pain, burning, and sclerosing. They may be chosen for their sclerosing effect rather than their antineoplastic effect (Cope, 2005).

    (3) Drugs that have a high local toxicity that causes pain and the tendency to create adhesions are not used for planned multiple-course therapies (Markman & Walker, 2006).

    (4) IP administration of biologic response modifiers is used for the enhancement of the immune system and for cytotoxic effect. They may be given alone

or in combination with chemotherapy (Hamilton et al., 2008; National Institutes of Health, 2007b).

E. Insertion procedures

1. External tunneled catheter (Rippe, 2007)

   a) The patient gives informed consent.

   b) Catheter can be placed at the time of the initial surgical exploration for the disease, laparoscopically under general anesthesia, or in a separate surgical procedure under local anesthesia, with or without IV sedation. Omentectomy is highly recommended if not already performed during the initial cancer surgery (Berek, 2004).

   c) The catheter is placed through the anterior abdominal wall at the level of the umbilicus.

   d) The external portion of the catheter should be placed in a downward direction to decrease the risk of infections by decreasing the collection of debris and fluid (O'Neill, Wasse, Asif, & Ash, 2007).

   e) The entire IP segment of the catheter, with its multiple exit holes or single lumen, must be placed in the peritoneum to avoid drug extravasation. The tip of the catheter is directed toward the cul-de-sac of the pelvis (Berek, 2004).

   f) After closure of the peritoneum, an SC tunnel is made to minimize infection and prevent catheter dislodgment.

   g) The external portion of the catheter is placed away from the initial puncture site and sutured in place until adequate healing around the cuff occurs.

   h) The external catheter is placed off to the side of the midline and away from the belt line to provide easy access for the patient.

   i) For peritoneal dialysis, Dacron cuffs are placed as previously described. Single Dacron cuff catheters are used primarily in oncologic situations because of the decreased length of time they will be used (usually less than a year) and because the surgical placement is much simpler. Both single- and double-cuff catheters have been shown to be equally effective in preventing infection in the peritoneal dialysis population (Rippe, 2007).

   j) Conversely, in gynecologic oncology clinical trials, Dacron cuffs and fenestrated catheters were found to increase catheter complications that include fibrin sheath development, increased infection, intestinal perforation, and adhesion formation, especially as late complications (Markman & Walk-

er, 2006). The difference in the two populations may be related to the extensive abdominal surgery that patients with cancer undergo at the time of initial diagnosis and the development of adhesions from this initial surgery. The use of chemotherapeutic agents that cause an inflammatory reaction in the abdominal cavity also may contribute to catheter complications.

2. Implanted SC port (Walker et al., 2006)

   a) The catheter can be placed during the initial surgical exploration for the disease, laparoscopically under general anesthesia, in a separate surgical procedure, or under local anesthesia with or without sedation in radiology. Prior omentectomy is recommended.

   b) The IP catheter portion of the device is placed as it is in the external catheter procedure with tip directed toward the cul-de-sac of the pelvis.

   c) After closure of the peritoneum, an SC tunnel is made to the selected port site, preferably over a bony prominence (usually a lower rib) to stabilize access.

F. Postoperative care

1. Assessment of the patient for surgical complications

   a) Pain at the exit site: Administer analgesics. Pain resolves in five to seven days.

   b) Bleeding into the peritoneum: The patient may have continuous exchanges of 1 liter of dialysate with no dwell time until the returned fluid is clear. Bleeding may be significant enough to require blood transfusions and/or surgery to remove or replace the catheter.

   c) Potential for bowel perforation: Assess the patient for severe abdominal pain, fever, and tense abdomen. Monitor bowel sounds.

   d) Peritonitis: Assess the patient for fever, nausea, vomiting, severe abdominal pain, and cloudy peritoneal fluid. If peritonitis is suspected, send cultures and administer antibiotics and analgesics as ordered.

2. Assessment of catheter complications (Marin et al., 2007)

   a) Leakage around the exit site of the external catheter: Chemotherapy is avoided for five to seven days to minimize leakage. The first course of chemotherapy may be placed in 1,000–1,200 ml of fluid, with subsequent treatments in 2,000 ml when the area has completely healed (Gynecologic Oncology Group, 2007).

   b) Tunnel or exit-site infection: Assess wound for drainage, erythema, and tenderness.

_____

Administer antibiotics as ordered. Maintain aseptic technique when caring for the catheter.

c) Catheter dislodgment: Assess the patient for abdominal pain. Assess exit site for absence of sutures on the external catheter or for the presence of a visible Dacron cuff exuding from the skin. Notify physician of dislodgment of catheter. Implanted port catheter dislodgment may be evidenced by an inability to flush. (It is common to be unable to drain off fluid from an implanted IP port.)

d) Nonfunctioning catheter: Assess ability to flush or withdraw peritoneal fluid. Reposition patient, and attempt to flush with sterile normal saline. Administer heparin flush (10–100 IU/ml). Notify physician of problem. Dye studies may be required to determine cause of problem.

e) Bleeding: Assess exit-site dressing for bleeding. Apply pressure if necessary. Notify physician of excessive amount. Assess peritoneal fluid for blood. The patient may require flushing of the peritoneal cavity with a few cycles of dialysate or normal saline solution containing heparin (500 IU/L) to minimize the chance of clotting in the catheter (Davies & Williams, 2007).

f) Bowel obstruction, perforation, or fistula: Assess the patient for signs of severe abdominal pain, fever, or leakage of IP fluid from vagina, bladder, or rectum. Notify physician immediately (Bilsel, Balik, Bugra, Yamaner, & Akyuz, 2005; Bryant, Shah, Triest, Schimp, & Morris, 2008; Walker et al., 2006).

3. Patient and family education (Hydzik, 2007)
a) For both catheters: Insertion and removal of the device, treatment regimen, rationale, side effects, signs of infection, and signs of complications, such as bowel perforation, obstruction, or fistula

b) For external catheters: Exit-site care, catheter care, frequency of dressing and cap changes, and frequency of flushing

G. Removal of devices
1. External catheters can be removed at the bedside or in the operating room with the patient under local anesthesia. Late complications of abscesses at the exit site from the retained Dacron cuff if removed at the bedside have been documented. Therefore, when therapy is completed, it is recommended that the catheter be completely removed surgically to prevent long-term complications of catheter migration, abscess, or persistent tunnel infections (Walker et al., 2006). Whether a trained RN or APN can remove short-term catheters depends on the individual state board of nursing. For states that do permit removal, training and competency records must be maintained.

2. Implanted SC ports require removal in the operating room with the patient under local anesthesia, and it is recommended that the catheter be removed as soon as therapy is complete to prevent long-term complications.

H. Maintenance care during IP treatments (Gynecologic Oncology Group, 2007) (see Appendix 10)
1. Sterile technique is required to prevent catheter tunnel infection and peritonitis. All equipment must be sterile. Use of sterile mask and gloves is highly recommended because of the vulnerability of the patient population to infection.

2. External catheters are accessed with a needleless (or needle-free) system.
a) Apply mask and then open supplies, including syringe, needleless connections, catheter cap and catheter clamp, gauze, and gloves, onto a sterile field.

b) Cleanse the exit site, catheter, and catheter cap using povidone-iodine swabs or 2% CHG/70% isopropyl alcohol swabs (ChloraPrep) in an outward spiral fashion, being careful not to go over the same area twice. Allow to air-dry. Long-term use of alcohol is not recommended, as it can cause discoloration as well as damage to the device. Acetone-based cleaning solutions should not be used because they are incompatible with the polymer material used to develop these catheters (Covidien, n.d.; Rosot Enterprises, Inc., n.d.).

c) Change the sterile needleless cap before connecting infusion tubing.

d) Flush catheter with 20 ml of sterile normal saline to ensure patency.

e) Withdraw peritoneal specimen for testing as ordered. Assess characteristics of fluid.

f) Connect the patient to infusion tubing; start infusion and assess for leakage, ease of flow, SC infiltration, and pain.

g) Apply occlusive dressing, and anchor tubing by taping with a stress loop, attaching to the abdomen to prevent excess pulling.

h) Administer treatment as ordered.

3. Implanted port requires noncoring needle to access (Gynecologic Oncology Group, 2007; Hydzik, 2007).

a) Apply mask and open supplies, including syringe, noncoring needle, catheter cap, gauze, and gloves, into a sterile field.

b) Draw up 20 ml of sterile normal saline aseptically (or use prefilled syringes), attach needleless cap to noncoring needle tubing, and prime with normal saline.

c) Cleanse access site with cleansing agent.

d) After inserting needle into port (see Section II.G: Implanted Ports), flush with 20 ml of sterile normal saline to ensure patency. Assess for leakage, ease of flow, SC infiltration, and pain. Withdraw peritoneal specimen as ordered. Often, peritoneal ports may not yield a specimen.

e) Connect patient to infusion tubing: Start infusion and assess for SC infiltration, leakage, ease of flow, and pain.

f) Apply occlusive dressing, and anchor tubing by taping with a stress loop, attaching to the abdomen to prevent excess pulling.

g) Administer treatment as ordered.

4. After treatment is complete, clamp the catheter. Fluid dwells in abdomen for the length of time ordered by the physician, usually four to six hours.

5. Fluid may be drained off or allowed to absorb per physician order. In patients with gynecologic cancer, the fluid is not drained off, to provide absorption into systemic circulation (Al-Hayki, Hopkins, & Le, 2006).

6. The external catheter is flushed aseptically with 20 ml of sterile normal saline. The implanted port is flushed with 20 ml of sterile normal saline, followed by heparinized saline (10–100 IU/ml) (Bard Access Systems, Inc., 2007a) or per institutional protocol. Tubing is disconnected.

a) The external catheter dressing remains in place for one week in the immediate postoperative period, unless excess soiling occurs. After the first week, dressings are changed three times a week; catheter caps and clamps are changed once a week.

b) A new sterile, occlusive pressure dressing is placed over the access site of the implanted port after the needle is removed and remains in place for 24–48 hours.

7. After the patient is disconnected from the treatment, turning from side to side every 15 minutes for one to two hours is recommended to allow distribution of the drug throughout the peritoneal cavity (Brueggen, Baird, & Meisheid, 2007).

I. General practice issues (Hydzik, 2007)

1. Administration of IP fluids and medications

a) Verify order and review patient laboratory work.

b) Explain the procedure to the patient.

c) If ordered, insert indwelling urinary catheter to facilitate monitoring of intake and output. If a urinary catheter is not ordered, request that the patient void before starting IP treatment.

d) Place the patient in semi-Fowler position to promote comfort.

e) Establish IV line and administer ancillary medication, including antiemetics and IV hydration. Although peritoneal drugs have fewer systemic effects than IV drugs, some of the drug crosses into the venous system, especially if the IP drug is allowed to be absorbed instead of drained. Controlling systemic effects with IV drugs allows for significant dose escalation (Berry et al., 2009).

f) If ascites is present, it may be possible to drain fluid prior to infusion of chemotherapy so that patients with a large volume of ascitic fluid may tolerate the therapy better. A peritoneal drainage bag will be needed for collection of fluid.

g) Warm IP fluid to body temperature to minimize cramping and shivering by soaking IP fluid with plastic sleeve intake in a bowl of warm water or with dry heat, such as a heating pad or in a blanket warmer.

(1) Although warming fluid has been recommended in both the renal and oncology nursing literature, no evidence-based research indicates that warmed solution is better tolerated than room-temperature solution.

(2) Warming blankets can be used if the patient becomes chilled (Hydzik, 2007).

(3) In addition, some recent concerns have arisen regarding the potential hazard of increased leakage of the toxin di(2-ethylhexyl) phthalate (DEHP) from the

warmed plastics in the IV fluid bags and tubing.

    (4) The FDA issued a safety announcement regarding caution in using warmed plastics in certain high-risk populations, such as male infants and pregnant females (FDA, 2002; Sattler, 2006) The FDA stated that the risk associated with DEHP is far less than the risks of forgoing the necessary critical procedures.

h) Access the device as previously described. Note that blood return is not expected, as the catheter is not in a vein.

i) Applying topical anesthetic cream over the port insertion site may aid in patient comfort. It is applied to the area 30 minutes before accessing the device (see Table 3).

j) Infuse fluid as ordered, usually over 30 minutes to two hours. In adult patients, a minimum of 1.5–2 liters of fluid is required to ensure distribution of drug throughout the peritoneal cavity. Chemotherapy, placed in 1 liter of fluid, and 1 liter of normal saline are connected to IV tubing. The infusion is begun with the main IV line by infusing 300 ml of normal saline. This allows the nurse to evaluate the ease of flow, presence of leakage, loculation, or extravasation. If no complications occur, the normal saline can be stopped, and the chemotherapy can be infused by connecting the tubing to the main IV line. The complete 1 liter of chemotherapy is given and followed by the remainder of the 1 liter of normal saline to flush the line. The last portion of IP fluid infusion can be adjusted for patient comfort (Markman & Walker, 2006).

    (1) Small-framed patients and older adults may require this adjustment. Using the patient's BSA, administering 1 liter of fluid per meter squared of BSA may be a useful target to determine the appropriate volume of fluid for an individual (NCI, 2006).

    (2) For infusions on sequential days, 1 liter of fluid is sufficient because the peritoneal space can absorb approximately 1 liter of fluid in 24 hours.

k) When fluid has infused, close clamp for the duration of dwell time, usually four to six hours. During that time, assist the patient to turn from side to side every 15–30 minutes to improve distribution throughout the abdomen. If the fluid will not be drained off, the catheter should be flushed and discon-

nected before the patient begins the turning procedures.

l) After dwell time, if ordered, open the drainage clamp and allow fluid to drain for 30 minutes to 2 hours. If fluid will not drain, attempt to reposition the patient, instruct the patient in Valsalva maneuver, apply manual pressure to abdomen, or irrigate the catheter with sterile normal saline. Drainage is more rapid with an external catheter, but the implanted port may or may not allow drainage of fluid.

m) Instruct patient, if an outpatient, to wear loose clothing with an expandable waistline and to arrange for transportation home.

n) Disconnect all tubing as previously described. Apply new dressing.

o) Be aware of the potential errors with IP administration related to mistakenly using the IP port for IV use—for example, to administer IV medications, IV chemotherapy, or blood products or to attempt to obtain serum laboratory specimens other than IP fluid from the IP port (Almadrones, 2007). Label tubing "peritoneal."

2. Palliative use of the IP catheter for drainage of ascites in selected patients: Patients and families may be taught how to perform this procedure in the home with the support of homecare or hospice services. External catheters provide the best means of draining ascites fluid (Winkelman, 2004). Sterile technique is required for the first 14 days following placement. Maintenance procedures after that can be done using an aseptic, no-touch technique (Redmond & Doherty, 2005).

a) Access the catheter as previously described.

b) Drain fluid, using a needleless system, into a drainage bag, via gravity or with the use of vacuum bottles.

c) Assess the patient's reaction to fluid drainage. A roller clamp may be used to adjust rate of drainage if the patient becomes orthostatic, as evidenced by complaints of light-headedness or dizziness, or experiences pain.

d) After drainage is complete, tubing is disconnected and occlusive dressing placed over the site, as previously described.

e) Education of the patient and family about the external catheter maintenance should include the following.

    (1) Exit-site, catheter, and cap care

    (2) Dressing change three times a week

    (3) Weekly cap and clamp change

(4) Implanted port does not require dressing change and access site cleaning when not in use. Family can be taught to access device.

(5) Signs and symptoms of infection

(6) Signs and symptoms that warrant calling physician

J. Complications: See Table 14.

K. Education and documentation: See Section X.

L. For a practicum on IP catheters, see Appendix 10.

M. Controversial issues regarding IP catheters

1. Heparin flush: Authors disagree on the need for flushing catheters with heparin after use. The IP catheter care was adapted from renal dialysis standards and policies for the external Tenckhoff catheter.

Table 14. Complications of Peritoneal Therapies and Interventions

Complication	Etiology	Signs/Symptoms	Interventions
Patient discomfort	Increased fluid volume in abdomen	Abdominal distention	Loosen clothing. Administer analgesics as ordered. Provide reassurance that problems are temporary. Evaluate patient's size and adjust fluid volume to 1 L/m² (Markman & Walker, 2006).
		Shortness of breath	Administer oxygen and elevate head of bed.
	Fluid loculation	Abdominal pain	Change patient's position.
	Fluid infusion rate too fast	Abdominal or rectal pressure	Administer analgesics as ordered.
		Increased urination	Insert urinary catheter if ordered.
		Diarrhea	Administer antidiarrheals as ordered.
		Esophageal reflux	Administer antacids.
		Anorexia	Provide small, frequent meals.
		Nausea and vomiting	Administer antiemetics as ordered.
		Anxiety	Provide reassurance that problems are temporary.
		Complaints of pain	Warm fluid before instillation. Slow the rate of infusion.
		Shivering, complaints of cold feeling	Use warming blanket. Offer warm oral (PO) fluids.
Inflow failure	Needle misplacement Implanted port flips over Fluid loculation	Inability to infuse solution or difficulty flushing	Assess port and needle placement.
	Catheter kinks Blood or fibrin clots in catheter Obstruction of catheter by abdominal adhesions or omental blockage Catheter migration Tumor progression	Inability to infuse solution or difficulty flushing	Reposition patient. Flush vigorously with normal saline (NS), repeat with 20 ml heparinized saline, 100 IU/ml if necessary. Prepare for dye study to check catheter position. If catheter is in place but unable to irrigate, instill tissue plasminogen activator (tPA). Let dwell for 2–4 hours (Davies & Williams, 2007). If still no success, catheter may need to be removed and therapy reevaluated.
Respiratory distress	Sudden rise in intra-abdominal pressure, which constricts diaphragm movement	Shortness of breath	Elevate head of bed to 45°. Administer oxygen per nasal cannula.

(Continued on next page)

Table 14. Complications of Peritoneal Therapies and Interventions *(Continued)*

Complication	Etiology	Signs/Symptoms	Interventions
		Dyspnea (severe)	Evaluate for hypersensitivity reaction. Stop infusion. Notify MD. Begin ABCs of resuscitation. Administer oxygen. Remain with patient. Provide reassurance. (Fung-Kee-Fung et al., 2007)
Outflow failure	Fibrin sheath formation creating a one-valve effect Omental adhesion or tumor causing outflow blockage of catheter Catheter migration	Inability to sample peritoneal fluid for diagnosis or specimen collection	Reposition patient; attempt to flush with 20 ml NS. If still unsuccessful, flush with 10 ml heparin, 100 IU/ml. Attempt to withdraw a fluid sample after 30 minutes. Notify physician if no improvement occurs.
		Inability to drain solution although able to infuse solutions	Assure patient that fluid will absorb at a rate of 1 liter in 24 hours.
		Ascites fluid may require paracentesis for removal.	Prepare patient for dye study to diagnose the problem. If catheter still infuses, future treatments may continue as ordered without the drainage of contents. tPA may be ordered.
Drug extravasation	Separation of port from catheter Dislodgment of port needle from septum Migration of catheter out of the peritoneum	Inability to aspirate fluid Poor rate of infusion and difficulty flushing Local swelling around exit site or port diaphragm Patient complains of pain Erythema at the site	Stop drug infusion. Notify physician. Attempt to aspirate drug if possible. Prepare patient for diagnostic studies to determine placement. Institute extravasation protocol for specific drug per Oncology Nursing Society guidelines (Polovich et al., 2009). Device will most likely be removed. Prepare patient for that possibility.
Exit-site infection	Break in aseptic technique when performing treatments, dressing changes, and catheter care Contamination of open area at exit site (usually from skin flora) Immunosuppressed patient Erosion of Dacron® (DuPont) cuff	Marked erythema or discharge from exit site Increased scab formation Local tenderness around exit site and over the outer cuff	Culture exudates. Administer PO or IV antibiotics as ordered. Increase local measures: Clean exit site once or twice a day, and apply new sterile dressing. If cuff erosion, catheter will have to be removed.
Tunnel infection	Same as for exit-site infection	Infection occurring between the two cuffs, manifesting as inflammation appearing along the tunnel line of the catheter	Same as for exit-site infection Decreased chance of resolution Catheter removal usually is required. Ultrasound will reveal fluid collection around the cannula.

(Continued on next page)

Table 14. Complications of Peritoneal Therapies and Interventions *(Continued)*

Complication	Etiology	Signs/Symptoms	Interventions
Peritonitis	Infection because of poor aseptic technique when accessing device, changing dressing, or performing therapies. Immunocompromised patients are at increased risk for infection. Less likely cause: Catheter erosion into small or large bowel	Fever and chills Abdominal tenderness to light palpation Rebound tenderness Cloudy fluid Positive cultures Peritoneal fluid with white blood cells greater than 100 cells/mm^3	Send cultures. Administer IV or intraperitoneal (IP) antibiotics as ordered. Administer analgesics. Catheter may need to be removed if infection does not resolve or recurs with same organism.
Slow infusion rate of solution	Kinks in catheter or tubing Fibrin sheath formation Obstruction of catheter by adhesions, omentum, or tumor	Increased time to infuse solution is more than 2 hr/L.	If using a port, check needle placement and gauge. Increase height of bag. Irrigate catheter with 20 ml NS. Change patient's position. Flush with 10 ml heparin, 100 IU/ml after the completion of treatment and let dwell until next treatment.
	Constipation	Pelvic pressure and discomfort	Administer laxative; prescribe stool softener.
Systemic toxicity of chemotherapy administered	Chemotherapy entering the systemic circulation via peritoneal membrane and the hepatic portal system	Nausea and vomiting	Administer antiemetics as ordered. Long-acting medications work best. Maintain hydration.
		Renal toxicity Electrolyte imbalance	Monitor complete blood counts, chemistry panel, and renal function. Administer diuretics as ordered. Provide symptom management as with IV chemotherapy. Provide supportive measures such as home health care for home hydration, electrolyte replacement (PO or IV), and colony-stimulating factors.
		Neurotoxicity	Administer IV amifostine.
Leakage at exit site	Incomplete healing of surgical wound Dislodgment of port needle from septum	Visible leakage of IP fluid around catheter or insertion site: Redness, local pain Dressings saturated	Stop the treatment immediately. Check needle placement. Notify MD. Perform sterile exit-site catheter care and place a new sterile dressing over the site. Send for dye study to verify catheter placement.
Chemical peritonitis	Irritation from chemotherapy agents, especially irritants and vesicants	Severe abdominal pain during infusion and afterward May have a fever and erythema but negative cultures, no rise in white blood cells (Berry et al., 2009)	May need to hold treatment for two weeks until adequate healing occurs. Check dose of drugs. Increase dilution of drugs if ordered. Warm fluid to body temperature. Administer analgesics as ordered. Slow the rate of infusion. Check for possible neutralizing agent, such as sodium thiosulfate, which may be given locally (Fung-Kee-Fung et al., 2007).

(Continued on next page)

Table 14. Complications of Peritoneal Therapies and Interventions *(Continued)*

Complication	Etiology	Signs/Symptoms	Interventions
Sclerosing encapsulating peritonitis (SEP) (Davies & Williams, 2007)	Late side effect of IP therapy, causing adhesions secondary to prolonged inflammation and sclerosing effect of agents used, or peritonitis or surgical complications from previous procedures. Dense abdominal adhesions, thickening, and fibrosis can result in bowel obstruction.	Inability to infuse or drain peritoneal fluid Abdominal pain Signs of bowel obstruction: Nausea, vomiting, fever, or abdominal distension	See interventions for inflow failure. If diagnosis is SEP, surgical repair of abdominal adhesions and/or bowel resection and removal of device will be necessary. Stop IP treatment. Provide emotional support and reassurance to patient. Prepare for surgery.
Catheter migration and erosion into other pelvic organs	Fistulization of catheter into pelvic organs: Small or large intestine, vagina, or bladder	Leakage of IP fluid from vagina, rectum, or bladder Abdominal/pelvic pain; urinary urgency	Stop infusion. Notify MD. Prepare patient for dye study and possible surgery to remove catheter. Provide emotional support.
Bleeding at exit site (external catheter)	Excessive movement of external tubing Removal of a crust (scab) before the natural separation has occurred	Bleeding when performing exit-site care, when dressing is removed Blood-stained gauze	Apply local pressure with sterile gauze. Anchor tubing to prevent movement when taping. Perform gentle exit-site care; do not pull or twist catheter.

a) The purpose of the heparin flush was to decrease fibrin formation, a major cause of inflow and outflow complications.

b) Review of the many manufacturers' brochures of implanted ports have always included and still include a heparin lock flush at the completion of therapy and every four weeks when not in use (Bard Access Systems, Inc., 2007a; Smiths Medical, 2005a, 2005b).

c) Recent review of IP nursing literature demonstrates normal saline flush only for both external and implanted IP catheters (Hydzik, 2007); heparin flush for implanted ports only (Marin et al., 2007); or no mention of flushing at all (Brueggen et al., 2007). The rationale for not using heparin is that the catheter is not in a vein; therefore, the catheter has a low risk of "clotting off" (Hydzik, 2007).

d) The International Society for Peritoneal Dialysis (Gokal et al., 1998) and Maaz (2004) recommended using heparin only if inflow/outflow problems arise.

e) It could be argued that the use of heparin flushes to prevent inflow/outflow failures caused by fibrin formation, in addition to the low cost of heparin and minimal risk to the patient, warrants its use. Nurses are encouraged to check the guidelines set forth by the individual institutions.

2. Catheter type: Single-lumen catheters versus fenestrated catheters: Walker et al. (2006) and Markman and Walker (2006) have identified the BardPort® (C.R. Bard, Inc.) 9.6 Fr single-lumen catheter as the preferred IP catheter, citing a decrease in catheter complications with its use.

a) Fenestrated catheters were associated with increased incidence of fibrin formation, infection, bowel perforation, and adhesion formation.

b) Conversely, Black et al. (2008) retrospectively reviewed their patient population and did not find an increase in complications when compared to the Walker et al. (2006) study.

c) Interestingly, it is not stated whether these catheters were routinely flushed with heparin. IP catheter choice will always be driven by physician preference. Nurses are in the unique position to make recommendations, as they are the ultimate first-line clinical care managers of the patient.

3. Warming of IP fluid: Throughout the oncology and renal nursing literature (Carpenito-Moyet, 2009; Marin et al., 2007; Potter & Held-Warmkessel, 2008), authors have recommended warming IP fluid for patient comfort. Hydzik (2007) identified that no evidence-based literature supports that treatment was better

tolerated with warm versus room-temperature fluid. In clinical practice, Hydzik recommended the use of warming blankets to comfort the patient.

a) The warming of fluid for IP dialysis continues to be done, not only for patient comfort but also to decrease the incidence of vasoconstriction in the peritoneal cavity that would hinder absorption of the dialysate and decrease heat loss of the patient (Richard, 1980). IP dialysis is done through external catheters that infuse fluid very quickly (2 liters in 10–15 minutes), whereas the infusion of chemotherapy through an implanted port takes 90–120 minutes. It is reasonable to conclude that the slower infusion rate may allow the patient to adapt to the fluid temperature.

b) Adding to the controversy was the concern over the safety of warmed fluid (Sattler, 2006). In 2002, the FDA made a safety announcement regarding the potential risk to the male reproductive system associated with the leakage of DEHP from warmed plastics such as IV tubing and IV bags. Other studies (Lucas & Brown, 2005) reviewed the actual amount of DEHP that leaks from IV bags and tubing and found the amount to be negligible.

c) Stuart, Knight, and Sugarbaker (2005) concluded that DEHP leaches after paclitaxel preparation and made the following statements regarding implications for nursing.

(1) Administer paclitaxel solution as soon as possible after preparation.

(2) Infuse drug as rapidly as possible.

(3) Clear the Tenckhoff catheter and extension tubing by draining ascites fluid through these tubes prior to subsequent IP infusions.

d) Non-DEHP tubing, bags, and filters have always been used for paclitaxel infusions in gynecologic oncology because of the known fact of DEHP leaching.

e) No standard exists as to how the fluid should be warmed. In the renal dialysis literature (Carpenito-Moyet, 2009), warming fluid using dry heat, such as with heating pads or incubators, is preferred over warm water baths. The concern is that warm water baths can cause contamination on the surface of the infusion bag, which in turn would cause infection in the patient. The gynecologic oncology literature has always suggested warm water baths, as long as the plastic sleeve of the IV fluid bag remains intact (Gynecologic Oncology Group, 2007).

f) External warming devices also have been used (Marin et al., 2007). Microwaving fluid is not recommended. More research is needed in this area. Again, nurses should refer to their institutional policy regarding this issue.

VIII. IMPLANTED PUMPS

A. History (Agency for Health Care Policy and Research, 1994)
   1. First implantable pumps were attempted in 1960s for insulin therapy.
   2. The need for chronic IV and SC infusions led to the further development of the implantable pump.
   3. Developments have led to specific drug therapy to specific body systems, such as the venous, arterial, and nervous systems.

B. Device description (see Table 15)
   1. An infusion device containing an intrinsic power source and refillable drug reservoir that allows long-term operation while being totally implanted subcutaneously.
   2. Designed for continuous, low-volume, long-term, site-specific drug therapy, as well as chronic IV or SC infusions. These therapies include intrathecal pain management (Ghafoor et al., 2007; Knight, Brand, Mchaourab, & Veneziano, 2007), intrathecal baclofen therapy (Barker, 2008), and hepatic artery infusion therapy (Osborne et al., 2006). Some experience exists with insulin therapy, but further testing is under way (Renard, 2008).
   3. Includes a pump and catheter
      a) Pump is composed of a pump body, septum or septums, reservoir, and intrinsic power source.
      b) Septum is parallel to skin surface, so percutaneous needlestick is perpendicular to skin.
      c) Suture sites are available around pump body.
      d) Catheter is attached at time of surgery or preattached and may terminate in artery, vein, or anatomic space. Most common sites for insertion are hepatic artery and intrathecal space. The catheter is radiopaque silicone.
   4. Pumps currently available
      a) SynchroMed® II (Medtronic, Inc.) drug infusion system: Energy is supplied by a lithium battery that powers a peristaltic roller pump, forcing the drug into the catheter. The settings for the pump are set and changed using a computer system with a wand that is placed over the pump. A sec-

Table 15. Implantable Pump Device Description

Characteristic	Codman® 3000 Constant Flow Implantable Pump[a]	SynchroMed® II Infusion System[b]
Pumping mechanism	Propellant separated from drug reservoir by accordion-like bellows. The gas places constant pressure on the bellows, causing drug to flow out of the chamber.	Positive displacement peristaltic pump; operated by noninvasive programmer and handheld telemetry wand that uses radio signals to relay information to pump
Energy source	Pressurized gas	Lithium battery; battery life depends on drug delivery rate; average life of three to four years
Weight	98–173 g	165–215 g
Pump reservoirs	16 ml, 30 ml, 50 ml	20 ml, 40 ml
Materials	Titanium pump, silicone catheter	Radiopaque titanium pump, silicone septum
Alarm feature	None	Low battery, low reserve volume, memory error
Shutdown	None	Battery or electrical module failure
Side port availability	None	Single side port
External influences on rate	Altitude, temperature, fluid viscosity	Not significantly dependent on external variables
Flow rates	0.3–3.6 ml/day depending on type of pump—high, medium, low, or ultra-low flow	0.048–24 ml/day Programmable
Catheter	Single lumen	Single lumen
Catheter material	Radiopaque silicone	Radiopaque silicone

[a] Manufactured by Codman & Shurtleff, Inc. [b] Manufactured by Medtronic, Inc.

Note. Based on manufacturers' product information.

ondary port is available for bolus injections of medication, which bypasses the reservoir.

b) Codman® 3000 (Codman & Shurtleff, Inc.): Divided into inner and outer chambers; the inner chamber contains the drug to be infused, and the outer chamber contains propellant permanently sealed inside. The patient's body temperature warms the propellant, which exerts pressure on the bellows, causing the drug to flow out of the chamber through a filter and flow restrictor and then slowly out of the catheter.

c) IsoMed® infusion system (Medtronic, Inc.): This system is no longer available, but patients may currently still have one in place.

5. Cost of pump and implantation: Approximately $20,000–$25,000

a) Pump placement is usually reimbursable.

b) Reimbursement for non-FDA–approved uses must be considered on a case-by-case basis with each patient's insurance company. The insurer considers the research base for the route and drug regimen as well as the patient's life expectancy.

C. Advantages and disadvantages (see Table 16)

1. Advantages of continuous infusion therapy

a) For all drugs, the peak-and-valley effect is eliminated, achieving constant drug administration.

b) Advantages for antineoplastic drugs include the following.

(1) Continuous drug administration over many cell cycles yields increased cell kill.

(2) A higher concentration of chemotherapy is delivered to the tumor that would

not be possible with systemic therapy (Elaraj & Alexander, 2004).

(3) Less acute systemic toxicity occurs because smaller doses are infused regionally (Codman & Shurtleff, Inc., n.d.; Elaraj & Alexander, 2004).

2. Advantages for baclofen and pain medications

a) Less medication required, therefore fewer side effects than if drug were taken orally (Barker, 2008)

b) Significant reductions in pain and drug toxicity (Smith & Coyne, 2005)

D. Patient selection and treatment criteria

1. The patient can be a young adult or adult.

2. The patient has sufficient body mass to hold implanted pump.

3. The patient has adequate performance status and ability to tolerate surgical procedure.

4. The patient has a disease or condition that responds to continuous infusion therapy (Elaraj & Alexander, 2004; Ethans, Schryvers, Nance, & Casey, 2005; Ghafoor et al., 2007; Knight et al., 2007).

a) Chronic, nonmalignant pain

b) Intractable cancer pain associated with a life expectancy of greater than three months

c) The patient has had a trial of intrathecal medication with a temporary catheter in the intrathecal or epidural space and has shown improvement of symptoms with trial of the medication (Knight et al., 2007).

d) Neuromuscular spasticity and dystonia

e) Hepatic metastasis of malignancy

5. Drugs used in an implanted pump must be FDA-approved for treatment of specific diseases.

Table 16. Advantages and Disadvantages of Implantable Pumps

Type of Pump	Advantages	Disadvantages
Implantable pump	• Totally implantable • Increased freedom to perform activities of daily living • Reduction/elimination of systemic side effects (Ethans et al., 2005; Knight et al., 2007) • Improvement of symptoms (Krach et al., 2006) • Higher response rates of unresectable hepatic disease than systemic therapy alone (Elaraj & Alexander, 2004) • Reduction of infections commonly associated with external access devices (Agency for Health Care Policy and Research, 1994) • Increased patient compliance and acceptance • Achieves continuous infusion therapy as well as bolus therapy • Magnetic resonance imaging scans permissible	• Potential discomfort with needlesticks • Higher initial cost of implantation • Special noncoring, single-use needle required for access • Limited volume for infusions • Single use of pump • Triggers metal detectors • Requires surgical insertion and removal • Pump mechanism increases in patients with fever.

a) FUDR is the most commonly used drug for intra-arterial use (Elajar & Alexander, 2004).

b) Examples of drugs approved for intrathecal infusion are morphine, clonidine, baclofen, and bupivacaine (Barker, 2008; Ghafoor et al., 2007; Smith & Coyne, 2005). These solutions must be preservative free.

6. Contraindications for pump implantation

   a) Large-volume infusions required

   b) Disseminated disease contraindicated for regional therapy

   c) Brief life expectancy

   d) Evidence of infection (Medtronic, Inc., 2005)

   e) Programmable pump contraindicated

     (1) When pump cannot be implanted less than 2.5 cm from surface

     (2) When patient has another implanted, programmable device, such as a pacemaker

7. Patient setting: Can be used by trained personnel in all settings (Barker, 2008; Ghafoor et al., 2007)

E. Insertion procedures and perfusion checks (Codman & Shurtleff, Inc., 2009a)

1. See Sections IV and VI for the insertion procedures of arterial and intrathecal catheters.

2. Pump implantation is performed in the operating room with the patient under anesthesia after obtaining informed consent.

3. Pumps are most commonly inserted through an open surgical procedure.

4. Pump reservoir is filled and catheter access port is flushed after connecting the catheter to the pump in the operating room.

5. Incision for pump pocket is approximately 8 cm long and is located in the lower left or right quadrant of the abdomen, below the umbilicus.

   a) The pump is placed in the SC pocket and sutured to the fascia with nonabsorbable sutures. To avoid stress on the suture line when the pump is accessed, the suture line should not transverse the center or secondary port septum.

   b) The incision is closed and covered with a sterile dressing or pressure dressing.

   c) Catheter placement and desired site of infusion are verified intraoperatively.

6. A perfusion check is performed.

   a) Catheter tip placement and desired site of infusion are verified intraoperatively.

   b) On postoperative days four through six and before drug therapy is initiated, a perfusion study or x-ray is done to verify region of perfusion and catheter tip placement.

F. Postoperative care

1. Assess implantation site for bleeding, drainage, swelling, or seroma.

2. Maintain pressure dressing for 24 hours or until no bleeding is present.

G. Removal: The pump is removed in the operating room with the patient under local anesthesia, and the catheter is removed subcutaneously.

H. Patient education

1. The patient should report any edema, fever, erythema, weakness of lower extremities, decreased sensation, or pain at site (Codman & Shurtleff, Inc., 2009a; Medtronic, Inc., 2005).

2. Provide the patient with a medical alert emblem, which alerts healthcare professionals in emergency situations, and a pump identification card for when the device triggers metal detectors.

3. General activity restriction: The patient should avoid sports or activities that might cause injury or dislodgment of pump.

4. Codman pump: The patient should avoid extended exposure to activities that may alter pump temperature and therefore pump flow rate (Codman & Shurtleff, Inc., n.d.).

I. General practice issues (Codman & Shurtleff, Inc., 2009b; Ethans et al., 2005; Medtronic, Inc., 2005)

1. The nurse should be familiar with the device and drug-related complications, and demonstrate implanted pump access competency. Education materials and clinical representatives are available from the manufacturer.

2. Identify the pump model number, reservoir size, and flow rate.

3. Use aseptic technique when accessing the pump septum.

4. Position the needle properly in the reservoir of the pump prior to drug instillation.

   a) Access the pump reservoir and not the secondary port.

   b) Improper injection through the secondary port (resulting in bolus administration) or into SC tissue may result in precipitation, overdose, or extravasation (Codman & Shurtleff, Inc., 2009b; Medtronic, Inc., 2005).

   c) Incorrect needle placement may damage the segment of the catheter in the pump pocket.

5. The pump must be refilled on a schedule. The interval depends on drug concentration, drug stability, pump reservoir volume, daily dose, and various treatment considerations. The pump should never become completely empty.

a) Drugs must be stable for the length of infusion time in the pump and compatible with the pump's composition material (Bianchi, Ginggen, & Tardy, 2008).

b) Plan refill schedule, taking into account any office closures and patient vacations and holidays. The pump usually requires a refill every two to eight weeks.

6. Overfilling the pump reservoir will result in overpressurization and overinfusion of medication.

7. Drug dose calculations are as follows.

a) Use manufacturer guidelines for calculating amount of drug needed to refill the pump.

b) Intra-arterial infusion will require liver function tests prior to calculating dose.

c) Calculate daily dosage needed.

d) Calculate next refill date.

8. Fluid should return immediately after accessing. If fluid is not obtained after accessing reservoir, do the following.

a) Verify the needle is through the septum and in the pump reservoir.

(1) Manually palpate pump features.

(2) Ensure the needle is against the stop.

(3) Check last refill date to ensure pump is not empty.

b) If the septum cannot be located, notify a physician. An x-ray of the pump can verify its location.

9. Inform physician of the following situations.

a) Inability to obtain fluid from the pump after access

b) Signs and symptoms of infection

c) Development of pump erosion or seroma

10. Document refill information.

a) Date and time of refill

b) Number of days since last refill

c) Return volume from pump after access

d) Infused volume (previous refill volume minus return volume)

e) Pump flow rate (infused volume divided by number of days since last refill)

f) Pump drug concentration

g) Drug refill volume

h) Injection via secondary port

i) Patient's response to procedure

J. Access procedures (see Figure 19 and Table 17)

1. Supply kit contents and access/refill procedures for the SynchroMed II pump and Codman pump are outlined in Table 17. A programmer is necessary to change the flow rate of the SynchroMed II pump. Adjusting the rate of and obtaining printouts on the SynchroMed pump are beyond the scope of this module. Contact the manufacturer for this information.

2. Solutions used for maintenance infusion or between drug intervals include the following.

a) Intra-arterial: Heparinized normal saline (1,000 IU/ml)

b) Intrathecal: Preservative-free normal saline

3. Both Codman & Shurtleff and Medtronic have clinician manuals and videos of pump refills available online.

a) www.codmanpumps.com

b) http://professional.medtronic.com

4. The pumps require the use of a 22-gauge noncoring needle to preserve the integrity of the septum.

5. Accessing the septum is similar to accessing an implantable port (see section II.G), with the exception that the supply kit contains alcohol and povidone-iodine swabs for cleansing the site.

6. Painful needlesticks: Apply topical anesthetic per health provider order (see Table 3).

K. Complications: See Table 18 for major complications.

L. Education and documentation: See Section X.

M. For a practicum on care of the implanted pump, see Appendix 11.

Figure 19. SynchroMed® Pump Being Accessed and Filled

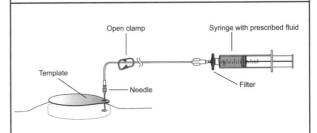

Note. From *SynchroMed® II Programmable Pumps Implant Manual* (p. 31), by Medtronic, Inc., 2007. Retrieved from http://professional.medtronic.com/downloads/itb/M221311A_a_014.pdf. Copyright 2007 by Medtronic, Inc. Reprinted with permission.

Table 17. Supplies and Access Procedures for Implantable Pumps

Pump	Supplies	Access Procedure
Codman® 3000 pump (Codman & Shurtleff, Inc.)	Supply kit from manufacturer (plus refill kit) Sterile gloves Syringe with appropriate refill solution 10 ml syringe of normal saline (NS)—preservative-free if intrathecal pump	1. Identify the pump model and reservoir volume size. 2. Confirm the refill volume of the prescribed drug in syringe does not exceed the reservoir size of the pump (16 ml, 30 ml, or 50 ml). 3. Place the patient in supine position, and palpate site to locate the raised septum. 4. Don sterile gloves, and prepare site. Place fenestrated drape over pump site. 5. Attach the needle and stopcock to the tubing set. Stopcock and clamp are in the open position. Attach the syringe in the kit to the stopcock. Tighten all connections. 6. Insert the noncoring needle perpendicular to the pump septum. 7. Allow the pump reservoir to empty—do not aspirate. 8. Close the stopcock, and record return volume. Discard syringe barrel and stopcock, leaving the needle and refill set in place. 9. Attach the syringe with the 10 ml NS and confirm needle is still in contact with the needle stop. Keep downward pressure on the needle and inject 5 ml of NS into the pump. 10. Release pressure on the plunger and allow the 5 ml to return into the syringe. 11. Expel air from the refill syringe. Attach the syringe to the refill set and, keeping downward pressure on the needle, begin to inject refill solution. 12. Release pressure every 5 ml and allow 1 ml of fluid to return into syringe. This will verify the needle is still in the correct place. 13. Continue to inject until the syringe is empty, and then clamp the refill set and pull the needle out of the pump septum. 14. Apply adhesive bandage to site.
SynchroMed® II pump (Medtronic, Inc.)	Supply kit from manufacturer: 20 ml syringe, pressure monitor with stopcock, extension tubing set with clamp (160 mcg volume), 22-gauge noncoring needle, 0.22 micron filter, template (optional), and fenestrated drape (optional) Not in kit/needs to be ordered/assembled separately: SynchroMed® Programmer (if pump is to be programmed), 4 × 4 gauze pads, site preparation materials, syringe containing 10 ml or 18 ml of prescribed drug depending on the reservoir size, sterile gloves, and adhesive bandage	1. Identify pump model and reservoir volume size. 2. Confirm that refill volume of prescribed drug in syringe does not exceed the reservoir size of the pump (20 ml or 40 ml). 3. Prepare site. 4. Place fenestrated drape over pump site (optional). 5. Assemble noncoring needle and tubing set, and empty 20 ml syringe. 6. Position template over pump (optional). Locate center of pump. 7. Insert needle through the template center hole and into the pump's septum until the needle touches the needle stop. 8. Open tubing clamp. 9. Withdraw the fluid from the reservoir using gentle, negative pressure. Empty the reservoir completely (i.e., until air bubbles are present in the tubing). The amount withdrawn should approximately equal the calculated residual volume. 10. Close the clamp and remove the 20 ml syringe. 11. Attach the filter to the syringe containing the prescribed fluid, and attach the pressure monitor to the filter. 12. Turn the pressure monitor to block the monitor tubing and purge all air from the filter/pressure monitor pathway. 13. Attach the syringe/filter/pressure monitor to the extension tubing set. 14. Open the clamp and slowly (1 ml/3 sec) inject fluid into the reservoir. Do not force injection. 15. Maintain pressure on syringe, and turn pressure monitor stopcock to SYRINGE OFF position. 16. Release syringe plunger pressure and check position of fluid meniscus in the pressure monitor. Use the top of the fluid level, not the bubble area. The meniscus must not go beyond the marked area of the pressure monitor tubing. 17. If the meniscus is beyond the mark, the pump reservoir has been overfilled and must be emptied. Close clamp and remove pressure monitor, filter, and syringe from tubing. Reattach only empty syringe to tubing, and empty pump completely. 18. Refill pump as mentioned earlier. 19. Close tubing clamp and carefully remove the needle from the pump septum. 20. Apply pressure to needle site, remove povidone-iodine if present, and apply adhesive bandage.

Note. Based on information from Codman & Shurtleff, Inc., 2009b; Medtronic, Inc., 2005.

Table 18. Implantable Pump Complications

Complication	Prevention	Presentation	Intervention
Seroma, hematoma	Instruct patient to avoid sports and other activities that may cause injury.	Tenderness, edema, fluid leakage, erythema occurring within 72 hours after surgery	Apply abdominal binder daily for one to two months (Knight, 2007). Reassure patient that both will reabsorb over time and with a pressure dressing in place.
Catheter occlusion • Thrombus • Catheter kinking/dislodgment (Krach et al., 2006) • Granuloma	Instruct patient to keep refill appointments. Do not let pump become completely empty.	Pump alarm, excess fluid remaining in pump, abdominal pain, medication withdrawal symptoms Lower extremity weakness Groin pain	Access catheter port and attempt to declot if necessary, following manufacturer instructions. Perform abdominal x-ray or catheter contrast study to confirm placement. Prepare patient for pump removal (rare) if occlusion cannot be cleared.
Equipment problems • Program problems • Incorrect setup • Improper rate	Confer with company technical support staff. Provide competency-based education.	Excess/less fluid remains in the pump, pump alarm, and systemic toxicity from incorrect drug dose infusion	Preprogram pump or remove reservoir and refill with proper concentration.
Infection (Borowski et al., 2008; Ethans et al., 2005; Krach et al., 2006) • Pocket • Sepsis • Spinal site	Use aseptic technique. Examine fluid for discoloration. Maintain closed system.	Tenderness, warmth, erythema, swelling, drainage at pump site Fever/chills Headache Neck pain	Culture site or fluid. Administer antibiotics as prescribed. Assess for signs of sepsis. Pump removal may be necessary; prepare patient for pump removal.
Pump inversion in subcutaneous pocket (Ethans et al., 2005)	Instruct patient to avoid sports and other activities that may cause injury. Ensure that patient maintains weight.	Unable to access pump	Perform x-ray to evaluate pump. Perform surgical intervention to reposition pump.
Skin necrosis over pump	Implant with sufficient tissue over pump. Ensure that patient maintains weight. Inspect skin over pump daily.	Erythema, pain, and skin breakdown	Apply semipermeable transparent dressing over skin to avoid friction with clothing. Prepare patient for pump removal. Remove pump and consider a new pump site.

Note. Based on information from Codman & Shurtleff, Inc., n.d.; Medtronic, Inc., 2005.

IX. AMBULATORY INFUSION PUMPS

A. History (Crowe, 2008; Saladow, 2004)

1. Watkins Chrono-Fusor, Inc., marketed the first ambulatory pump in the late 1950s to infuse the chemotherapy agent 5-fluorouracil. Lightweight pumps were created to allow treatment outside the hospital.

2. A mechanical keyed wind-up watch motor was used as the power source with a rotary peristaltic mechanism.

3. Over the next two decades, pump manufacturers developed smaller, more cost-effective pumps. In the early 1980s, the computerized ambulatory drug delivery system pump was developed. Use of home infusion therapy grew, and manufacturers introduced ambulatory infusion pumps.

4. In early 1990s, multiple-therapy pumps were developed to be programmed to administer various infusions.

5. By the 2000s, new breeds of "smart" pumps were developed with the ability to store dosing guidelines and to provide warnings to clinicians for potentially unsafe infusions.

6. In 2006, Medicare Part D broadened to allow coverage of the ambulatory pump and medications administered.

B. Description and types (Dodd, 2007; Donmez, Araz, & Kayhan, 2005; Emergency Care Research Institute [ECRI], 2008a, 2008b; Remerand et al., 2008; Saladow, 2007; Skryabina & Dunn, 2006)

1. Deliver parenteral agents by three delivery systems: Peristaltic, syringe driven, and elastomeric.

2. Small size of pump allows patient to carry or wear in a pouch.
   a) Peristaltic pumps: 1–3 pounds
   b) Syringe pumps: 1–7 pounds
   c) Elastomeric pumps: 0.5–2 pounds

3. Provide continuous or intermittent infusion for medications and nutrition

4. Pumps are designed for small volumes, such as an antibiotic, or for large volumes, such as TPN.

5. Available in varying flow rates from 0.02–300 ml/hr

6. Reservoirs are available as bags, cassettes, elastomeric balloons, or syringes

7. Are used in patient's home, which gives the patient ability to perform activities of daily living while receiving prescribed therapy

8. Elastomeric pumps consist of an elastomeric membrane containing the drug inside a protective shell (conformable elastomer or rigid plastic).
   a) Membranes are made of natural and synthetic material, such as isoprene rubber, latex, and silicone.
   b) Membranes can be single or multiple layers.

9. Syringe pumps typically are used to administer highly concentrated drugs or antibiotics.

10. Cost: Reimbursement varies with different insurance companies for pump, tubing, and connectors.
    a) Rental fee: A monthly fee is charged for pump use.
    b) Medicare coverage is dependent on type of therapy and patient diagnosis.
    c) Peristaltic: Approximately $1,200–$3,500 for pump cost
    d) Syringe: Approximately $3,000–$8,000 for pump cost
    e) Elastomeric: Approximately $30–$86 for disposable pump

C. Advantages and disadvantages: See Table 19.

D. Patient selection (Dodd, 2007; ECRI, 2008b; Skryabina & Dunn, 2006)

1. Patient age: Pumps can be used for all ages. Special consideration should be given for the following.
   a) Children: Smaller, less-obtrusive pump devices may be an advantage for enabling participation in school activities or outdoor activities.
      (1) Neonatal and pediatrics primarily use syringe pumps.
      (2) Accurate volume delivery and consistent flow for small volumes
   b) Older adults: Consider weight of pump and reservoir for the patient.
   c) Consider ability of the patient or significant other to provide pump care and troubleshooting for complications.
   d) Consider the type of access device inserted, such as venous, arterial, epidural, or SC.

2. Disease states appropriate for treatment administered by an ambulatory pump
   a) Gastrointestinal diseases such as Crohn disease, malabsorption, and ulcerative colitis
   b) HIV/AIDS
   c) Cancer
   d) Infections
   e) Diabetes mellitus
   f) Chronic intractable pain
   g) Cystic fibrosis

3. Type of therapy (Mentz, Ruiz-Razura, Newall, & Patronella, 2005; Moore, Espeleta, & McMenamin, 2008; Remerand et al., 2008; Saladow, 2007): Medications can be delivered by

Table 19. Advantages and Disadvantages of Ambulatory Infusion Pumps

Type of Pump	Advantages	Disadvantages
Peristaltic	Provides intermittent and continuous infusions Used for all types of therapy Alarm features Wide range of infusion rates and volumes Easy-to-read display for adjustments and troubleshooting Pump memory available Smart pump technology	Requires programming Carrying pouch can be cumbersome and heavy when full. Free-flow risk Labor intensive
Syringe	Lightweight and portable Cost-effective Easy for patients to use No dose calculations Little or no maintenance Ability to visualize drug flow Alarm features Disposable syringe Smart pump technology	Device can fracture or break if dropped. Limited volumes Not for large-volume infusions Drug stability factor Requires adequate manual dexterity to maintain syringe and tubing Free-flow risk
Elastomeric	Lightweight, portable, and concealable Easy for patients to use No programming No maintenance Reservoir and tubing attached Disposable Simple directions	Difficult to fill, especially those with multilayer membranes Admixture considerations Drug stability factor Requires calculation of concentrations and volumes Limited infusion rates Not for large-volume infusions Not all insurances reimburse No alarms Poor flow accuracy

Note. Based on information from Baxter International Inc., 2008; Cardinal Health, 2008; CME America LLC, 2009; Emergency Care Research Institute, 2008a, 2008b; InfuSystem, Inc., 2008; Smiths Medical, 2008; WalkMed Infusion LLC, 2009.

an ambulatory pump to enter the epidural, venous, SC, or perineural systems.

   a) TPN: Continuous therapy for 24 hours a day and cyclic infusions for 6–12 hours a day

   b) Antibiotics

   c) Pain management: Continuous narcotic infusion into the venous or intrathecal system with the capability of patient-activated bolus or patient-controlled analgesia for breakthrough pain. Pulse oximetry available on most patient-controlled analgesia pumps to monitor oxygen saturation.

   d) Chemotherapy: Primarily for continuous infusions; however, can be used for intermittent protocols

   e) Insulin

   f) Hydration

E. Operational procedures: How to use and operate (Baxter International Inc., 2008; Cardinal Health, 2008; CME America LLC, 2009; Dodd, 2007; InfuSystem, Inc., 2008; Remerand et al., 2008; Saladow, 2007; Skryabina & Dunn, 2006; Smiths Medical, 2008; WalkMed Infusion LLC, 2009)

1. Source of power

   a) Peristaltic pumps

      (1) Two to four AA alkaline batteries

      (2) Rechargeable battery packs

      (3) Nine-volt batteries

   b) Syringe pumps: Provide constant force to plunger, creating constant pressure within the syringe

      (1) Non-electronic with constant flow with no bolus, no free-flow features

      (2) Lithium-ion battery

   c) Elastomeric balloon: Uses elastomeric membrane to generate infusion pressure

2. Method of infusion/rate regulation: Flow rates should remain within 5% of the set flow rate provided by manufacturer (ECRI, 2008a).

   a) Linear peristaltic/rotary peristaltic

      (1) Mechanism propels fluid forward using appendages that move in a wave-like motion.

      (2) Rotary rotates the tubing between a cam (or disk) and cylinder to move fluid forward with specific rocking or reciprocating motion.

(3) Rate is programmed into pump as continuous or intermittent. Some have optional programmed bolus feature.

(4) 1–3,000 ml/day delivery capability with program flexibility available with milliliters, milligrams, or micrograms

(5) Dual-channel for simultaneous infusion available

b) Syringe infusions

(1) Motor-driven lead screw or gear mechanism propels fluid by forcing plunger or piston on syringe barrel.

(2) Rate is regulated by the size of the syringe and speed of the motor.

c) Elastomeric

(1) Elastomeric membrane generates infusion pressure when filled with fluid. As gravity or positive pressure causes membrane to deflate, fluid is forced out.

(2) Rate regulation is controlled by an in-line orifice or flow restrictor within the administration set and is affected by the pressure gradient across the flow restrictor and by fluid viscosity.

(3) The type of membrane determines the pressure generated on the fluid when stretched. Multilayer membranes can generate higher pressure compared with single layer.

(4) Infuse at rates of 0.5–500 ml/hr.

3. Alarm system

a) Peristaltic pumps: Available with audible and/or visual alarms for occlusion, air in line, low reservoir volume, low battery, and pump malfunction

b) Syringe pumps: Intermittent audible tone when infusion ends or with occlusion

(1) Authors of a study evaluating two types of syringe pumps with more than 560 alarm-time measurements revealed that occlusion alarm activation was longer with the use of lower infusion rates and larger syringes (Donmez et al., 2005).

(2) Authors recommended using smaller-sized, low-compliant syringes with reduced compressibility to reduce the time before an occlusion alarm.

c) Elastomeric: No alarm system

4. Administration sets/medication reservoirs: Administration tubing available from manufacturer for each type of pump

a) Peristaltic: Bag or cassette change may be daily or every 7–10 days depending on drug,

drug stability, and reservoir size. Reservoir covers are available.

b) Syringe: Use 5–60 ml syringe depending on pump. Change syringe every 12–24 hours or at end of infusion.

c) Elastomeric balloons: Available tubing with or without filters. Filling device is available to fill pump with drug. Dispose of after use.

5. Drug calculations

a) Assess the drug concentration required to place the drug's dose in a reservoir to allow for drug stability.

b) Room temperature stability: Drug must be stable for duration of infusion.

c) Rate of infusion is programmed into the pump according to concentration of drug in reservoir.

d) Dose error reduction systems (DERSs) are available and often referred to as "smart pumps" on syringe and peristaltic pumps (ECRI, 2008a).

(1) DERSs provide guided manual programming using pump-based software.

(2) Drug libraries are downloaded to the pump.

(3) The software checks programmed doses against preset limits stored in drug libraries.

(4) Alerts are given if programmed doses exceed preset limits, which require confirmation before infusion (referred to as *soft limits*) or the pump will not infuse (referred to as *hard limits*).

F. Maintenance and care

1. Continuous infusion minimizes necessity to disconnect the system, which obviates requirement to flush the access device.

2. Intermittent infusion requires the access device to be flushed with 10–20 ml of normal saline after drug completion and appropriate lock solution administered.

a) For some devices, such as the syringe and elastomeric device, the patient or significant other may need to disconnect the pump after flushing.

b) Patient teaching is necessary to ensure proper disconnection from pump.

3. Tubing and reservoir changes

a) Elastomeric devices are disposable with each dose.

b) The patient and significant other can be taught to change the cassette or syringe or connect the elastomeric devices.

c) Reservoirs, syringes, or elastomeric devices may necessitate one home visit or clinic visit per day to change drug reservoir or may be changed every three to seven days depending on the drug and treatment plan. Some patients may need to go into the clinic to have the pump reservoir changed; this is dependent on insurance coverage or the ability to care for pump.

d) Tubing for TPN is recommended to be changed every 24 hours.

4. Elastomeric pumps can be routinely weighed several times a day to detect potential infusion abnormalities, because alarms are not available (Remerand et al., 2008).

a) Device dysfunction can occur. After studying 430 elastomeric pumps used for postoperative regional anesthesia, 20.5% (88) of the pumps did not deflate correctly.

b) Authors suggested weighing the devices every three hours to ensure pump is infusing as prescribed.

c) Scale may be sent home with the patient so that the patient or significant other can weigh the device.

5. Pump data logs should be available to record pump settings, setting changes, and alarm activations. Log should include when batteries are changed or charged (ECRI, 2008a).

G. Complications

1. Occlusion

a) An empty reservoir can cause an occlusion and increase the risk of clot formation. Patient should be instructed on how to disconnect the pump or to return to the clinic to have pump disconnected.

b) Kinked tubing: The extension tubing should be looped and secured to prevent kinking and occlusion.

c) IV catheter infiltration: Patient should be taught signs of infiltration and how to stop the pump from continuing to infuse. The clinic should be called immediately.

d) Pump malfunction: The patient should be taught about alarms and instructed to call pump provider. A phone number should be given to the patient.

(1) Most troubleshooting can be conducted over the phone. If the pump malfunction cannot be corrected, the patient should be instructed to return to the clinic for a backup pump.

(2) Some pump companies will allow a second pump to be kept at the patient's home to be used as a backup.

2. Incorrect programming of pump (ECRI, 2008b; Eisenberg, 2009; Saladow, 2007)

a) Causes: Bypassing alert messages, bypassing potential safeguards of the pump, and input of incorrect pump settings

b) Pump information should be verified with another nurse to ensure pump setting is correct prior to connecting to patient.

c) Use of barcode technology on the drug bag, cassette, or syringe allows information to be compared with the patient's prescribed information.

d) Use of customized therapy protocol library for patient care reinforces correct dose.

e) Label each syringe, cassette, or bag with drug, rate of infusion, and patient name.

f) ECRI (2008a) strongly recommends the use of "smart pump" technology to minimize the risk of incorrect dosing.

(1) Technology warns users of incorrect medicine orders, calculation errors, and misprogramming.

(2) Soft limits require confirmation prior to initiating the infusion if preset limits differ from program.

(3) Hard limits will not allow infusion if preset limits differ from program.

(4) Some pumps are available to store alerts and log information, which can be analyzed to improve drug libraries and subsequent clinical practice.

g) Pumps should be checked frequently to ensure pump is infusing correctly and no occlusion is present. The patient and significant other must be taught how to monitor this in the home setting.

3. Incorrect flow rate of elastomeric pump (Remerand et al., 2008; Skryabina & Dunn, 2006)

a) Back pressure in pump can occur as a result of vertical displacement of the device to the infusion set. Keep device steady in carrying case.

b) Underfilling or overfilling of the device: Use filling device to measure medication accurately.

c) Variations in atmospheric pressure: Instruct patient to monitor infusion.

d) Temperature changes affect the rate. Manufacturers recommend to maintain temperature of calibration, which is usually at skin temperature. In general, an increase or decrease in flow rate can occur by 2%–3% for every 1° of temperature increase or decrease for water-based solutions.

e) Increased viscosity of the drug will decrease the flow rate. Monitor infusion.

H. Education and documentation: See Section X.

X. EDUCATION AND DOCUMENTATION ISSUES FOR ACCESS DEVICES

A. Education

1. Patient or significant other education about the access device is documented in the healthcare record.

   a) Indications for access device

   b) Type of device inserted

   c) Potential complications of access device (see Tables 5, 9, 14, and 18 for examples)

   d) Signs and symptoms of access device complication to report to the healthcare team

   e) Demonstration of self-care skills related to access device care, as appropriate

   f) Community resources for supplies and emergency care related to access device, if appropriate

   g) Care and maintenance of device, such as dressing change, flushing procedure, or follow-up appointments to receive care (see Tables 1 and 8 for examples)

   h) Type of instruction used (e.g., verbal explanation, demonstration, return demonstration, written instructions, educational video, Web sites, online instructions) (see Appendix 12 for an example of written instructions for patients)

   i) Patient teaching checklist used, signed, and dated by the nurse and the patient or significant other

   j) Consideration of factors that can affect learning (e.g., age, physical condition, emotional state, educational level, caregiver abilities, financial resources or insurance to cover supplies)

   k) Referral to home care, physician's office, or hospital

2. Nurse education and competency in caring for patients with access devices should be documented in the nurse's personnel record.

   a) Nursing educational activities should address the following (Pieger-Mooney, 2005).

      (1) Content on specific access devices, as many new products and procedures are available

      (2) Insertion and access procedures

      (3) Care and maintenance: Assessment of site, dressing change, and flushing procedure

      (4) Assessment of catheter function, potential complications, and interventions

      (5) Elements of patient and family education about access devices

   b) Comprehensive skill forms are used to validate training and evaluation. Skills include

placement, assessment, and interventions used for complications (Pieger-Mooney, 2005).

   c) Nurses participate in annual or biannual continuing education opportunities to maintain knowledge.

   d) Clinical competency in access device technology should be considered annually to ensure adherence to procedures.

   e) Staff training and education help to improve access device care (CDC, in press; Morris & Tay, 2008).

B. Nursing documentation (Gorski, 2007, 2009; Higuchi, Edwards, Danseco, Davies, & McConnell, 2007; Morris & Tay, 2008)

1. Assessment

   a) Assess need for access device and type of device needed. Include the patient/caregiver in decision process (Macklin, 2005).

   b) Systemic assessment of the patient to include type, purpose, and duration of therapy, previous access device problems, and other health problems (Higuchi et al., 2007).

2. Interventions

   a) Insertion

      (1) Informed consent for procedure with patient's signature, if appropriate

      (2) Date, time, and setting of insertion

      (3) Type of device inserted (need to include name, manufacturer, lot or serial number, and size)

      (4) Location of insertion site for device (specify vein or artery if appropriate)

      (5) Preparation of insertion site

      (6) Presence of blood return or other body fluid such as peritoneal or CSF; ability to flush

      (7) Complications of insertion procedure

      (8) Method used to secure device and type of dressing used

      (9) Confirmation of catheter placement (i.e., x-ray if appropriate)

   b) Use of access device

      (1) Date, time, and purpose for which device was used

      (2) Methods used to evaluate proper functioning of device prior to use

      (3) Complications noted with use

      (4) Notification of appropriate member of the healthcare team

      (5) Strategies used to manage complications

      (6) The Joint Commission (2006) listed risk-reducing strategies that can be adapted to the practice of access de-

vice use. Recommendations include the following.

(a) Color-label all fluid bags, tubing, and catheters to distinguish type of access used such as IP, epidural, intrathecal, and arterial.

(b) Trace all tubing to point of origin with every use before connecting infusions.

(c) Recheck all tubing and trace all connections to point of origin again upon arrival in new settings or services, such as transfers to other care units.

(d) Route tubing having different purposes in different directions or different sides of the bed or chair.

(e) Inform nonclinical staff, patients, and families to seek help from the nurse if there is a perceived need to connect or disconnect infusion tubing (this should never occur for chemotherapy administration).

(f) Educate all nurses during orientation and chemotherapy training with regard to the importance of accessing the appropriate route (e.g., IV, IP, or other route).

(g) Educate patients and caregivers about the difference between IV and other access devices and purposes of each.

c) Care and maintenance of access device
   (1) Dressing change—type of dressing and procedure used
   (2) Flushing procedure: Type of flush, volume, frequency, difficulties encountered
   (3) Cap change: Type of cap and frequency of changes
   (4) Use of clamps on the device or extension tubing
   (5) Date of assessment of insertion site and exit site, intactness of device, and subjective information

d) Removal of access device
   (1) Indication for removal
   (2) Date and time of device removal
   (3) Type of device removed and description of device after removal
   (4) Procedure used for removal and observations of complications during device removal
   (5) Patient teaching about post-removal care and potential complications of what to report to healthcare team

3. Patient response to the intervention
   a) Verbalizes the purpose, care, and possible complications of access device
   b) Asks appropriate questions
   c) Can demonstrate care and maintenance of device if going home with device in place or accessed

XI. SPECIAL CONSIDERATIONS FOR IMMUNOSUPPRESSED PATIENTS WITH ACCESS DEVICES

(Moran & Camp-Sorrell, 2002; Polovich et al., 2009)

A. Patients undergoing therapy with chemotherapeutic agents often require placement of VADs to minimize frequent venipunctures and ensure safe administration of chemotherapeutic agents.

B. Immunosuppression from disease states and therapies increases the risk of access device–related infections. Myelosuppression is the suppression of bone marrow activity and includes neutropenia, anemia, and thrombocytopenia. Immunosuppression is an alteration in the body's immune response.

C. Because normal immune response may be inadequate to prevent infection, the use of additional or alternative methods to supplement the host's defense mechanisms is necessary to reduce mortality and morbidity from catheter-related infections in an immunosuppressed patient.

D. Catheter-related infections in immunosuppressed patients generally require aggressive antimicrobial therapy or early removal of the catheter, which translates to greater potential toxicity to the patient, antimicrobial resistance, and an increase in healthcare-associated costs (Chambers et al., 2005).

E. Patient/caregiver factors that increase infection risk in immunosuppressed patients (Elihu & Gollin, 2007; Worth, Seymour, & Slavin, 2009): Severe neutropenia (absolute neutrophil count less than 500) at time of catheter insertion, prolonged episode of immunosuppression, type of malignancy (solid tumor versus hematologic), type of treatment, mucositis, prior catheter infection, fibrin sheath or thrombus on catheter, lack of patient/ caregiver education to recognize complications, poor nutritional status, poor hand hygiene, and poor aseptic technique during catheter insertion and maintenance

F. Catheter factors that contribute to increased infection risk (Sariosmanoglu et al., 2008): Polyvinyl chloride material, insertion site in chest or groin, type of catheter (nontunneled versus implanted port), multiple catheter lumens, and frequent catheter manipulations through use and maintenance

G. Common infectious pathogens in patients with hematologic malignancies (Boersma, Jie, Verbon, van Pampus, & Schouten, 2008): Coagulase-negative *Staphylococcus*, *Staphylococcus aureus*, gram-negative bacilli such as *Enterobacteriaceae*, *Escherichia coli* and *Pseudomonas* spp., and *Candida* spp.

H. Strategies to prevent infections in immunosuppressed patients: Implement central line care bundles (IHI, n.d.).
1. Choice of catheter
   a) Tunneled catheter or implanted port
   b) Use of silicone material
   c) Use of catheter with as few lumens as possible
2. Avoid femoral insertion site.
3. Use maximal sterile barrier precautions during insertion, such as sterile gloves, sterile barriers, sterile gowns, and sterile mask.
4. Use maximal precautions for access device maintenance. Adhere to strict aseptic guidelines. To date, no research provides an evidence base for using sterile technique except for devices used in peritoneal, epidural, intraventricular, and intrathecal systems.
5. Catheter maintenance (CDC, in press)
   a) Perform adequate hand hygiene prior to catheter care or manipulation.
   b) Use chlorhexidine-based antiseptic for cleansing. Apply for 30 seconds and allow to dry.
   c) Use standardized protocol for cleansing catheter hubs and injection ports when utilizing device.
   d) The optimal dressing type and frequency of site care requires more research. No current recommendations exist for the use of sterile versus nonsterile gloves during dressing changes (CDC, in press; Pratt et al., 2007). Use of a no-touch technique with sterile or nonsterile gloves is recommended to prevent bacterial contamination (Pratt et al., 2007).
   e) Minimize frequency of catheter manipulations.
6. Novel approaches to decrease risk of infection
   a) Use of antibiotic/antiseptic lock or flush protocol to prevent infection requires more

research; however, it may be appropriate for catheter salvage when used together with systemic antibiotics (Mermel et al., 2009).

b) Use of antiseptic/antibiotic-impregnated dressing, such as a chlorhexidine-impregnated sponge, has been shown to decrease the incidence of catheter-related tunnel and exit-site infections in neutropenic patients but probably does not decrease the risk of catheter-related sepsis or bacteremia (Chambers et al., 2005). More research is needed for recommendations.

c) Use of antibiotic/antiseptic-impregnated catheter seems to correlate with a reduced risk of infection, especially in immunosuppressed patients; however, the optimal antimicrobial/antiseptic agent to be used requires more research (Jaeger et al., 2005; Maaskant, De Boer, Dalesio, Holtkamp, & Lucas, 2009).

d) Thrombolytic/heparin solutions for routine flush may be appropriate to minimize biofilm (a microbial environment that adheres to the surface of the VAD) that may promote growth of virulent bacteria. Urokinase and other antithrombolytics are not currently recommended by the Infectious Diseases Society of America as adjunct treatment for catheter-related infections. The interrelationship between thrombosis and infection requires more research. It is currently hypothesized that many catheter-related infections are preceded by formation of a fibrin sheath that may harbor microorganisms. Potentially minimizing the fibrin sheath could lead to a reduction in catheter-related infections (Boersma et al., 2008).

e) If the patient is neutropenic at the time of device insertion, consider administering a systemic prophylactic antibiotic.

f) Perform daily assessment of device to ascertain the necessity for antibiotics.

7. Removal of catheter (also see p. 49)
a) When no longer indicated for treatment
b) Infection identified that requires removal (see Table 20)

8. Adequate patient/caregiver education
a) Appropriate catheter site care (e.g., hand hygiene, aseptic or no-touch technique for catheter care)
b) Signs of complications, erythema, fever greater than 100.5°F (38°C), chills, exudates/bleeding from site, discomfort, ede-

ma, inability to flush catheter, inability to withdraw blood, or pain with infusing solution
c) The system to notify healthcare professional if complication is suspected

9. Infection rate surveillance using a standard formula (INS, 2006)

$$\frac{\text{Number of catheter-related infections}}{\text{Total number of catheter days}} \times 1,000 = \text{Number of catheter-related infections per 1,000 catheter days}$$

10. Use of a combined modality protocol or "bundle" procedure may be most effective at preventing infection in the immunocompromised population (Galpern, Guerrero, Tu, Fahoum, & Wise, 2008). A bundle procedure is a combination of evidence-based procedures that together form a protocol. When used consistently together, they may decrease infection rates. Examples of bundle procedures:
a) Staff education, maximal barrier precautions, hand washing, skin preparation with chlorhexidine, use of a central line cart, and avoidance of femoral lines
b) Use of a central line cart with CVC insertion and maintenance supplies. Required procedure followed by all personnel that manage CVCs.

11. Identification and management of infection (see Table 20)
a) Rapid identification of signs of infection is crucial to minimize morbidity and mortality in this population.
b) The decision to remove a catheter should be made after assessing the clinical condition of the patient, response to therapy, and outcome of microbiologic results, if available.

Table 20. Initial Management of Suspected Catheter-Related Infections in Neutropenic Patients

Considerations	Exit-Site Infection	Tunnel/Pocket Infection	Catheter-Related Bloodstream Infection
Treat with catheter in place?	Yes	Yes (unless tracking is evident, then catheter should be removed)	Yes
Culture method	Culture of site exudate	Paired peripheral and central blood cultures	Paired peripheral and central blood cultures
Empiric treatment	Topical antibiotics if nonpurulent drainage from site Empiric therapy with vancomycin if purulent drainage or patient is febrile Daily surveillance of the area Daily cleaning with chlorhexidine and gauze and tape	Empiric therapy with vancomycin until organism is identified Daily surveillance of the area Daily cleaning with chlorhexidine and gauze and tape	Empiric therapy with vancomycin until organism is identified Gram-negative organism coverage Consider empiric antifungal coverage. Daily surveillance of the area Daily cleaning with chlorhexidine and gauze and tape
Duration of therapy	10–14 days*	10–14 days*	10–14 days*

* Treatment duration may be significantly longer (4–6 weeks) in presence of known infection with *Staphylococcus aureus* or other infectious complications such as septic thrombosis, endocarditis, or osteomyelitis.

Note. Based on information from Bishop et al., 2007; Boersma et al., 2008; Mermel et al., 2009; Raad et al., 2007; Sariosmanoglu et al., 2008; Wolf et al., 2008.

XII. CONTROVERSIAL ISSUES

(See Table 21 for a summary of studies related to access devices.)

A. Dressing types

1. Transparent dressings versus gauze dressings

   a) Until prospective, multisite randomized studies are conducted in which the cleansing protocols, frequencies of dressing changes, differences in transparent dressing brands, patient characteristics, and outcome variables are standardized, determining which type of dressing and maintenance care protocol will result in the least number of complications will be difficult.

   b) A systematic review was conducted to compare gauze and tape and transparent polyurethane CVC dressings in terms of catheter-related infection, catheter security, tolerance to dressing material, and dressing condition in hospitalized adults and children (Gillies et al., 2003). The authors analyzed six studies, with results indicating no difference in the incidence of infectious complications among any of the dressing types. The authors concluded that all of the studies reported a small patient sample, and the lack of difference between dressing types may be the result of a lack of adequate data.

   c) Past studies, using both retrospective and prospective designs, support and refute the use of gauze and transparent dressings (see Table 21).

      (1) Many of the studies had methodologic flaws and insufficient power to detect significant differences in infection rates; therefore, drawing conclusions regarding differences in infection is difficult.

      (2) There was heterogeneity in the operational definition of catheter-related infections, varying measures of outcome, and different patient populations, cleansing protocols, frequency of dressing changes, and types of catheters as well as catheter dwell time.

      (3) Studies in which prospective designs were used revealed an increase in catheter tip and exit-site infections with transparent occlusive dressings when compared to dry gauze dressings.

   d) Investigators who conducted studies in which infection rates were higher with transparent dressings concluded that the transparent dressings did not allow for adequate evaporation of perspiration, leading to increased colonization of bacteria at the catheter exit site. Most studies were done with older versions of dressings. Current dressings are available that may reduce the rate of organism colonization.

   e) Newer versions of transparent dressings with semipermeable and highly permeable membranes that allow for increased moisture vapor transmission rates can remove up to eight times more moisture from the exit site than other transparent dressings.

   f) The cost of transparent dressings, even when the frequency of dressing changes is considered, remains higher than the cost of dry gauze dressings.

2. No dressing versus gauze dressing: One study investigated CVC-related sepsis, comparing no dressing or gauze dressing for newly inserted CVCs in transplant recipients (Olson et al., 2004). Findings suggested that no significant difference existed in catheter-related sepsis between the no-dressing and dressing groups; however, the gauze dressing group had a significantly shorter time interval to the development of sepsis.

3. The most recent recommendations from the CDC (in press) suggested that the choice of dressing could be a matter of preference.

B. Cleansing agents

1. Before catheter insertion and for catheter site care/dressing changes: The CDC recommends a 2% chlorhexidine-based preparation; however, tincture of iodine, an iodophor, or 70% alcohol can be used (CDC, in press). No recommendations can be made for the use of chlorhexidine in infants younger than two months of age (CDC, in press). Additional skin cleansing recommendations from the CDC include application of the solution with friction, allowing 30 seconds of air-dry time without wiping the solution.

   a) The efficacy of skin disinfection for catheter site care with CHG versus povidone-iodine was investigated in a meta-analysis to evaluate risk for catheter-related bloodstream infections (Chaiyakunapruk et al., 2002). The eight studies analyzed included central venous, peripheral venous, peripheral arterial, pulmonary arterial, PICC, introducer sheath, and hemodialysis catheters. Types of dressings included sterile gauze, semiocclusive, and transparent.

Dressing changes and site care were conducted every 48–72 hours. Several types of CHG solution were used, including 0.5% or 1% CHG alcohol solution and 0.5% or 2% CHG aqueous solution. Results suggested that the incidence of bloodstream infection was significantly reduced with CHG versus povidone-iodine for insertion-site skin disinfection.

2. Before epidural catheter placement: The best skin disinfection prior to epidural catheter placement has yet to be determined (see Table 21).

a) Spray disinfection with a 2-propanol and benzalkonium chloride solution was found to be as efficacious as swab disinfection with the same solution (Debreceni, Meggyesi, & Mestyan, 2007).

b) DuraPrep™ (3M Health Care), an iodophor-in-isopropyl alcohol solution, was found to decrease the number of positive skin cultures and decrease bacterial growth in comparison to povidone-iodine (Birnbach et al., 2003).

c) In 2006, the American Society of Regional Anesthesia and Pain Medicine recommended chlorhexidine (Hebl, 2006).

3. Before needle puncture of a protective catheter cap: A disinfectant is used routinely to cleanse the protective cap of a catheter prior to puncture with a needle. The best disinfectant to use to reduce microbial contamination of the hub has yet to be determined.

a) Results of an in vitro study suggested that a 15-second scrub using a 70% alcohol or a 3.15% chlorhexidine/70% alcohol solution produced bactericidal effects in four different types of injection access caps (Kaler & Chinn, 2007).

b) Several studies have suggested that use of a novel antiseptic barrier/connector cap significantly decreased the risk of microorganism transmission (Buchman, Spap-

peri, & Leopold, 2009; Menyhay & Maki, 2006, 2008). Further research is needed. No conclusions can be drawn to affect practice.

c) The CDC (in press) recommends cleansing injection ports with 70% alcohol or iodophor before accessing the system.

4. Skin disinfection prior to port access: No studies have been conducted to investigate cleansing agents and protocols for skin cleansing prior to implanted port access. It may be inferred that port access is similar to catheter insertion in causing a break in skin integrity. Therefore, CDC recommendations and use of 2% CHG may be considered. Further research is needed.

5. Large, prospective, randomized clinical trials investigating different cleansing agents, with dressing types controlled, are needed to determine the most appropriate cleansing agent.

C. Flushing agents

1. Central venous lines

a) The effectiveness of dilute heparin solution and of normal saline in flushing and maintaining the patency of CVCs is disputed. Analyses of research about heparinized versus nonheparinized vascular lines found no evidence to support the use of heparinized saline over normal saline (Kannan, 2008). Cesaro et al. (2009) compared standard flushing of Broviac-Hickman CVCs with heparin solution or normal saline. Results suggested a higher incidence of catheter occlusion and bacteremia with normal saline flushing; however, the authors recommended further research to clarify whether the results were related to saline flushes or to once-a-week flushing.

b) The issues of volume and frequency of flushing continue to be controversial among institutions across the country. Multisite, randomized prospective studies examining the relationship of these variables with factors such as patency, type of device, patient characteristics, infection, and cost will help to standardize protocols used in multiple institutions.

2. No evidence exists on flushing access devices in patients with heparin-induced thrombocytopenia. Consideration should be given to insert devices with valves and use normal saline flush.

3. Venous implantable ports

a) In a retrospective study, administration of 1,000 IU of heparin flush every six weeks was compared to 500 IU of heparin flush every four weeks in 89 patients with cancer who had completed chemotherapy (Kefeli et al., 2009). Ports were maintained for one year. No differences in port-related infection or thrombosis were found between the groups.

   b) Similar results were found in a retrospective study exploring Port-A-Cath accession intervals for catheter maintenance (Kuo et al., 2005). The study included a total of 73 patients with gynecologic carcinomas. Seven patients had no blood return during routine catheter accession. No statistically significant difference was found between the average accession intervals in patients with no blood return (79 days) versus those patients with no difficulty in catheter accession (63 days).

4. Arterial pressure lines
   a) Recent research focusing on patency and monitoring arterial pressure lines is limited with mixed results. Del Cotillo, Grane, Llavore, and Quintana (2008) investigated the efficacy of heparinized (1 IU/ml) versus saline flushes in arterial catheter maintenance. Results suggested no significant difference in function or duration of the arterial catheters in comparison to normal saline flushes. Whitta, Hall, Bennetts, Welman, and Rawlins (2006) compared normal saline and heparinized saline (3 ml/hr as a continuous flush) on the function of arterial lines. Results indicated that heparin as a continuous flush did not improve the function of arterial lines as compared to normal saline. In a literature review of arterial line maintenance care, Lapum (2006) found saline was as effective as heparin in maintaining patency in one study; however, four studies concluded that a heparinized solution was more effective in maintaining patency of arterial lines. As the author noted, critical appraisal of these studies found that research rigor was questionable, and further research is needed that evaluates confounding variables.
   b) The use of heparinized flushes to maintain patency remains controversial and carries the increased risk of coagulopathies and heparin-induced thrombocytopenia. Hall, Bennetts, Whitta, Welman, and Rawlins (2006) found that the use of heparin in normal saline as a continuous flush for an arterial catheter did not alter platelet counts. However, Del Cotill et al. (2008) found significant alterations in activated partial thromboplastin time. The risks of nonpatency must be weighed against the risks of heparin-induced thrombocytopenia, especially for long-term arterial catheters (Glass & Spitrey, 2009; Leeper, 2006).

D. VAD without blood return: No studies to date have provided a research-based answer as to when to give medications through a device without a blood return.
   1. It generally is recommended in various clinical settings that prior to administering medications through VADs in which no blood return exists, placement verification should be accomplished through either x-ray or dye studies. Peripheral and midline catheters should be reinserted if there is no blood return (Gorski, Perucca, & Hunter, 2010; Hamilton, 2006; Rosenthal, 2007).
   2. Administration of vesicants should be prohibited unless catheter tip placement, catheter body intactness, and catheter patency are determined. If the catheter tip is determined to have a fibrin sheath or clot resulting in backflow, vesicants should not be administered. Backtracking of a vesicant can result in extravasation (Sauerland, Engelking, Wickham, & Corbi, 2006; Schulmeister & Camp-Sorrell, 2000; Polovich et al., 2009). A physician order should be obtained to use a VAD when there is no blood return if the VAD is determined to be intact, in the correct position, patent, and without backflow.

E. Catheter occlusion
   1. The use of alteplase for catheter occlusion has been found to be safe and effective (Blaney et al., 2006; Davis, Vermeulen, Banton, Schwartz, & Williams, 2000; Ng, Li, Tu, & Semba, 2004; Timoney et al., 2002).
   2. Reteplase currently is indicated for the management of acute myocardial infarction for the improvement of ventricular function, reduction of congestive heart failure, and reduction of mortality associated with acute myocardial infarction. A preliminary study investigating reteplase for catheter occlusion has suggested it is a safe and effective thrombolytic agent for VADs (Liu et al., 2004). Further research is needed.
   3. Studies investigating different catheter and flushing protocols to prevent catheter thrombosis are limited. Recent studies investigating CVC occlusion and different types of catheters found no significant reduction

in risk of catheter occlusion with heparin-bonded catheters (Shah & Shah, 2007). However, CVCs capped with a single-valve or positive-pressure–valve needleless connector device were found to have lower complete catheter occlusion rates (Schilling, Doellman, Hutchinson, & Jacobs, 2006). Two studies investigating flushing protocols and catheter occlusion found a higher incidence of catheter occlusion and bacteremia with normal saline flushing via a positive-pressure cap (Cesaro et al., 2009) and with lepirudin flushing (Horne et al., 2006) compared to heparin flushing.

4. Several meta-analyses and literature reviews have been conducted recently to investigate the use of low-dose warfarin and thrombus formation in patients with cancer who have CVCs (Akl et al., 2007; Chan, Iannucci, & Dager, 2007; Chaukiyal, Nautiyal, Radhakrishnan, Singh, & Navaneethan, 2008; Cunningham, White, Hollywood, & O'Donnell, 2006; Kuter, 2004; Rawson & Newburn-Cook, 2007). Findings suggest that the incidence of catheter-related thrombosis is not significantly reduced with the use of prophylactic warfarin. The prophylactic use of SC unfractionated heparin or low-molecular-weight heparin in patients with cancer who have CVCs has also shown no significant reduction in catheter-related thrombus (Akl et al., 2007; Verso et al., 2005). Prophylactic warfarin was found to be effective in preventing catheter-related thrombus in patients with CVCs undergoing high-dose chemotherapy followed by peripheral blood stem cell transplantation (Magagnoli et al., 2006). The American College of Chest Physicians does not recommend routine use of low-dose warfarin or low-molecular-weight heparin to prevent thrombosis related to venous access devices in patients with cancer (Geerts et al., 2004).

5. Risk factors associated with CVC thrombosis in patients with cancer include an inadequate position of the CVC tip in the upper half of the superior vena cava, left-sided CVC insertion, and chest radiotherapy (Verso et al., 2008).

F. Infection/infection control

1. The presence of bacterial biofilms or deposits on the surfaces of vascular catheters is of unknown clinical importance. However, their presence has the potential to serve as a nidus (focus) for infection and bacteremia (Aslam, 2008). The value of the routine use of thrombolytic agent instillation to cleanse the internal lining of slime-enclosed biofilms is unknown.

2. The value of scheduled replacement of peripheral IV catheters is unknown. Restarted catheters in 72 hours have shown a greater risk of complications than catheters maintained for 96 hours. INS (2006) recommends that peripheral catheters be rotated every 72 hours, and the CDC (in press) recommends rotation every 72–96 hours.

3. The value of scheduled replacement of nontunneled CVCs has been controversial in the past, with studies showing mixed results (Safdar & Maki, 2005; Smith et al., 2008). Routine replacement of CVCs is not supported (CDC, in press).

4. The use of different types of intravascular devices and the risk of bloodstream infections is unknown. One study found higher rates of bloodstream infections with short-term noncuffed and nonmedicated CVCs compared to IV catheters and midline catheters, while arterial catheters and PICCs had bloodstream infection rates similar to CVCs (Maki et al., 2006). Previous studies have not clearly answered this question because of the numerous variables. Ports usually are inserted in patients with solid tumors receiving less aggressive regimens; therefore, the patients do not have prolonged nadirs. However, tunneled catheters, usually multilumen, are placed in patients with hematologic cancers who receive aggressive regimens that result in prolonged nadirs. Further research is needed that includes the type of device, therapy, maintenance protocols, and the patient's disease, comorbidities, age, and manual dexterity.

5. The value of coating a catheter with an antimicrobial agent prior to insertion for the prevention of catheter-associated infections is controversial. Findings from several studies have either supported or refuted the use of antimicrobial agents (Hockenhull et al., 2008, 2009; Niel-Weise et al., 2007).

   a) Investigators have compared the efficacy of chlorhexidine and silver sulfadiazine–impregnated catheters with nonimpregnated catheters for the prevention of catheter-related infections and have found mixed results (Jaeger et al., 2001; Kalfon et al., 2007; Khare et al., 2007; Osma et al., 2006).

   b) Studies have found a lower rate of infection with minocycline and rifampin-impregnated catheters in comparison to chlorhexidine and silver sulfadiazine–

impregnated catheters (Falagas, Fragoulis, Bliziotis, & Chatzinikolaou, 2007; Fraenkel et al., 2006; Yucel et al., 2004).

c) A lower rate of infection has been found with benzalkonium chloride–coated catheters in comparison to a non-antiseptic catheter.

6. The value of using an antibiotic lock technique in the port reservoir to prevent catheter-related sepsis is controversial. A review of antibiotic lock technique suggests utility in the prevention of VAD removal associated with catheter-related sepsis (Bestul & VandenBussche, 2005; Mermel, 2009). The CDC does not recommend an antibiotic lock as a routine prevention measure; however, antibiotic lock use is recommended for high-risk patients (CDC, in press).

7. The use of antimicrobial ointment at the insertion site periodically falls out of favor for lack of evidence supporting its use in preventing infection. However, the contribution of these topical ointments to the incidence of infection (especially fungemia) has been questioned (CDC, in press). No recent studies have been conducted. The CDC has recommended no ointment.

8. The use of chlorhexidine-impregnated dressing/sponges at the insertion site releases CHG over several days. Studies suggest that the use of chlorhexidine-impregnated dressing/sponges significantly reduces the rates of central venous and epidural catheter–related infections (Banton, 2006; Ho & Litton, 2006; Levy et al., 2005; Ruschulte et al., 2009; Timsit et al., 2009).

9. The issue of selecting the best site of catheter insertion to decrease the risk of infection is controversial. One randomized controlled trial was found comparing internal jugular, subclavian, and cephalic veins for CVC placement (Biffi et al., 2009). Results indicated no difference in risk of infection among any of these catheter insertion sites. One prospective study found an association between catheter contamination and femoral CVC sites (Goetz, Wagener, Miller, & Muder, 1998). Further research is needed to compare specific sites of catheter insertion, the type of device, and insertion protocols.

10. One retrospective descriptive study investigated infection rate in 62 patients using an aseptic technique for accessing and deaccessing implantable ports using nonsterile gloves (Camp-Sorrell, 2009). Results indicated only two of the six infections that occurred could be attributed to the aseptic nonsterile glove technique for accessing and deaccessing implantable ports.

11. Study findings investigating the relationship between needleless access devices and bloodstream infection rates suggested no association, whereas other studies have found an increase in bloodstream infection rates associated with needleless devices (Field et al., 2007; Salgado, Chinnes, Paczesny, & Cantey, 2007). An increased risk of bloodstream infection also was found when the devices were changed every six to seven days (Toscano et al., 2009).

12. Although no research has been conducted on the benefits of routine surveillance of access catheters, it has been suggested to monitor the catheter sites visually or by palpation through the intact dressing on a regular basis, depending on the clinical situation of individual patients (CDC, in press).

13. Additional references related to catheter infection include Aslam, 2008; Esteve et al., 2007; Mermel, 2007; Mermel et al., 2009; Opilla, 2008; Raad et al., 2007; Ramritu et al., 2008; Safdar & Maki, 2005, 2006; Worthington & Elliott, 2005; Yoshida et al., 2008.

G. Removal of CVCs: Deciding when to remove CVCs in the presence of catheter-related bacteremia is difficult (see Table 21).

1. Immunosuppressed and thrombocytopenic patients are placed at higher risk for infections and bleeding if the existing catheter is removed and a new one is placed.

2. No recent studies were found investigating VAD removal in the presence of bacteremia. Nonetheless, it generally is recommended that the catheter be removed when VAD-related septicemia is confirmed, tunnel infection exists, signs and symptoms of septicemia persist despite antibiotics, or the causative organism is fungi, bacilli, or pseudomonas (Bishop et al., 2007; Mermel et al., 2009; Raad et al., 2007; Vescia et al., 2008).

3. The Centers for Medicare and Medicaid Services implemented a new payment system on October 1, 2008. Preventable conditions, which include vascular catheter–associated infections, will not be reimbursed to Medicare and Medicaid–certified hospitals unless the conditions were present on admission. Measures to prevent catheter-related infections in hospitalized patients are critical. Medicare has not given suggestions regarding prevention of infections (Centers for Medicare and Medicaid Services, 2008).

H. Blood sampling from CVCs
   1. Accessing and obtaining blood cultures from an implantable port with clinical signs of an infection is controversial because of the risk of hematogenous seeding; however, this may be necessary to isolate the causative microorganism for specific antibiotic treatment (Camp-Sorrell, 2007; Marschall et al., 2008; Moran & Camp-Sorrell, 2002).
      a) A recent meta-analysis was conducted to compare diagnostic test characteristics of blood cultures obtained from intravascular catheters and peripheral veins (Falagas, Kazantzi, & Bliziotis, 2008). Six studies were included in the analysis. Findings indicated that a culture obtained from an intravascular catheter is a diagnostic test for bacteremia with better sensitivity and better negative predictive value but less specificity and lower positive predictive value compared to a culture obtained from a peripheral venipuncture.
      b) In a prospective study, blood cultures were obtained from CVCs 100 days after placement, even in the absence of signs and symptoms of infection, to evaluate sensitivity, specificity, positive predictive value, and negative predictive value for the diagnosis of bacteremia (Chatzinikolaou et al., 2006). Results suggested that quantitative cultures of organisms from blood collected

through CVCs were highly sensitive, specific, and predictive of bacteremia.
   2. Studies investigating coagulation testing from heparinized VADs compared with peripheral samples have had mixed results. International normalized ratio (INR) specimens from heparinized CVCs and activated partial thromboplastin time specimens obtained from PICCs have shown no significant difference compared to samples obtained from peripheral venipuncture (Boyd, Dunne, Townsend, & Pai, 2006; Rondina, Markewitz, Kling, Nohavec, & Rodgers, 2007). Past research, however, found that coagulation testing from heparinized tunneled VADs and Hickman catheters was significantly different compared to peripheral samples (see Table 21).
   3. In a prospective comparison study, coagulation tests consisting of prothrombin time, activated partial thromboplastin time, and INR were obtained from peripheral venipuncture and a VAD after discarding 6 ml, 9 ml, and 12 ml of blood (Lin, Fowler, Dise, & Bustami, 2009). Results indicated a high correlation between peripheral venipuncture and all VAD blood samples. No differences were found between the three VAD samples, indicating that 6 ml was an adequate discard volume.
   4. One study found similar laboratory results with the push-pull method and the discard method of obtaining blood samples from CVCs (Barton et al., 2004). However, previous research suggested not reinfusing the discard blood collection because of the presence of clots and because the push-pull method can increase the risk of hemolysis with the agitation of blood (Frey, 2003).
   5. Further research investigating blood sampling and blood collection methods in different types of VADs is needed.

I. Power injection of contrast media
   1. Power injection VADs have become increasingly popular in oncology clinical practice. Studies investigating different catheter types and sizes and power injection of contrast media for CT studies are limited.
   2. One in vitro study found that a 7 Fr multilumen CVC can be used safely to give contrast media at injection rates of 3–5 ml/s (Sanelli, Deshmukh, Ougorets, Caiati, & Heier, 2004).
   3. One in vitro study found that 5 Fr single-lumen and double-lumen PICCs were able to tolerate power injection of contrast media for CT examinations at a rate of 2 ml/s (Coyle et al., 2004). Only use power ports for power in-

jections; otherwise, hand inject using 10 ml or greater syringe (FDA, 2009).

4. VADs should not be used if the device does not flush easily or if the device is known to have complications, as this increases pressure and risk of rupture.

5. Although no studies are available on power ports or catheters and the use of power injections, numerous radiographic suites will only use VADs specifically designed for power injection, such as the PowerPort® (C.R. Bard, Inc.).

6. Power injection of contrast media should only be used by healthcare professionals who clearly understand power injection of contrast media (Brown, Papadouris, Davis, Vedantham, & Pilgram, 2005; Coyle et al., 2004; Salis et al., 2004; Zamos, Emch, Patton, D'Amico, & Bansal, 2007). The power injector must be programmable to the catheter manufacturer's pressure specifications. Other variables that affect or increase the pressure are internal diameter, outer diameter, partial/complete occlusion, catheter material, and catheter length.

J. Controversial issues related to nursing practice

1. Suturing of PICCs by RNs is defined by each State Board of Nursing's scope of practice. Several states permit "trained" RNs to stabilize a PICC with sutures. No research has been conducted investigating RN suturing of PICCs, although one study was found exploring efficacy of advanced clinical nurses' suturing dermal lacerations in emergency department settings following a standardized training program (Middleton, 2006). Results suggested that nurses were capable of providing high-quality care for patients with dermal lacerations with no wound healing complications. Unfortunately, opinions on training requirements for insertion of PICCs vary from state to state and institution to institution, and a lack of uniformity exists regarding certification criteria for inserting these catheters. Training received in one state is not necessarily transferable to another. Further research is needed to investigate the RN scope of practice in suturing PICCs.

2. Removal of tunneled catheters by RNs

   a) Several State Boards of Nursing allow a trained RN to remove tunneled catheters.

   b) Further research is needed to investigate the RN scope of practice in removing tunneled catheters.

3. Role of assistive personnel in the care of VADs

   a) It is unclear whether assistive personnel may perform procedures such as accessing or flushing VADs or obtaining blood samples. Training requirements may vary depending on state or institution.

   b) Nurses in supervisory positions should review the State Board of Nursing Practice Act and establish appropriate policies and procedures for the care of VADs by assistive personnel within their institution.

   c) Further research is needed to investigate the role of assistive personnel in caring for VADs.

Table 21. Summary of Studies Related to Access Devices

Issue Studied	Study	Study Design, Sample, Purpose	Intervention/Variables Examined	Findings
Dressing types	Conly et al., 1989	*Study Design:* Prospective *Sample:* 79 medical, surgical, or pediatric patients with indwelling central venous catheters (CVCs) randomly assigned to two dressing groups: transparent, n = 58, and gauze, n = 57 (some patients received more than one CVC) *Purpose:* To compare incidence of insertion-site colonization, local catheter-related infections, and CVC-related sepsis	Gauze and transparent dressing site care protocol (same for both) 15-second hand scrub with 10% povidone-iodine or 2% chlorhexidine by employee CVC exit-site scrub with 70% isopropyl alcohol (IPA), followed by 10% povidone-iodine Dressings changed every 48 hours	Significantly greater colonization was observed after 48 hours in transparent dressings. More local CVC infections occurred in transparent dressing (62%) than in gauze dressing (24%). More catheter-related bacteremia occurred in transparent dressing (16.6%) than gauze dressing (0). No differences related to disease, purpose of catheter, or duration of catheterization were observed. Difference in cleansing method was not discussed.

(Continued on next page)

Table 21. Summary of Studies Related to Access Devices *(Continued)*

Issue Studied	Study	Study Design, Sample, Purpose	Intervention/Variables Examined	Findings
Dressing types *(cont.)*	Dickerson et al., 1989	*Study Design:* Prospective Phase I: 80 subclavian catheters Three dressing types were used: Transparent, n = 36 Gauze, n = 33 Combination, n = 11 Phase II: 81 subclavian catheters Two dressing types were used: Gauze covered by transparent, n = 77 Gauze covered by tape, n = 4 *Sample:* Patients from critical care, general medicine, and oncology *Purpose:* To examine differences in clinically significant infections	Phase I dressings: Transparent Gauze Combination Phase II dressings: Gauze covered by transparent Gauze covered by tape Site-care protocol not discussed	Phase I findings: More catheter-related infections occurred with transparent dressing (8.3%) compared to gauze (3%) (not statistically significant, no mention of third dressing). Phase II findings: No distinction made between dressing types used when reporting infection rates. Unclear if differences exist in dressing change frequencies between phases I and II. Although authors state that their data add to evidence that transparent dressings have higher infection rates, no conclusion can be drawn from this study.
	Hoffmann et al., 1992	*Study Design:* Meta-analysis of infection risks associated with transparent versus gauze dressings *Sample:* CVC studies (n = 15) Peripheral catheter studies (n = 12)	CVC outcome variables: Catheter tip infection Bacteremia Catheter sepsis Peripheral catheter outcome variables: Phlebitis Infiltration Skin colonization Catheter tip infection	Transparent dressings were associated with an increased risk of catheter tip infections in both CVCs and peripheral catheters and a statistically significant trend toward increases in bacteremias and catheter sepsis in CVCs. However, the difference in rates of catheter-related bloodstream infections (BSIs) was not statistically significant. Analysis confounders include durations of catheter use, frequency of dressing changes, use of antiseptic ointment, and subject characteristics.
	Laura et al., 2000	*Study Design:* Prospective *Sample:* 399 bone marrow transplant (BMT) recipients with indwelling CVCs randomly assigned to two different time interval protocols for dressing changes: Group A, n = 230 Group B, n = 169 *Purpose:* To compare two different time interval protocols for CVC dressings to assess local infections and toxicity	Dressing changes: Group A—every 5 or 10 days Group B—every 2 or 5 days	No significant difference in the rate of local infections. Significant increase in local skin toxicity in dressings changed every two days. Significant reduction in costs associated with longer dressing change intervals.
	Madeo et al., 1997	*Study Design:* Prospective *Sample:* 80 patients with peripheral IVs randomized into two groups: Gauze, n = 31 Transparent, n = 49 *Purpose:* To compare security of fixation, dressing condition, skin condition, and rates of inflammation	Sterile gauze dressing Transparent polyurethane dressing	Dressing condition and adherence significantly better in transparent group. No other significant differences found.

(Continued on next page)

Table 21. Summary of Studies Related to Access Devices *(Continued)*

Issue Studied	Study	Study Design, Sample, Purpose	Intervention/Variables Examined	Findings
Dressing types *(cont.)*	Olson et al., 2004	*Study Design:* Prospective *Sample:* 78 patients with cancer stratified by gender and transplant status with newly inserted CVCs randomly assigned to receive either a gauze dressing or no dressing *Purpose:* To compare gauze dressing and no dressing and risk of CVC-related sepsis and incidence of rehospitalization rates	Sterile gauze dressing No dressing	No significant difference was reported in CVC-related sepsis or rehospitalization rates. Gauze dressing group developed CVC-related sepsis significantly sooner than no-dressing group.
	Petrosino et al., 1988	*Study Design:* Prospective *Sample:* 52 patients with cancer with indwelling CVCs randomly assigned to four groups of dressings Two observation times: n = 41 for first observation n = 28 for second observation *Purpose:* To determine CVC exit-site infection rates among four dressing types	Dressing groups: Tegaderm™ (3M Health Care) transparent OpSite® (Smith & Nephew) transparent Gauze No dressing Site cleansing solution: Hydrogen peroxide (H_2O_2), alcohol, and povidone-iodine (plus povidone-iodine ointment to site) Transparent dressings changed every three days Gauze dressings changed every day	When cleansing solutions are controlled, a nonstatistically significant trend toward a higher infection rate in transparent dressings exists; however, the sample size may affect the power of the analyses. No conclusion can be drawn.
	Shivnan et al., 1991	*Study Design:* Prospective *Sample:* 98 BMT patients randomized into two groups: Gauze, n = 47 Transparent, n = 51 *Purpose:* To compare incidence and severity of complications, patient comfort, and calculation of nursing time	Dressing changes: Both dressings changed every four days Site care: H_2O_2 Povidone-iodine × 2 Protective skin barrier (for gauze dressing only)	No significant differences related to infections or complications were observed between the two dressings. Skin irritation was more prevalent in gauze dressings. Transparent dressings were more cost and time effective. Transparent dressings were more comfortable for patients.
	Treston-Aurand et al., 1997	*Study Design:* Retrospective *Sample:* 3,931 CVCs evaluated for three types of dressings: Tape and gauze, n = 1,374 Transparent, n = 880 Highly permeable transparent, n = 1,677 *Purpose:* To compare dressing type with CVC infection rates and staff satisfaction	Tape and gauze dressing changed every 48 hours Transparent dressing changed every 48 hours Highly permeable transparent dressing changed every 48 hours	The highly permeable transparent dressing resulted in a 25% decrease in catheter-related infections and an 88% staff satisfaction compared to 28% with the tape and gauze dressing.
	Tripepi-Bova et al., 1997	*Study Design:* Prospective *Sample:* 229 patients with peripheral IVs randomized into two groups: Gauze, n = 121 Transparent, n = 108 *Purpose:* To compare frequency of phlebitis, infiltration, and catheter dislodgment	Sterile gauze dressing Transparent polyurethane dressing	Frequency of catheter dislodgment was significantly higher with the gauze dressing. A trend toward lower frequencies of phlebitis and infiltration was noted with the transparent dressings.

(Continued on next page)

Table 21. Summary of Studies Related to Access Devices *(Continued)*

Issue Studied	Study	Study Design, Sample, Purpose	Intervention/Variables Examined	Findings
Cleansing agents	Birnbach et al., 2003	*Study Design:* Prospective *Sample:* 60 women requiring epidural analgesia *Purpose:* To evaluate the antisepsis with DuraPrep™ (3M Health Care) compared with povidone-iodine	Disinfection with DuraPrep Disinfection with povidone-iodine	A significant decrease was reported in the number of positive skin cultures, bacterial regrowths, and colonization of the epidural catheters with DuraPrep compared to povidone-iodine.
	Buchman et al., 2009	*Study Design:* Prospective *Sample:* In vitro model of hub contamination with *Staphylococcus aureus, Staphylococcus epidermidis, Pseudomonas aeruginosa,* and *Candida albicans* *Purpose:* To compare antimicrobial catheter cap, positive control caps, and negative control caps in reducing catheter-related infection	Saline infused through antimicrobial cap following hub contamination on days 1, 3, 5, and 7 Negative control caps not contaminated Positive control caps were contaminated and lacked cleaning solution. Effluent fluid collected from efferent end	Antimicrobial catheter significantly decreased likelihood of catheter-related infection in comparison to positive control caps.
	Debreceni et al., 2007	*Study Design:* Prospective *Sample:* 70 patients who received epidural analgesia *Purpose:* To compare the efficacy of conventional swab disinfection with spray disinfection prior to epidural catheterization	Disinfection with swabs containing 2-propanol and benzalkonium chloride Disinfection with spray of the same solution	No significant difference was observed in colonization rate of catheters following removal between the groups.
	Hibbard et al., 2002	*Study Design:* Randomized, parallel group *Sample:* Healthy subjects (N = 85) Abdominal sites cleansed with CHG (n = 43) plus IPA (n = 42) Inguinal sites cleansed with CHG plus IPA (n = 26), IPA (n = 28), or CHG (n = 20) *Purpose:* To compare the immediate and persistent antimicrobial effect of CHG plus IPA with IPA alone and CHG alone	Cleansing protocol: Skin microbial counts obtained prior to cleansing. Antiseptics applied for 30 seconds on abdomen and for 1 minute on the groin. Allowed to dry for 30 seconds on abdomen and 1 minute on groin. Outcome variables: Skin microbial counts and skin assessment at 10 minutes, 6 hours, and 24 hours after antiseptic application	No skin irritations were reported. CHG plus IPA showed significantly greater antimicrobial activity at 24 hours on the abdomen than IPA or CHG alone. No differences were found in the groin sites.

(Continued on next page)

Table 21. Summary of Studies Related to Access Devices *(Continued)*

Issue Studied	Study	Study Design, Sample, Purpose	Intervention/Variables Examined	Findings

Cleansing agents *(cont.)*	Jones, 1987	*Study Design:* Quasiexperimental
		Sample: 57 patients with hematologic cancers
		Purpose: To compare indwelling CVC infection rates in a shorter site care protocol than existing protocol
			Existing protocol:
			  2.5 minute Betadine® (Purdue Frederick) hand scrub by nurse
			  Masks worn by nurse and patient
			  Gloves worn by nurse
			  Cleansing with alcohol and iodine swabs six times
			Shorter protocol:
			  No time specification for hand scrub
			  Masks worn by nurse and patient
			  Gloves worn by nurse
			  Cleansing with alcohol and iodine swabs twice
			  Daily gauze dressing changed, heparin irrigation, and blood withdrawal for both groups
				Most patients were immunosuppressed.
				No significant differences in CVC-related infections existed between the groups.
				Major limitations of study:
				  Lack of randomization
				  Existing protocol sample consisted of patients with previously inserted catheters.
				  Shorter protocol sample consisted of patients who were going to have CVC inserted.
				  Small sample size

	Kasuda et al., 2002	*Study Design:* Randomized controlled trial
		Sample: Patients undergoing epidural catheter insertion with povidone-iodine cleanse (n = 28) or chlorhexidine ethanol cleanse (n = 34)
		Purpose: To determine the rate of catheter colonization associated with short-term epidural catheter placement using 0.5% chlorhexidine ethanol compared to 10% povidone-iodine
			Cleansing protocol:
			  Skin cleansed twice with either povidone-iodine or chlorhexidine ethanol before sterile drape is placed. No antibiotic or antiseptic ointment was applied. No dressing change until catheter was removed.
			Outcome variables:
			  Cultures
			  Gloves
			  Catheter tip
				Nine glove cultures found *Staphylococcus epidermidis* and micrococcus.
				Six catheter tip cultures found *S. epidermidis.*
				No difference found between the two groups.

	Kinirons et al., 2001	*Study Design:* Randomized controlled trial
		Sample: Pediatric patients requiring an epidural catheter cleansed with chlorhexidine (n = 52) or povidone-iodine (n = 44)
		Purpose: To compare 0.5% chlorhexidine and 10% povidone-iodine in decreasing catheter colonization associated with short-term epidural catheter placement
			Cleansing protocol:
			  Skin cleansed twice prior to application of sterile drape. No topical antibiotic or antiseptic was applied. No dressing change until catheter was removed.
			Outcome variables:
			  Catheter tip culture
				Chlorhexidine was found to reduce the risk of catheter colonization before epidural catheter insertion.

(Continued on next page)

Table 21. Summary of Studies Related to Access Devices *(Continued)*

Issue Studied	Study	Study Design, Sample, Purpose	Intervention/Variables Examined	Findings
Cleansing agents *(cont.)*	Mann et al., 2001	*Study Design:* Randomized controlled trial *Sample:* Women undergoing elective gynecologic surgery with epidural catheter placement *Dressing:* Biopatch® (Ethicon, Inc.) (n = 29) Control group with unknown type of dressing (n = 26) *Purpose:* To determine the efficacy of Biopatch, a chlorhexidine-impregnated dressing, in reducing the incidence of bacterial colonization at the exit site	Cleansing protocol: Biopatch placed on exit site and then covered with transparent dressing Outcome variables: Exit-site skin swab culture after catheter is removed	Biopatch was found to be effective in reducing rate of bacterial colonization.
	Menyhay & Maki, 2006	*Study Design:* Prospective *Sample:* 105 needleless Luer-activated valve connectors *Purpose:* To evaluate needleless catheter connector disinfection with 70% alcohol compared to antiseptic cap	All device septums contaminated with *Enterococcus faecalis* 15 devices not disinfected 30 devices disinfected with 70% alcohol 60 devices with antiseptic barrier cap threaded onto connector causing chlorhexidine-impregnated sponge to saturate surface	Antiseptic barrier cap significantly decreased microorganism entry in comparison to 70% alcohol.
	Menyhay & Maki, 2008	*Study Design:* Prospective *Sample:* 15 precontaminated positive control connectors not disinfected before entry 30 connectors disinfected with 70% alcohol 60 needle-free connectors disinfected with antiseptic barrier cap *Purpose:* In vitro study comparing effectiveness of standard disinfection of needleless Luer-activated valve connectors with 70% alcohol and effectiveness of an antiseptic barrier cap that sterilizes surface	Standard disinfection with 3–5 second swabbing using a sterile pledget of 70% IPA Antiseptic barrier cap that is threaded onto a Luer-adaptable needleless connector causing spike to rupture capsule containing 0.25 ml of 2% chlorhexidine gluconate (CHG) in 70% alcohol, saturating sponge	Antiseptic barrier significantly decreased transmission of microorganisms.
	Nikoletti et al., 1999	*Study Design:* Randomized controlled trial *Sample:* Patients requiring multilumen CVC (N = 132) *Purpose:* To determine the frequency of skin colonization, hub colonization, and CVC colonization in transparent hydrocolloid dressings compared to standard polyurethane dressings	Outcome variables: Cultures from skin insertion site, catheter hub, catheter tip, and blood samples	Skin and hub cultures found no significant difference in colonization. The hydrocolloid group had a significantly (p = 0.048) higher rate of catheter colonization than the polyurethane group. There was a significantly (p = 0.03) higher frequency of positive blood cultures in the polyurethane group.

(Continued on next page)

Table 21. Summary of Studies Related to Access Devices *(Continued)*

Issue Studied	Study	Study Design, Sample, Purpose	Intervention/Variables Examined	Findings
Cleansing agents *(cont.)*	Paice et al., 1999	*Study Design:* Experimental *Sample:* Five DuPen® (Bard Access Systems) epidural catheters *Purpose:* To determine whether three epidural catheter port cleansing techniques used to apply a povidone-iodine solution differed with respect to the introduction of this solution through the epidural catheter on insertion	Cleansing protocol: Five DuPen epidural catheters each were randomly cleansed twice in a laboratory setting with a 10% povidone-iodine swabstick, a pledget impregnated with 10% povidone-iodine, and a gauze pad saturated with 10% povidone-iodine. Each solution was used to clean the port for 10 seconds and allowed to dry for 30 seconds. After the port cleansing, water was injected, and the solution from the tip of the catheter was analyzed.	A statistically significant ($p = 0.02$) difference existed between the cleansing techniques, with the pledget yielding the lowest values of povidone-iodine contamination of the epidural catheter.
Flushing agents	Cesaro et al., 2009	*Study Design:* Prospective *Sample:* 203 pediatric patients with newly placed Broviac-Hickman CVCs *Purpose:* To compare standard flushing with heparin versus flushing with normal saline via a positive-pressure cap	Standard flushing with heparin solution Normal saline flushing via a positive pressure cap	Significantly higher incidence of occlusion ($p = 0.0002$) and bacteremia ($p = 0.01$) with normal saline flushing was reported. No difference was found in either the cause or frequency of premature removal of the CVCs.
	Del Cotillo et al., 2008	*Study Design:* Prospective *Sample:* 133 hospitalized patients with arterial catheters *Purpose:* To compare effectiveness of heparinized solution versus saline solution for the maintenance of arterial catheters and analyze changes in activated partial thromboplastin time and platelet count in samples taken from both groups	Flushing with heparinized solution (1 IU/ml) Flushing with saline solution Arterial catheter assessed every 8 hours for patency, reliability of arterial pressure, and curve quality Blood drawn from arterial catheter and from venous catheter with 7.5 ml discard	No difference was reported between heparin and saline flushing in maintaining arterial catheter. Heparin flush significantly ($p = 0.001$) altered activated partial thromboplastin time (aPTT).
	Hall et al., 2006	*Study Design:* Prospective *Sample:* 65 hospitalized patients with arterial catheters *Purpose:* To compare heparinized saline versus normal saline via a continuous flush device on platelet counts	30 arterial catheters with continuous normal saline flush 35 arterial catheters with 500 IU heparin flush	No significant difference in platelet counts reported.

(Continued on next page)

Table 21. Summary of Studies Related to Access Devices *(Continued)*

Issue Studied	Study	Study Design, Sample, Purpose	Intervention/Variables Examined	Findings

Flushing agents *(cont.)*	Kelly et al., 1992	*Study Design:* Descriptive (Prospective, 1989; Retrospective, 1987–1988)
		Sample: 82 patients with 89 catheter insertions receiving chemotherapy (various cancer types; several bone marrow transplants) via indwelling CVCs (87 double-lumen Raff® [Quinton Instrument] catheters, two Silastic® [Dow Corning] Cook® [Cook Co.] catheters)
		Purpose: To determine the rates of infection and alteration in patency in patients using the once weekly flushing protocol; to compare findings with those in the literature
			Protocol: Flushing technique with 5 ml of heparin 10 IU/ml weekly	Infection rate was 19.1% (comparable to range reported in literature for weekly flushing: 12%–30%). *Staphylococcus epidermis* was isolated in 10 of 17 infections; comparable to a review of 17 articles in a five-year period where *S. epidermis* was predominant.
				Six exit-site infections were reported:
				  3 *Staphylococcus* coagulase negative
				  2 *S. aureus* (1 followed by an infection with *S. epidermis*)
				  1 *Pseudomonas*
				Comparable to pathogens identified by authors of review of 17 articles
				Alterations in patency was 13.5%, requiring change in flushing protocol from weekly to every three days for 1–26 weeks (mean duration 4.2 weeks) until catheter dysfunction cleared. No lines removed due to patency dysfunction; no total line occlusions required use of streptokinase or urokinase. (Comparison to literature findings was not included in the study discussion.)

	Stephens et al., 1997	*Study Design:* Experimental
		Sample: 78 patients with cancer undergoing apheresis collection for peripheral blood stem cells
		Purpose: To examine the incidence of thrombotic occlusions in CVCs using heparin flush versus saline flush
			Flushing protocol:
			  Saline flush 10 ml
			  Heparin flush 5 ml (100 IU/ml of saline)
			Variables examined:
			  Apheresis flow rate
			  Urokinase use for thrombolysis
			  Radiographic evidence of catheter thrombosis
				No significant differences were found for any study variables between the two groups.

	Tuten & Gueldner, 1991	*Study Design:* Quasiexperimental, nonequivalent control group, post-test-only design
		Sample: 77 gynecologic and orthopedic surgery inpatients with 114 peripheral intermittent IV devices (PIIDs)
		Purpose: To determine if the patency of PIIDs can be maintained as effectively with sodium chloride as with dilute heparin and if fewer local complications occur with sodium chloride
			Flushing protocol:
			  Device flushed every eight hours and after medication administration using positive-pressure technique
			  1 ml 0.9% sodium chloride (experimental)
			  1 ml of 100 IU heparin in 1 ml 0.9% sodium chloride (control)
			Variables examined:
			  Demographics
			  Needle insertion date
			  PIID insertion date
			  Needle type and gauge
			  Reason for device
			  Frequency of use
			  Date and reason for discontinuation
				No site loss occurred due to coagulation in either group.
				Control group had two incidences of phlebitis; experimental group had none.
				Control group had five infiltrations; experimental group had two.

(Continued on next page)

Table 21. Summary of Studies Related to Access Devices *(Continued)*

Issue Studied	Study	Study Design, Sample, Purpose	Intervention/Variables Examined	Findings
Flushing agents *(cont.)*	Whitta et al., 2006	*Study Design:* Prospective *Sample:* 65 hospitalized patients with arterial catheters *Purpose:* To evaluate arterial lines for function and blood sampling with normal saline flush versus heparin flush	35 arterial catheters flushed with normal saline 30 arterial catheters flushed with heparinized saline (3 ml/hr continuous flush)	No significant difference between normal saline flush and heparinized flush was observed.
Catheter occlusion	Blaney et al., 2006	*Study Design:* Prospective *Sample:* 310 pediatric patients with occluded central vascular access devices (VADs) *Purpose:* To evaluate incidence of intracranial hemorrhage and efficacy of alteplase in restoration of catheter function with maximum of two doses (less than or equal to 2 mg per dose) of alteplase	Assessment of function conducted 30 and 120 minutes after each dose	No significant adverse events were reported. Cumulative rate of restoration of catheter function was 82.9%.
	Boraks et al., 1998	*Study Design:* Retrospective *Sample:* Patients with anticoagulation (n = 108) Patients without anticoagulation (n = 115) All patients had hematologic malignancies. *Purpose:* To evaluate the use of anticoagulation therapy to prevent CVC thrombosis	Protocol: Patients given warfarin 1 mg/day at time of catheter insertion Outcome variables: Catheter thrombosis	Significant reduction (p = 0.03) in catheter thrombosis in patients given warfarin. Five percent of those receiving warfarin developed thrombosis compared to 13% who did not receive anticoagulants.
	Bowers et al., 2008	*Study Design:* Prospective *Sample:* 102 patients with single-lumen PICCs with positive-pressure Luer-activated devices *Purpose:* To compare normal saline flush and heparinized saline flush for their effect on occlusion rates	50 PICCs flushed with normal saline 52 PICCs flushed with heparinized saline	No significant difference in occlusion rates was observed.
	Carr & Rabinowitz, 2000	*Study Design:* Retrospective *Sample:* Chart review prior to physician education (n = 39) Chart review after physician education (n = 35) Chart review after physician-independent protocol (n = 43) *Purpose:* To assess compliance rate of prophylactic low-dose warfarin prescription in patients with cancer with a CVC	Physician-independent protocol: Nurse practitioner assigned to warfarin prescribing at time of catheter insertion Outcome variables: Compliance rate Catheter-related thrombosis	Prior to physician education, 10% of patients were prescribed warfarin. After physician education, 20% of patients were prescribed warfarin. After physician-independent protocol, 95% of patients were prescribed warfarin. Thrombotic complications occurred in 11% of patients on prophylactic anticoagulation compared to 21% not on anticoagulation therapy.

(Continued on next page)

Table 21. Summary of Studies Related to Access Devices (Continued)

Issue Studied	Study	Study Design, Sample, Purpose	Intervention/Variables Examined	Findings
Catheter occlusion (cont.)	Davis et al., 2000	*Study Design:* Prospective *Sample:* Pediatric and adult patients (N = 58) *Purpose:* To assess dosage and efficacy of alteplase for clearing CVC access occlusions	Protocol: Alteplase 0.5 mg with dose escalation to 1 and 2 mg sequentially until catheter clearance Outcome variables: Catheter patency Bleeding episodes	Fifty (86%) catheters were cleared with alteplase 0.5 mg. Five (8.6%) were cleared with 1 mg. One (1.7%) was cleared with 2 mg. Two (3.4%) catheter failures occurred. No bleeding episodes related to alteplase administration were reported.
	Harter et al., 2002	*Study Design:* Prospective *Sample:* Silver sulfadiazine-coated catheter (n = 120), standard catheter (n = 113) *Purpose:* To assess a silver sulfadiazine-coated CVC for risk of catheter-related thrombosis	Outcome variables: Catheter thrombosis	No difference was found in catheter thrombosis in silver sulfadiazine-coated and standard CVCs.
	Heath & Jones, 2001	*Study Design:* Prospective *Sample:* 102 catheters with elastomeric continuous infusion device, 89 catheters with saline, administration of medication, saline, heparin (SASH) procedure *Purpose:* To evaluate the elastomeric continuous infusion device	Protocol: Elastomeric device attached to existing infusion device: Continuous infusion of 0.9% sodium chloride at rate of 0.5 ml/hr SASH procedure outcome variables: Incidence of occlusions Number of device restarts secondary to occlusion Nursing time Patient costs	A 50% reduction occurred in catheter patency loss, and a 53% reduction occurred in patient charges with continuous infusion device. Decrease in nursing time for catheter maintenance was observed.
	Horne et al., 2006	*Study Design:* Prospective *Sample:* 49 adult patients undergoing BMT for hematologic malignancies or metastatic solid tumors *Purpose:* To evaluate efficacy of lepirudin flushes in comparison to heparinized saline flushes to prevent withdrawal occlusion of central venous access devices	24 patients received heparin 100 IU/ml per catheter lumen at least once per day 25 patients received lepirudin 100 mcg/ml per catheter lumen at least once per day	No difference was found between lepirudin and heparin flushes.
	Liu et al., 2004	*Study Design:* Prospective *Sample:* 139 patients with cancer with CVC occlusion *Purpose:* To evaluate efficacy and safety of reteplase for CVC occlusion	Reteplase 0.4 IU instilled into each catheter lumen with dwell time of 30 minutes and additional dwell time of 30 minutes if no function. Second dose repeated at 60 minutes after the first dose if catheter occlusion persisted.	First attempt success rate after 30 minute dwell time was 66.9%. The cumulative success rates at 60, 90, and 120 minutes were 88.5%, 94.7%, and 94.7%, respectively.
	Magagnoli et al., 2006	*Study Design:* Retrospective *Sample:* 228 patients with CVC treated with high-dose chemotherapy *Purpose:* To evaluate efficacy and safety of minidose warfarin	Prophylactic oral warfarin of 1 mg/day starting on the day of CVC insertion	Four thrombotic events were reported with three occurrences directly related to the catheter and one deep saphenous-vein thrombosis.

(Continued on next page)

Table 21. Summary of Studies Related to Access Devices (Continued)

Issue Studied	Study	Study Design, Sample, Purpose	Intervention/Variables Examined	Findings
Catheter occlusion (cont.)	Minassian et al., 2000	*Study Design:* Retrospective *Sample:* Gynecologic patients (N = 268) Indwelling catheters: Infuse-A-Port® (AngioDynamics, Inc.) (n = 162) Peripheral access (n = 75) Hickman (n = 68) *Purpose:* To evaluate the safety of three different long-term indwelling catheters	Outcome variables: Catheter thrombosis	Infuse-A-Ports and peripheral access ports had a lower risk of infection and longer catheter duration than Hickman catheters. Patients were significantly (p = 0.004) less likely to develop thrombosis when receiving prophylactic anticoagulation therapy.
	Ng et al., 2004	*Study Design:* Prospective *Sample:* 240 patients with single- or double-lumen peripherally inserted central catheters (PICCs) *Purpose:* To evaluate safety and efficacy of alteplase treatment	Alteplase (2 mg/2 ml) instilled and catheter assessed at 30 and 120 minutes Second dose instilled if catheter occlusion persisted	No significant adverse events were reported. Cumulative rate of restoration of catheter function was 92.9%.
	Schilling et al., 2006	*Study Design:* Prospective *Sample:* CVC lumens capped with one of three needleless connector devices with a four-group design *Purpose:* To evaluate efficacy of single-valve or positive-pressure valve needleless connector device to reduce CVC occlusion rates in comparison to standard device	Group 1: Lumens capped with a standard device Group 2: Single-valve device Group 3: Positive-pressure valve device flushed with heparinized saline Group 4: Positive-pressure valve device flushed with saline	CVCs capped with a single-valve or positive-pressure valve needleless connector device has lower catheter occlusion rates than those capped with a standard device. No difference was found between heparinized flush and saline flush; however, a trend occurred toward lower infection rates with the use of heparinized saline.
	Timoney et al., 2002	*Study Design:* Prospective *Sample:* Attempted catheter clearances (N = 168) in patients with transcutaneous, SC, or peripheral indwelling central catheters (n = 121) *Purpose:* To determine the safety and efficacy of cryopreserved solutions of the thrombolytic agent alteplase for occluded central VADs	Protocol: Alteplase 1 mg/ml prepared in 2.5 ml aliquots and stored at –20°C Alteplase solution instilled and allowed to dwell for 30 minutes. Aspiration attempts every 30 minutes until catheter is cleared. Aspiration of 4–5 ml to remove alteplase and residual clot. Outcome variables: Catheter clearance	Successful clearance of 136 catheters (81%) of the 168 catheter clearance attempts were reported.
	Verso et al., 2005	*Study Design:* Prospective *Sample:* 385 patients with CVCs *Purpose:* To evaluate efficacy of enoxaparin in prevention of venous thromboembolism	Enoxaparin 40 mg every day subcutaneously (SC) starting two hours before CVC insertion lasting for six weeks Placebo	No difference was found in the rate of CVC-related venous thromboembolism.

(Continued on next page)

Table 21. Summary of Studies Related to Access Devices *(Continued)*

Issue Studied	Study	Study Design, Sample, Purpose	Intervention/Variables Examined	Findings
Catheter occlusion *(cont.)*	Verso et al., 2008	*Study Design:* Prospective *Sample:* 310 patients with CVCs *Purpose:* To identify the risk factors for CVC-related thrombosis in patients included in a randomized, double-blind, placebo-controlled study aimed at assessing the efficacy and safety of enoxaparin for the prophylaxis of CVC-related thrombosis	Study was only done to identify risk factors.	Incidence of CVC-related thrombosis was 16.1%. Risk factors for thrombosis were presence of distant metastases, CVC tip misplaced in the upper half of superior vena cava, left-sided CVC insertion, and chest radiotherapy.

Infection	Aufwerber et al., 1991	*Study Design:* Retrospective examination of bacteriologic data for all patients with a CVC-tip culture
		Sample: 542 CVC tips obtained from 453 patients
		Catheter types:
		Subclavian, jugular, or femoral
		Port-A-Cath® (SIMS Deltec, Inc.)
		Swan-Ganz catheter
		Purpose: Comparison of semi-quantitative cultures (SQCs) with blood cultures to detect or predict infection associated with CVC
			CVC catheter removed and tip sent to laboratory for culture
			Peripheral blood cultures drawn using an SQC solid agar technique
			When catheter tip cultures found, patient data examined for blood cultures drawn 14 days before and after catheter removal
				Thirty-two percent of tips were positive for bacterial growth.
				Catheter infection discovered in 137 of 174 positive cultures.
				Blood culture results available in 93/174 catheter tip culture episodes, of which 30 proved positive.
				Seventeen catheter-associated bacteremias occurred.
				Sixty-eight percent of tips were positive for bacterial growth.
				Blood cultures were drawn in 121 of these cases, of which 29 were positive (14 considered contaminated).
				Positive predictive value:
				    Bacteremia of growth on catheter tip (32%)
				    Catheter infection (36%)
				    Catheter-associated bacteremia (18%)
				    Absence of bacteremia of a negative culture (76%)
				    Negative SQC (77%)
				Conclusion: SQC techniques yield low predictive values for bacteremias; therefore, quantitative cultures drawn through the line may be more effective.

	Bonawitz et al., 1991	*Study Design:* Randomization of surgical intensive care patients with subclavian CVCs into four groups
		Purpose: To evaluate routine catheter changes and implantable collagen cuff in reducing catheter-related infections in critically ill patients
			Four groups:
			Group 1: Collagen cuff, catheter changed every three days
			Group 2: Collagen cuff, catheter changed every seven days
			Group 3: No cuff, catheter changed every three days
			Group 4: No cuff, catheter changed every seven days
			Outcome variables:
			    Culture tip cultures
			    Exit-site skin cultures
			    Peripheral blood cultures
			    Fever
			    Tachycardia
			    Leukocytosis
				No statistically significant differences in catheter colonization or catheter infection rates were observed between three-day and seven-day catheter changes or between cuff or no cuff.

(Continued on next page)

Table 21. Summary of Studies Related to Access Devices *(Continued)*

Issue Studied	Study	Study Design, Sample, Purpose	Intervention/Variables Examined	Findings
Infection *(cont.)*	Carratala et al., 1999	*Study Design:* Randomization of patients with hematologic malignancies *Sample:* 117 patients with nontunneled multilumen CVCs undergoing chemotherapy *Purpose:* To determine the efficacy of an antibiotic-lock technique in preventing endoluminal catheter-related infection with gram-positive bacteria in patients with neutropenia	Two groups: Group 1: Heparin 10 IU/ml instilled in catheter lumen and allowed to dwell for one hour every two days Group 2: Heparin 10 IU/ml and vancomycin 25 mg/ml instilled in catheter lumen and allowed to dwell for one hour every two days Outcome variables: Catheter hub cultures Catheter-related bacteremia	Catheter-related bacteremia was found in four (7%) patients receiving heparin compared to none in patients receiving heparin and vancomycin. Patients receiving heparin and vancomycin had significantly longer time to catheter hub colonization (p = 0.004) and catheter-related bacteremia (p = 0.06) than patients with heparin only.
	Cook et al., 1997	*Study Design:* Systematic literature review *Sample:* Randomized trials of catheter replacement over a guidewire or at a new site (N = 12). *Purpose:* To evaluate the effect of guidewire exchange and use new site replacement strategies on the frequency of catheter colonization, infection, catheter-related bacteremia, and mechanical complications	Literature review on guidewire exchange and new site replacement From a pool of 151 randomized controlled trials on CVC management, 12 relevant randomized trials of catheter replacement over a guidewire or at a new site were identified.	As compared to new site replacement, guidewire exchange is associated with a trend toward higher rates of catheter colonization, exit-site infection, and bacteremia and lower rates of mechanical complications.
	Darouiche et al., 1999	*Study Design:* Randomized controlled trial *Sample:* Patients with CVCs with dwell time greater than three days (N = 865) *Purpose:* To determine the use of CVCs impregnated with minocycline and rifampin and chlorhexidine and silver sulfadiazine in reducing rates of catheter-related BSI and colonization in comparison to nonimpregnated catheters	Catheter tips and SC segments cultured after catheter removal Blood cultures obtained when clinically indicated	CVCs impregnated with minocycline and rifampin had a lower rate of catheter colonization and BSI compared to chlorhexidine and silver sulfadiazine.
	Douard et al., 1999	*Study Design:* Prospective *Sample:* Examination of 170 removed venous access ports (VAPs) for confirmed or suspected related infections *Purpose:* To analyze the relationship between the septum deposits and the occurrence of VAP-related infections	Paired quantitative blood cultures: Peripheral specimen Port specimen Catheter tip cultures VAP septum cultures	Paired quantitative blood cultures were 77% sensitive and 100% specific and had a positive predictive value of 100% for diagnosing VAP-related infections. Septum culture was 93.3% sensitive with a 46% sensitivity for tip culture.
	Fraenkel et al., 2006	*Study Design:* Prospective *Sample:* 646 CVC insertions *Purpose:* To compare infection rates of silver-platinum-carbon–impregnated catheters with rifampicin-minocycline–coated catheters	327 silver-platinum-carbon–impregnated catheters 319 rifampicin-minocycline–coated catheters	Rifampicin-minocycline–coated catheters had a lower colonization rate in comparison to silver-platinum-carbon–impregnated catheters.

(Continued on next page)

Table 21. Summary of Studies Related to Access Devices *(Continued)*

Issue Studied	Study	Study Design, Sample, Purpose	Intervention/Variables Examined	Findings
Infection *(cont.)*	Goetz et al., 1998	*Study Design:* Prospective *Sample:* CVCs (N = 300), patients (N = 204) *Purpose:* To determine the influence of catheter type and site on infection rates	Outcome variables: Clinical infection Catheter contamination	Seventy percent of the catheters were inserted in upper body sites, and 30% were inserted in the femoral vein. Forty-five percent were triple-lumen catheters. Bacteremia occurred in 2.7% of the insertions. Catheter contamination was associated with the femoral site.
	Heard et al., 1998	*Study Design:* Randomized, controlled trial *Sample:* Patients requiring CVC randomized to one of two groups Group A: Uncoated triple-lumen catheter (n = 157) Group B: Catheter coated with chlorhexidine and silver sulfadiazine (n = 151) *Purpose:* To evaluate the efficacy of triple-lumen CVCs coated with chlorhexidine and silver sulfadiazine to reduce the incidence of catheter-related infection and catheter-related bacteremia	Catheters were removed when no longer needed or with suspected infection. Tip and 5 cm segment of the catheter were cultured. Blood cultures obtained when clinically indicated. The remaining segments of coated catheters were incubated on an agar plate with *Staphylococcus aureus* and enterococcus.	Coated catheters reduced the incidence of significant bacterial growth on the tip and intradermal segment of the catheter but had no effect on the incidence of catheter-related infections.
	Homer & Holmes, 1998	*Study Design:* Retrospective	Outcome variables: IV start date Termination date and reason Number of restarts	The probability of a complication was lowest in first 24 hours, increased slightly in 24–48 hours, and decreased in 48–96 hours. The restarted catheter had a significantly (p = 0.02) higher risk of complications in the first 24 hours than the initial catheter.
	Jaeger et al., 2001	*Study Design:* Prospective, randomized trial evaluating benzalkonium chloride–impregnated CVC to prevent catheter-related infection in patients undergoing chemotherapy *Patients:* Acute leukemia (n = 28) Lymphoma (n = 17) Solid tumors (n = 5) *Sample:* Antiseptic-impregnated catheter (n = 25) Standard triple-lumen catheter (n = 25) *Purpose:* To compare the incidence of catheter-related colonization and catheter-related bacteremia with benzalkonium chloride-impregnated CVC with standard triple-lumen CVC	Catheter colonization Catheter-related bacteremia	Catheter-related colonization was proven in four (16%) cases, and catheter-related bacteremia was proven in one (4%) case in both groups. No significant differences were found between the study group and the control group.

(Continued on next page)

Table 21. Summary of Studies Related to Access Devices *(Continued)*

Issue Studied	Study	Study Design, Sample, Purpose	Intervention/Variables Examined	Findings
Infection *(cont.)*	Kalfon et al., 2007	*Study Design:* Prospective *Sample:* 577 patients with 617 multilumen CVCs *Purpose:* Comparison of silver-impregnated and standard multilumen CVCs	320 silver-impregnated multilumen CVCs 297 standard multilumen CVCs	No difference was found in rate of colonization between silver-impregnated and standard multilumen CVCs.
	Khare et al., 2007	*Study Design:* Prospective *Sample:* 246 CVC insertions *Purpose:* To evaluate the effect of a silver zeolite-impregnated catheter on catheter-related colonization and infection	122 silver-impregnated CVCs 124 nonimpregnated CVCs	Colonization rate was significantly ($p < 0.025$) lower in the silver zeolite-impregnated CVC tips compared with the control CVC tips.

	Longuet et al., 2001	*Study Design:* Experimental
		Sample: 12 HIV-positive and 8 patients with cancer with VAP-related bacteremia
		Purpose: To describe the rate of response to an antibiotic-lock technique in the treatment of VAP-related bacteremia and to analyze the role of the reservoir in the persistence of infection
			Blood cultures:
			  Peripheral vein
			  Catheter blood draw
			Catheter culture:
			  Tip
			  Reservoir
				Response to the antibiotic lock technique revealed 31% cured, 12.5% cured but had recurrent infection with another microorganism, and 56% had persistent positive blood and catheter cultures. Authors concluded that the limited efficacy of the antibiotic-lock technique could be explained by the presence of fibrin deposits that have bacteria clusters inside the port reservoir.

	Martinez et al., 1999	*Study Design:* Prospective *Sample:* Adult patients undergoing BMT or intensive chemotherapy with positive blood cultures after two days of antimicrobial therapy (N = 19) *Purpose:* To evaluate the safety and efficacy of CVC exchange by guidewire after unsuccessful antimicrobial therapy	Blood cultures: Catheter tip culture	Clinical symptoms of sepsis resolved in less than 24 hours in all cases.
	Moss et al., 2000	*Study Design:* Prospective *Sample:* Triple-lumen CVCs: Coated with benzalkonium chloride (n = 117) Polyurethane nonantiseptic (n = 118) *Purpose:* To evaluate incidence of catheter-associated colonization with benzalkonium chloride compared to nonantiseptic catheter	Outcome variables: Microbial colonization	Benzalkonium chloride catheter significantly ($p = 0.0016$) reduced incidence of catheter-associated colonization.
	Osma et al., 2006	*Study Design:* Prospective *Sample:* 133 patients requiring central venous catheterization *Purpose:* To evaluate the impact of CVCs impregnated with chlorhexidine and silver sulfadiazine on the incidence of colonization and catheter-related BSIs	64 antiseptic-impregnated triple-lumen catheters 69 standard triple-lumen catheters	No difference was found in rate of catheter colonization or catheter-related BSI between antiseptic-impregnated catheters and standard catheters.

(Continued on next page)

Table 21. Summary of Studies Related to Access Devices *(Continued)*

Issue Studied	Study	Study Design, Sample, Purpose	Intervention/Variables Examined	Findings
Infection *(cont.)*	Raad & Bodey, 1992	*Study Design:* Retrospective surveillance of indwelling CVC sepsis *Sample:* 70 patients with catheter-related coagulase-staphylococcal bacteremia	Peripheral blood Culture for coagulase-staphylococci CVC tip culture CVC blood cultures	Patients were successfully treated with antibiotics without removal of CVC. An 11% mortality rate existed irrespective of catheter removal. A 20% bacteremia recurrence rate existed, compared to 3% of those removed.
	Rubin et al., 1999	*Study Design:* Prospective *Sample:* 43 port-related infections in pediatric patients with hematologic cancer *Purpose:* To determine the efficacy of antibiotic treatment of catheter-related infections without port removal	IV antibiotics given through the port for a median of 11 days. Outcome variables: Blood cultures immediately afterward and 30 days post-treatment	Seventy-eight percent cure rate occurred with two of four relapses cured with a second course of antibiotics.
	Safdar & Maki, 2005	*Study Design:* Prospective *Sample:* 115 hospitalized patients with 251 PICCs placed *Purpose:* To determine the risk of PICC-related BSI	Incidence of BSI	PICCs used in high-risk hospitalized patients are associated with a rate of catheter-related BSI similar to conventional CVCs placed in the internal jugular or subclavian veins.
	Smith et al., 2008	*Study Design:* Retrospective *Sample:* Cases of catheter-associated BSIs in PICCs in infants *Purpose:* To evaluate risk of bloodstream infection associated with PICC dwell time in infants	1,540 PICCs placed over 27-month period	No increased risk of catheter-associated BSI was observed with increased catheter dwell time.
	Veenstra et al., 1999	*Study Design:* Meta-analysis Randomized trials from 1966–1998 comparing chlorhexidine-silver sulfadiazine–impregnated CVCs with nonimpregnated catheters *Sample:* Catheter colonization (N = 2,611); catheter-related BSI (N = 2,603) *Purpose:* To evaluate the efficacy of chlorhexidine-silver sulfadiazine–impregnated CVCs in the prevention of catheter-related BSIs	Catheter colonization Catheter-related BSIs	CVCs impregnated with chlorhexidine and silver sulfadiazine appeared to reduce the incidence of catheter colonization and catheter-related BSIs in patients at high risk for catheter-related infections.
	Yucel et al., 2004	*Study Design:* Prospective *Sample:* 223 patients with CVCs *Purpose:* Comparison of miconazole-rifampicin–modified CVCs and standard triple-lumen CVCs in reducing catheter colonization and infection	118 miconazole-rifampicin CVCs 105 standard CVCs	Significantly lower risk was reported for catheter colonization (p < 0.001) and catheter-related infections (p = 0.002) with miconazole-rifampicin–modified CVCs in comparison to standard triple-lumen CVCs.

(Continued on next page)

Table 21. Summary of Studies Related to Access Devices *(Continued)*

Issue Studied	Study	Study Design, Sample, Purpose	Intervention/Variables Examined	Findings
Chlorhexidine-impregnated sponges/dressings	Garland et al., 2001	*Study Design:* Prospective *Sample:* 705 neonates with CVCs *Purpose:* To compare povidone-iodine dressing with CHG-impregnated dressing for prevention of CVC-related infections	355 chlorhexidine dressings replaced weekly 370 skin disinfection with povidone-iodine, redressing the site every 3–7 days	No difference in efficacy was reported in preventing catheter-related BSIs among the dressing protocols.
	Levy et al., 2005	*Study Design:* Prospective *Sample:* 145 pediatric patients with CVCs *Purpose:* To compare chlorhexidine-impregnated dressing versus transparent polyurethane dressing for the reduction of CVC colonization and CVC-associated BSI	71 patients with transparent polyurethane dressing 74 patients with chlorhexidine-impregnated dressing	The chlorhexidine-impregnated dressing significantly ($p = 0.0446$) reduced the rate of CVC colonization.
	Ruschulte et al., 2009	*Study Design:* Prospective *Sample:* 601 patients with CVCs admitted for chemotherapy *Purpose:* To compare chlorhexidine-impregnated dressing versus sterile dressing for the reduction of CVC-related infections	301 patients with sterile dressings 300 patients with chlorhexidine-impregnated dressings	Chlorhexidine-impregnated dressings significantly ($p = 0.016$) reduced the incidence of CVC-related infections.
	Timsit et al., 2009	*Study Design:* Prospective *Sample:* 1,636 patients with CVCs *Purpose:* To compare chlorhexidine-impregnated dressing versus standard dressing for the reduction of CVC infections	Chlorhexidine-impregnated dressing Standard dressing	Chlorhexidine-impregnated dressings significantly ($p = 0.03$) reduced the risk of catheter-related infection.
Catheter insertion site	Biffi et al., 2009	*Study Design:* Prospective *Sample:* 401 patients with CVCs *Purpose:* To compare central venous insertion sites and risk of catheter-related infection	132 internal jugular 136 subclavian vein 133 cephalic vein	No significant difference was observed in risk of catheter-related infections between insertion sites.
Needleless access devices	Do et al., 1999	*Study Design:* Case-control, prospective cohort *Sample:* Case patients with CVC or midline catheter (N = 53) Study period IV catheter days (98,483) *Purpose:* To evaluate the infection control practices and BSIs associated with the use of needleless devices	Needleless device end caps were cleansed with alcohol before flushing and administering IV medications. End cap changed from once per week to once every two days. Outcome variables: BSIs Risk factors for BSIs	Risk factors for BSI included lower education level, younger age, having a CVC with multiple ports, or having a tunneled CVC. Patients with a tunneled CVC who were allowed to shower at home had an increased risk of BSI. Changing the needleless device end cap every two days in comparison to once weekly decreased the BSI rate.
	McDonald et al., 1998	*Study Design:* Retrospective, case control *Sample:* Pediatric patients in three intensive care units with BSI (N = 8) *Purpose:* To determine risk factors for BSIs and use of needleless access devices	Outcome variables: BSIs Needleless access device replacement protocol	An increased risk of BSI was associated with intermittent IV therapy and needleless device replacement every six days. Decreased risk of BSI associated with replacement of entire device, valve, and end cap every 24 hours.

(Continued on next page)

Table 21. Summary of Studies Related to Access Devices *(Continued)*

Issue Studied	Study	Study Design, Sample, Purpose	Intervention/Variables Examined	Findings
Needle-less access devices *(cont.)*	Salgado et al., 2007	*Study Design:* Retrospective *Sample:* Needleless split-septum device and needleless mechanical valve device *Purpose:* To analyze catheter-related BSIs with needleless split-septum devices and needleless mechanical valve device	Needleless split-septum device (n = 83) Needleless mechanical valve device (n = 62)	A significant (p < 0.001) increase was reported in catheter-related BSIs with needleless mechanical valve device.
	Seymour et al., 2000	*Study Design:* Prospective *Sample:* CVC connector: Needleless (n = 105) Conventional (n = 132) *Purpose:* To evaluate the microbial contamination of a needleless connector compared to a conventional connector	Outcome variables: Microbial contamination of connectors after removal of CVC	No significant difference was found of microbial contamination in needleless connectors compared to conventional connectors.
Blood sampling	Barton et al., 2004	*Study Design:* Prospective *Sample:* 28 pediatric patients with CVCs *Purpose:* To compare push-pull method and discard method in blood sampling CVCs	438 pairs of blood samples	No significant difference in blood sample results was reported.
	Chatziniko-laou et al., 2006	*Study Design:* Prospective *Sample:* 165 quantitative blood cultures collected through CVCs *Purpose:* Evaluation of quantitative blood cultures collected from CVCs in differentiating between contamination and BSI	–	Quantitative cultures from CVCs were found to be highly sensitive, specific, and predictive of bacteremia.
	Cosca et al., 1998	*Study Design:* Pretest/post-test *Sample:* Adult patients with cancer (N = 50) *Purpose:* To determine the presence of clots in the 10 ml blood discard from VADs prior to blood sampling and the presence of clots formed in the discarded blood specimen during the five-minute dwell time while obtaining blood samples	Sampling protocol: Two 5 ml discard samples drawn in separate syringes Syringe #1 filtered Syringe #2 filtered after five-minute dwell time Outcome variables: Presence of clots	50% of syringe #1 had clots present. 4% of syringe #2 had clots present. Reinfusion of discard blood from VADs not recommended.
	Hinds et al., 2002	*Study Design:* Descriptive comparative *Sample:* Pediatric patients with tunneled VADs (N = 53) *Purpose:* To compare prothrombin time (PT), aPTT, and fibrinogen results collected from heparinized tunneled VADs and venipuncture	Sampling protocol: Blood collected from catheter within seconds of venipuncture collection. Blood (3 ml) discarded from catheter, then three sequential samples of 3 ml each Outcome variables: PT aPTT Fibrinogen 6 ml, 9 ml, and 12 ml; discard samples	A significant difference (sample 1: p = 0.0001; sample 2: p = 0.0001; sample 3: p = 0.0008) was found in results of PT, aPTT, and fibrinogen from heparinized VAD and venipuncture samples.

(Continued on next page)

Table 21. Summary of Studies Related to Access Devices *(Continued)*

Issue Studied	Study	Study Design, Sample, Purpose	Intervention/Variables Examined	Findings
Blood sampling *(cont.)*	Holmes, 1998	*Study Design:* Prospective *Sample:* Patients with CVCs requiring complete blood count and chemistry profile samples (N = 25) *Purpose:* To compare the push-pull method versus the discard method of obtaining blood samples from CVCs	Sampling methods: Push-pull: Catheter flushed with 5 ml 0.09% sodium chloride in 10 ml syringe. Without removal of syringe, 6 ml of blood aspirated and pushed back into catheter. Process repeated three times. Empty syringe removed and blood collection conducted. Catheter then flushed with 20 ml of 0.09% sodium chloride. Discard: Catheter flushed with 5 ml 0.09% sodium chloride in 10 ml syringe. Blood (6 ml) aspirated and discarded. Blood collection conducted and catheter flushed with 20 ml of 0.09% sodium chloride.	Similar laboratory blood results were found with both collection methods.
	Rondina et al., 2007	*Study Design:* Prospective *Sample:* 41 patients with PICCs *Purpose:* To compare aPTTs measured from blood drawn from PICCs and from peripheral vein	41 blood samples from PICCs 41 blood samples from peripheral vein	No significant difference in aPTT results was found.
Power injection of contrast media	Coyle et al., 2004	*Study Design:* Prospective *Sample:* 110 PICCs *Purpose:* To evaluate patient safety, catheter rupture rates, and computed tomography (CT) quality with power injection of CT contrast media through PICCs	Single-lumen and double-lumen PICCs in vivo with injection rates ranging from 1–4 ml/s	Contrast media was safely injected at a rate of 2 ml/s with satisfactory image quality.
	Herts et al., 2001	*Study Design:* Prospective, randomized trial *Sample:* Patients receiving CT exams with contrast media through CVC (n = 174) or peripheral IV (n = 51) *Purpose:* To evaluate the feasibility, safety, and efficacy of power injecting contrast media through a CVC	Outcome variables: Feasibility: Successful injection of contrast media through randomized access route Safety: Reported complications Efficacy: Comparison of enhancement of thoracic aorta, pulmonary artery, abdominal aorta, and liver	No statistical difference was found in complications between the CVC and peripheral IV access. Enhancement was greater in the thoracic aorta, pulmonary artery, and liver for the peripheral IV access group.
	Sanelli et al., 2004	*Study Design:* Prospective *Sample:* 104 in vivo cases *Purpose:* To determine safety and feasibility of using a CVC for rapid contrast injections	Rapid contrast injections, 3–5 ml/s in 104 cases with 7 French (Fr) Arrow-Howes™ (Teleflex Inc.) multilumen CVCs	No immediate or early patient or catheter complications were observed.

(Continued on next page)

Table 21. Summary of Studies Related to Access Devices *(Continued)*

Issue Studied	Study	Study Design, Sample, Purpose	Intervention/Variables Examined	Findings
Power injection of contrast media *(cont.)*	Williamson & McKinney, 2001	*Study Design:* Descriptive *Sample:* 50 silicone PICCs in three single-lumen sizes (3–5 Fr) and two double-lumen sizes (6 Fr and 7 Fr) and two lengths: 35 and 45 cm *Purpose:* To determine the tolerance of silicone PICCs to power injection of contrast media	Protocol: Uniform volume of 74% ioversol injected at increasing rates by power injector Outcome variables: 　Flow rate 　Volume 　Peak pressure	The 3 Fr catheters were not adequate. The 4 Fr single-lumen and 6 Fr double-lumen catheters were marginal for CT studies. The 5 Fr single-lumen and 7 Fr double-lumen catheters tolerated power injection adequate for CT studies. For each catheter, 35 cm length withstood higher flow rates than 45 cm length.
Suturing	Middleton, 2006	*Study Design:* Prospective *Sample:* 80 patients requiring sutures *Purpose:* To evaluate efficacy of advanced clinical nurses suturing skin lacerations	Nurses completed a standardized training program in wound management and repair.	No wound healing complications were reported.

REFERENCES

Adlard, K. (2008). Examining the push-pull method of blood sampling from central venous access devices. *Journal of Pediatric Oncology Nursing, 25,* 200–207. doi:10.1177/1043454208320975

Agency for Health Care Policy and Research. (1994, January). External and implantable infusion pumps [AHCPR Pub. No. 94-0013]. Retrieved from http://www.ncbi.nlm.nih.gov/bookshelf/br.fcgi?book=hs archive&part=A43810

Ahmed, F., Salhab, K., Stergiopoulos, K., Seifert, F., & Baram, D. (2009). Intramural hematoma of the aorta: Delayed pericardial tamponade. *Thoracic and Cardiovascular Surgeon, 57,* 112–114. doi:10 .1055/s-2008-1038846

Aiello-Laws, L., & Rutledge, D.N. (2008). Management of adult patients receiving intraventricular chemotherapy for the treatment of leptomeningeal metastasis. *Clinical Journal of Oncology Nursing, 12,* 429–435. doi:10.1188/08.CJON.429-435

Aitken, D.R., & Minton, J.P. (1984). The "pinch-off sign": A warning of impending problems with permanent subclavian catheters. *American Journal of Surgery, 148,* 633–636.

Akl, E.A., Kamath, G., Yosuico, V., Kim, S.Y., Barba, M., Sperati, F., ... Schunemann, H.J. (2008). Thromboprophylaxis for patients with cancer and central venous catheters: A systematic review and a meta-analysis. *Cancer, 112,* 2483–2492. doi:10.1002/cncr.23479

Akl, E.A., Yosuico, V.E.D., Kim, S.Y., Barba, M., Sperati, F., Cook, D., ... Kamath, G. (2007). Anticoagulation for thrombosis prophylaxis in cancer patients with central venous catheters. *Cochrane Database of Systematic Reviews* 2007, Issue 3. Art. No.: CD006468. doi: 10.1002/14651858.CD006468.pub2

AlHayki, M., Hopkins, L., & Le, T. (2006). Intraperitoneal chemotherapy for epithelial ovarian cancer. *Obstetrical and Gynecological Survey, 61,* 529–534. doi:10.1097/01.ogx.0000228777.15365.32

Almadrones, L. (2007). Patient safety and intraperitoneal therapy. *Journal of Gynecologic Oncology Nursing, 17,* 6–7.

Anderson, N.R. (2004). Midline catheters: The middle ground of intravenous therapy administration. *Journal of Infusion Nursing, 27,* 313–321. doi:10.1097/00129804-200409000-00005

Anderson, S.L., & Shreve, S.T. (2004). Continuous subcutaneous infusion of opiates at end-of-life. *Annals of Pharmacotherapy, 38,* 1015–1023. doi:10.1345/aph.1D395

AngioDynamics. (2009). Vortex® ports (LP, MP, TR & VX). Retrieved from http://www.angiodynamics.com/products/vortex-ports/vascular

Anton, N., Cox, P.N., Massicotte, M.P., Chait, P., Yasui, Y., Dinyari, P.M., ... Mitchell, L.G. (2009). Heparin-bonded central venous catheters do not reduce thrombosis in infants with congenital heart disease: A blinded randomized, controlled trial. *Pediatrics, 123,* e453–e458. doi:10.1542/ peds.2008-1508

Arai, Y., Takeuchi, Y., Inaba, Y., Yamaura, H., Sato, Y., Aramaki, T., ... Seki, H. (2007). Percutaneous catheter placement for hepatic arterial infusion chemotherapy. *Techniques in Vascular and Interventional Radiology, 10,* 30–37. doi:10.1053/j.tvir.2007.08.007

Armstrong, D.K., Bundy, B., Wenzel, L., Huang, H.Q., Baergen, R., Lele, S., ... Burger, R.A. (2006). Intraperitoneal cisplatin and paclitaxel in ovarian cancer. *New England Journal of Medicine, 354,* 34–43. doi:10.1056/NEJMoa052985

Arrow International, Inc. (2007). Epidural catheter care guidelines. Retrieved from http://www.arrowintl.com/documents/pdf/education/ epdcg-s0407.pdf

ASHP Commission on Therapeutics. (2006). ASHP therapeutic position statement on the institutional use of 0.9% sodium chloride injection to maintain patency of peripheral indwelling intermittent infusion devices. *American Journal of Health-System Pharmacy, 63,* 1273–1275. doi:10.2146/ajhp060094

Askegard-Geismann, J.R., Caniano, D.A., & Kenney, B.D. (2009). Rare but serious complications of central line insertion. *Seminars in Pediatric Surgery, 18,* 73–83. doi:10.1053/j.sempedsurg.2009.02.003

Aslam, S. (2008). Effect of antibacterials on biofilms. *American Journal of Infection Control, 36,* S175.e9–S175.e11. doi: 10.1016/j.ajic.2008.10.002

Aufwerber, E., Ringertz, S., & Ransjo, U. (1991). Routine semiquantitative cultures and central venous catheter-related bacteremia. *Acta Pathologica, Microbiologica, et Immunologica Scandinavica, 99,* 627–630. doi:10.1111/j.1699-0463.1991.tb01237.x

Bacchetti, S., Pasqual, E., Crozzolo, E., Pellarin, A., & Cagol, P.P. (2009). Intra-arterial hepatic chemotherapy for unresectable colorectal liver metastases: A review of medical devices complications in 3172 patients. *Medical Devices: Evidence and Research, 2,* 31–40.

Bader, S.G., Balke, P., Jonkers-Schuitema, C.F., Tas, T.A.J., & Sauerwein, H.P. (2006). Evaluation of 6 years of sodium hydroxide solution to clear partially occluded central venous catheters. *Clinical Nutrition, 26,* 141–144. doi:10.1016/j.clnu.2006.09.008

Bamgbola, O.F., del Rio, M., Kaskel, F., & Flynn, J.T. (2005). Recombinant tissue plasminogen activator infusion for hemodialysis catheter clearance. *Pediatric Nephrology, 20,* 989–993. doi:10.1007/s00467 -004-1797-1

Banton, J. (2006). Techniques to prevent central venous catheter infections: Products, research, and recommendations. *Nutrition in Clinical Practice, 21,* 56–61. doi:10.1177/011542650602100156

Barber, F.D., Mavligit, G., & Kurzrock, R. (2004). Hepatic arterial infusion chemotherapy for metastatic colorectal cancer: A concise overview. *Cancer Treatment Reviews, 30,* 425–436. doi:10.1016/j.ctrv.2004.04.002

Bard Access Systems. (2007a). Instructions for use. Retrieved from http:// www.bardaccess.com/ifus.php

Bard Access Systems. (2007b). PowerPort implanted port with open-ended catheter: Nursing guide. Retrieved from http://www.bardnordic.com/ inc/getFile.asp?fileId=53&filetype=file

Barker, E. (2008). Managing spasticity with intrathecal drug delivery. *RN, 71*(4), 24–29.

Barton, S.J., Chase, T., Latham, B., & Rayens, M.K. (2004). Comparing two methods to obtain blood specimens from pediatric central venous catheters. *Journal of Pediatric Oncology Nursing, 21,* 320–326. doi:10.1177/1043454204269604

Baxter International Inc. (2008). Flo-Gard GSP syringe pump [Brochure]. Deerfield, IL: Author.

Berek, J.S. (2004). Surgical techniques. In J.S. Berek & N.F. Hacker (Eds.), *Practical gynecologic oncology* (4th ed., pp. 739–782). Philadelphia, PA: Lippincott Williams & Wilkins.

Bering, E.A., Jr., Rall, D.P., Walker, M., Leventhal, C., & Ommaya, A. (1969). Intrathecal chemotherapy of gliomas: Rationale and current status. *Annals of the New York Academy of Sciences, 159,* 599–602. doi:10.1111/j.1749-6632.1969.tb48309.x

Berry, E., Matthews, K.S., Singh, D.K., Buttin, B.M., Lurain, J.R., Alvarez, R.D., & Schink, J. (2009). An outpatient intraperitoneal chemotherapy regimen for advanced ovarian cancer. *Gynecologic Oncology, 113,* 63–67. doi:10.1016/j.ygyno.2008.12.035

Bertino, J.R. (2008). Implantable pump for long-term chemotherapy administration via the hepatic artery: Has it fulfilled its promise? *Journal of Clinical Oncology, 26,* 4528–4529. doi:10.1200/JCO.2008.18.0117

Bestul, M.B., & VandenBussche, H.L. (2005). Antibiotic lock techniques: Review of the literature. *Pharmacotherapy, 25,* 211–227. doi:10.1592/ phco.25.2.211.56947

Bianchi, F., Ginggen, A., & Tardy, Y. (2008). Stability and compatibility of drug mixtures in an implantable infusion system. *Anaesthesia, 63,* 972–978. doi:10.1111/j.1365-2044.2008.05516.x

Biffi, R., Orsi, F., Pozzi, S., Pace, U., Bonomo, G., Monfardini, L., ... Goldhirsch, A. (2009). Best choice of central venous insertion site for the prevention of catheter-related complications in adult patients who need cancer therapy: A randomized trial. *Annals of Oncology, 20,* 935–940. doi:10.1093/annonc/mdn701

Bilsel, Y., Balik, E., Bugra, D., Yamaner, S., & Akyuz, A. (2005). A case of protrusion of an intraperitoneal chemotherapy catheter through rectum. *International Journal of Gynecological Cancer, 15,* 171–174. doi:10.1111/j.1048-891X.2005.14427.x

Birnbach, D.J., Meadows, W., Stein, D.J., Murray, O., Thys, D.M., & Sordillo, E.M. (2003). Comparison of povidone iodine and DuraPrep, an iodophor-in-isopropyl alcohol solution, for skin disinfection prior to epidural catheter insertion in parturients. *Anesthesiology, 98,* 164–169. doi:10.1097/00000542-200301000-00026

Bishop, L., Dougherty, L., Bodenham, A., Mansi, J., Crowe, P., Kibbler, C., ... Treleaven, J. (2007). Guidelines on the insertion and management of central venous access devices in adults. *International Journal of Laboratory Hematology, 29,* 261–278. doi:10.1111/j.1751-553X .2007.00931.x

Black, D., Levine, D.A., Nicoll, L., Chou, J.F., Iasonos, A., Brown, C.L., ... Barakat, R.R. (2008). Low risk of complications associated with the fenestrated peritoneal catheter used for intraperitoneal chemotherapy in ovarian cancer. *Gynecologic Oncology, 109,* 39–42. doi:10.1016/j. ygyno.2007.12.004

Blaney, M., Shen, V., Kerner, J.A., Jacobs, B.R., Gray, S., Armfield, J., & Semba, C.P. (2006). Alteplase for the treatment of central venous catheter occlusion in children: Results of a prospective, open-label, single-arm study (the Cathflo Activase Pediatric Study). *Journal of Vascular and Interventional Radiology, 17,* 1745–1751. doi:10.1097/01.RVI .0000241542.71063.83

Blom, J.W., Doggen, C.J.M., Osanto, S., & Rosendaal, F.R. (2005). Malignancies, prothrombotic mutations, and the risk of venous thrombosis. *JAMA, 293,* 715–722. doi:10.1001/jama.293.6.715

Boersma, R.S., Jie, K.-S.G., Verbon, A., van Pampus, E.C.M., & Schouten, H.C. (2008). Thrombotic and infectious complications of central venous catheters in patients with hematological malignancies. *Annals of Oncology, 19,* 433–442. doi:10.1093/annonc/mdm350

Bonawitz, S.C., Hammell, E.J., & Kirkpatrick, J.R. (1991). Prevention of central venous catheter sepsis: A prospective randomized trial. *American Surgeon, 57,* 618–623.

Boodhan, S., Maloney, A.M., & Dupuis, L.L. (2006). Extent of agreement in gentamicin concentration between serum that is drawn peripherally and from central venous catheters. *Pediatrics, 118,* e1650–e1656. doi:10.1542/peds.2006-0023

Boraks, P., Seale, J., Price, J., Bass, G., Ethell, M., Keeling, D., ... Marcus, R. (1998). Prevention of central venous catheter associated thrombosis using minidose warfarin in patients with haematological malignancies. *British Journal of Haematology, 101,* 483–486. doi:10.1046/ j.1365-2141.1998.00732.x

Borowski, A., Shah, S.A., Littleton, A.G., Dabney, K.W., & Miller, F. (2008). Baclofen pump implantation and spinal fusion in children: Techniques and complications. *Spine, 33,* 1995–2000. doi:10.1097/ BRS.0b013e31817bab42

Borschel, D.M., Chenoweth, C.E., Kaufman, S.R., Hyde, K.V., VanDerElzen, K.A., Raghunathan, T.E., ... Saint, S. (2006). Are antiseptic-coated central venous catheters effective in a real-world setting? *American Journal of Infection Control, 34,* 388–393. doi:10.1016/j.ajic.2005.08.004

Bowe-Geddes, L.A., & Nichols, H.A. (2005). An overview of peripherally inserted central catheters. *Topics in Advanced Practice Nursing eJournal, 5.* Retrieved from http://www.medscape.com/viewarticle/508939

Bowers, L., Speroni, K.G., Jones, L., & Atherton, M. (2008). Comparison of occlusion rates by flushing solutions for peripherally inserted central catheters with positive pressure Luer-activated devices. *Journal of Infusion Nursing, 31,* 22–27. doi:10.1097/01.NAN.0000308542.90615.c2

Boyd, A., Dunne, A., Townsend, K., & Pai, A.B. (2006). Sampling for international normalized ratios in patients on hemodialysis with central venous catheters. *Nephrology Nursing Journal, 33,* 408–411.

Brashear, A., & Lambeth, K. (2009). Spasticity. *Current Treatment Options in Neurology, 11,* 153–161. doi:10.1007/s11940-009-0018-4

Bregenzer, T., Conen, D., Sakmann, P., & Widmer, A.F. (1998). Is routine replacement of peripheral intravenous catheters necessary? *Archives of Internal Medicine, 158,* 151–156. doi:10.1001/archinte.158.2.151

Brill, S., Gurman, G.M., & Fisher, A. (2003). A history of neuraxial administration of local analgesics and opioids. *European Journal of Anaesthesiology, 20,* 682–689. doi:10.1097/00003643-200309000-00002

Brown, D., Papadouris, D., Davis, R., Vedantham, S., & Pilgram, T. (2005). Power injection of microcatheters: An in vitro comparison. *Journal of Vascular and Interventional Radiology, 16,* 101–106. doi:10.1097/01. RVI.0000141718.12025.2C

Brown, D.B., Cardella, J.F., Sacks, D., Goldberg, S.N., Gervais, D., Rajan, D.J., ... Towbin, R.B. (2006). Quality improvement guidelines for transhepatic arterial chemoembolization, embolization, and chemotherapeutic infusion for hepatic malignancy. *Journal of Vascular and Interventional Radiology, 17,* 225–232.

Brueggen, C., Baird, G., & Meisheid, A. (2007). Pseudomyxoma peritonei syndrome of appendiceal origin: An overview. *Clinical Journal of Oncology Nursing, 11,* 525–532. doi:10.1188/07.CJON.525-532

Brun-Buisson, C., Doyon, F., Sollet, J.-P., Cochard, J.-F., Cohen, Y., & Nitenberg, G. (2004). Prevention of intravascular catheter-related infection with newer chlorhexidine-silver sulfadiazine-coated catheters: A randomized controlled trial. *Intensive Care Medicine, 30,* 837–843. doi:10.1007/s00134-004-2221-9

Bryant, C.S., Shah, J.P., Triest, J.A., Schimp, V.L., & Morris, R.T. (2008). Bladder erosion by an intraperitoneal chemotherapy catheter resulting in catheter protrusion through the external urethral meatus. *Gynecologic Oncology, 111,* 552–554. doi:10.1016/j.ygyno.2007.12.029

Bryant, J., Clegg, A.J., Sidhu, M.K., Brodin, H., Royle, P., & Davidson, P. (2004). Clinical effectiveness and costs of the Sugarbaker procedure for the treatment of pseudomyxoma peritonei. *Health Technology Assessment, 8*(7), iii, 1–54.

Buchman, A.L., Spapperi, J., & Leopold, P. (2009). A new central venous catheter cap: Decreased microbial growth and risk for catheter-related bloodstream infection. *Journal of Vascular Access, 10,* 11–21.

Bullock-Corkhill, M. (2010). Central venous access devices: Access and insertion. In M. Alexander, A. Corrigan, L. Gorski, J. Hankins, & R. Perucca (Eds.), *Infusion nursing: An evidence-based approach* (3rd ed., pp. 480–494). St. Louis, MO: Elsevier Saunders.

Camp-Sorrell, D. (2004). Implantable ports: Skin erosion. *Clinical Journal of Oncology Nursing, 8,* 309–310. doi:10.1188/04.CJON.309-310

Camp-Sorrell, D. (2007). Clinical dilemmas: Vascular access devices. *Seminars in Oncology Nursing, 23,* 232–239. doi:10.1016/j. soncn.2007.05.008

Camp-Sorrell, D. (2009). Accessing and deaccessing ports: Where is the evidence? *Clinical Journal of Oncology Nursing, 13,* 587–590. doi:10.1188/09.CJON.587-590

Cardinal Health. (2008). Alaris® CC syringe pump [Brochure]. Retrieved from http://www.carefusion.com/products-and-services/product-brands/ Alaris-index.aspx

Carpenito-Moyet, L.J. (2009). *Nursing care plans and documentation: Nursing diagnoses and collaborative problems* (5th ed.). Philadelphia, PA: Lippincott Williams & Wilkins.

Carr, K.M., & Rabinowitz, I. (2000). Physician compliance with warfarin prophylaxis for central venous catheters in patients with solid tumors. *Journal of Clinical Oncology, 18,* 3665–3667.

Carratala, J., Niubo, J., Fernandez-Sevilla, A., Juve, E., Castellsague, X., Berlanga, J., ... Gudiol, F. (1999). Randomized, double-blind trial of an antibiotic-lock technique for prevention of gram-positive central venous catheter-related infection in neutropenic patients with cancer. *Antimicrobial Agents and Chemotherapy, 43,* 2200–2204.

Casey, J., Davies, J., Balshaw-Greer, A., Taylor, N., Crowe, A.V., & McClelland, P. (2008). Inserting tunnelled hemodialysis catheters using elective guidewire exchange from nontunneled catheters: Is there a greater risk of infection when compared with new-site replacement? *Hemodialysis International, 12,* 52–54. doi:10.1111/j.1542-4758.2008.00240 .x

Catton, J.A., Dobbins, B.M., Kite, P., Wood, J.M., Eastwood, K., Sugden, S., ... Wilcox, M.H. (2005). In situ diagnosis of intravascular catheter-related bloodstream infection: A comparison of quantitative culture, differential time to positivity, and endoluminal brushing. *Critical Care Medicine, 33,* 787–791. doi:10.1097/01.CCM.0000157968.98476.F3

Centers for Disease Control and Prevention. (in press). Guidelines for the prevention of intravascular catheter-related infections. *Morbidity and Mortality Weekly Report.*

Centers for Medicare and Medicaid Services. (2008, August 4). Medicare takes new steps to help make your hospital stay safer [Fact sheet]. Retrieved from http://www.cms.hhs.gov/apps/media/fact_sheets.asp

Cesaro, S., Tridello, G., Cavaliere, M., Magagna, L., Gavin, P., Cusinato, R., ... Carli, M. (2009). Prospective, randomized trial of two different modalities of flushing central venous catheters in pediatric patients with cancer. *Journal of Clinical Oncology, 27,* 2059–2065. doi:10.1200/JCO.2008.19.4860

Chaiyakunapruk, N., Veenstra, D.L., Lipsky, B.A., & Saint, S. (2002). Chlorhexidine compared with povidone-iodine solution for vascular catheter-site care: A meta-analysis. *Annals of Internal Medicine, 136,* 792–801.

Chambers, S.T., Sanders, J., Patton, W.N., Ganly, P., Birch, M., Crump, J.A., & Spearing, R.L. (2005). Reduction of exit-site infections of tunneled intravascular catheters among neutropenic patients by sustained-release chlorhexidine dressings: Results from a prospective randomized controlled trial. *Journal of Hospital Infections, 61,* 53–61. doi:10.1016/j.jhin.2005.01.023

Chan, A., Iannucci, A., & Dager, W.E. (2007). Systemic anticoagulant prophylaxis for central catheter-associated venous thrombosis in cancer patients. *Annals of Pharmacotherapy, 41,* 635–641. doi:10.1345/aph.1G714

Chang, L., Tsai, J.-S., Huang, S.-J., & Shih, C.-C. (2003). Evaluation of infectious complications of the implantable venous access system in a general oncologic population. *American Journal of Infection Control, 31,* 34–39. doi:10.1067/mic.2003.29

Chatzinikolaou, I., Hanna, H., Darouiche, R., Samonis, G., Tarrand, J., & Raad, I. (2006). Prospective study of the value of quantitative culture of organisms from blood collected through central venous catheters in differentiating between contamination and bloodstream infection. *Journal of Clinical Microbiology, 44,* 1834–1835. doi:10.1128/JCM.44.5.1834-1835.2006

Chau, D.L., Walker, V., Pai, L., & Cho, L.M. (2008). Opiates and elderly: Use and side effects. *Clinical Interventions in Aging, 3,* 273–278.

Chaukiyal, P., Nautiyal, A., Radhakrishnan, S., Singh, S., & Navaneethan, S.D. (2008). Thromboprophylaxis in cancer patients with central venous catheters. A systematic review and meta-analysis. *Thrombosis and Haemostasis, 99,* 38–43. doi:10.1160/TH07-07-0446

Clayton, J., Vloeberghs, M., Jaspan, T., Walker, D., MacArthur, D., & Grundy, R. (2008). Intrathecal chemotherapy delivered by a lumbar-thecal catheter in metastatic medulloblastoma: A case illustration. *Acta Neurochirurgica, 150,* 709–712. doi:10.1007/s00701-008-1577-y

CME America LLC. (2009). CMExpress infusion pump [Brochure]. Retrieved from http://www.cmeamerica.com/cmexpress.html

Codman & Shurtleff, Inc. (2009a). Patient education: Codman 3000 pump. Retrieved from http://codmanpumps.com/Patient_chemo_pump.asp

Codman & Shurtleff, Inc. (2009b). Refill kit Codman 3000 series instruction sheet. Raynham, MA: Author.

Codman & Shurtleff, Inc. (n.d.). Patient education: HAI therapy. Retrieved from http://codmanpumps.com/Patient_chemo_responsibilities.asp

Compton, C.N., & Raaf, J.H. (2006). Vascular access devices. In F.E. Johnson, K.S. Virgo, T.C. Lairmore, & R.A. Audisio (Eds.), *The bionic human: Health promotion for people with implanted prosthetic devices* (pp. 561–585). Totowa, NJ: Humana Press.

Conly, J.M. (2005). Infectious complications of intravascular access devices used in critical care. In J.B. Hall, G.A. Schmidt, & L.D.H. Wood (Eds.), *Principles of critical care* (3rd ed., pp. 815–822). New York, NY: McGraw-Hill.

Conly, J.M., Grieves, K., & Peters, B. (1989). A prospective, randomized study comparing transparent and dry gauze dressings for central venous catheters. *Journal of Infectious Diseases, 159,* 310–319.

Cook, D., Randolph, A., Kernerman, P., Cupido, C., King, D., Soukup, C., & Brun-Buisson, C. (1997). Central venous catheter replacement strategies: A systematic review of the literature. *Critical Care Medicine, 25,* 1417–1424. doi:10.1097/00003246-199708000-00033

Cope, D.G. (2005). Malignant effusions and edema. In C.H. Yarbro, M.H. Frogge, & M. Goodman (Eds.), *Cancer nursing: Principles and practice* (6th ed., pp. 839–842). Sudbury, MA: Jones and Bartlett.

Cosca, P.A., Smith, S., Chatfield, S., Meleason, A., Muir, C.A., Nerantzis, S., ... Williams, S. (1998). Reinfusion of discard blood from venous access devices. *Oncology Nursing Forum, 25,* 1073–1076.

Couban, S., Goodyear, M., Burnell, M., Dolan, S., Wasi, P., Barnes, D., ... Anderson, D.R. (2005). Randomized placebo-controlled study of low-dose warfarin for the prevention of central venous catheter–associated thrombosis in patients with cancer. *Journal of Clinical Oncology, 23,* 4063–4069. doi:10.1200/JCO.2005.10.192

Covidien. (n.d.). Quinton™ Curl Cath™ peritoneal catheters and kits. Retrieved from http://www.kendallhealthcare.com/kendallhealthcare/pageBuilder.aspx?topicID=76840&breadcrumbs=0:121623,81037:0,76205:0

Coyle, D., Bloomgarden, D., Beres, R., Patel, S., Sane, S., & Hurst, E. (2004). Power injection of contrast media via peripherally inserted central venous catheters for CT. *Journal of Vascular and Interventional Radiology, 15,* 809–814.

Crowe, M.B. (2008, November/December). Infusion technology: Past, present, and future. *ALN Magazine.* Retrieved from http://www.alnmag.com/article/infusion-technology-past-present-and-future

Cummings-Winfield, C., & Mushani-Kanji, T. (2008). Restoring patency to central venous access devices. *Clinical Journal of Oncology Nursing, 12,* 925–934. doi:10.1188/08.CJON.925-934

Cunningham, M.S., White, B., Hollywood, D., & O'Donnell, J. (2006). Primary thromboprophylaxis for cancer patients with central venous catheters—a reappraisal of the evidence. *British Journal of Cancer, 94,* 189–194. doi:10.1038/sj.bjc.6602917

D'Silva, K.J., Dwivedi, A.J., Shetty, A., & Ashare, R. (2005) Pinch-off syndrome: A rare complication of totally implantable venous devices. *Breast Journal, 11,* 83–84. doi:10.1111/j.1075-122X.2005.21565.x

Damascelli, B., Patelli, G., Ticha, V., Di Tolla, G., Frigerio, L.F., Garbagnati, F., ... Zunino, F. (2007). Feasibility and efficacy of percutaneous transcatheter intraarterial chemotherapy with paclitaxel in albumin nanoparticles for advanced squamous-cell carcinoma of the oral cavity, oropharynx, and hypopharynx. *Journal of Vascular and Interventional Radiology, 18,* 1395–1403. doi:10.1016/j.jvir.2007.06.009

Danks, L.A. (2006). Central venous catheters: A review of skin cleansing and dressing. *British Journal of Nursing, 15,* 650–654.

Darouiche, R.O., Raad, I.I., Heard, S.O., Thornby, J.I., Wenker, O.C., Gabrielli, A., ... Mayhall, G. (1999). A comparison of two antimicrobial-impregnated central venous catheters. *New England Journal of Medicine, 340,* 1–8. doi:10.1056/NEJM199901073400101

Dasgupta, M., Binns, M., & Rochon, P. (2000). Subcutaneous fluid infusion in a long-term care setting. *Journal of the American Geriatrics Society, 48,* 795–799.

Dauerman, H.L., Applegate, R.J., & Cohen, D.J. (2007). Vascular closure devices: The second decade. *Journal of the American College of Cardiology, 50,* 1617–1626. doi:10.1016/j.jacc.2007.07.028

Davies, J., Casey, J., Li, C., Crowe, A.V., & McClelland, P. (2004). Restoration of flow following haemodialysis catheter thrombus: Analysis of rt-PA infusion in tunnelled dialysis catheters. *Journal of Clinical Pharmacy and Therapeutics, 29,* 517–520. doi:10.1111/j.1365-2710.2004.00581.x

Davies, S.J., & Williams, J.D. (2007). Complications of peritoneal dialysis. In J. Feehally, J. Floege, & R.J. Johnson (Eds.), *Comprehensive clinical nephrology* (3rd ed., pp. 991–1000). Philadelphia, PA: Elsevier Mosby.

Davis, S.N., Vermeulen, L., Banton, J., Schwartz, B.S., & Williams, E.C. (2000). Activity and dosage of alteplase dilution for clearing occlusions in venous-access devices. *American Journal of Health-System Pharmacy, 57,* 1039–1045.

Dayani, P.N., Gould, J.E., Brown, D.B., Sharma, K.V., Linette, G.P., & Harbour, J.W. (2009). Hepatic metastasis from uveal melanoma: Angiographic pattern predictive of survival after hepatic arterial chemoembolization. *Archives of Ophthalmology, 127,* 628–632. doi:10.1001/archophthalmol.2009.45

de Graff, J., Bras, L., & Vos, J. (2006). Early transaction of a central venous catheter in a sedated ICU patient. *British Journal of Anaesthesia, 97,* 832–834. doi:10.1093/bja/ael255

Debreceni, G., Meggyesi, R., & Mestyan, G. (2007). Efficacy of spray disinfection with a 2-propanol and benzalkonium chloride containing solution before epidural catheter insertion—A prospective, randomized, clinical trial. *British Journal of Anaesthesia, 98,* 131–135. doi:10.1093/bja/ael288

DeChicco, R., Seidner, D.L., Brun, C., Steiger, E., Stafford, J., & Lopez, R. (2007). Tip position of long-term central venous access devices used for parenteral nutrition. *Journal of Parenteral and Enteral Nutrition, 31,* 382–387. doi:10.1177/0148607107031005382

Deer, T.R., Raso, L.J., & Garten, T.G. (2007). Inflammatory mass of an intrathecal catheter in patients receiving baclofen as a sole agent: A report of two cases and a review of the identification and treatment of the complication. *Pain Medicine, 8,* 259–262. doi:10.1111/j.1526-4637 .2006.00150.x

Del Cotillo, M., Grane, N., Llavore, M., & Quintana, S. (2008). Heparinized solution vs. saline solution in the maintenance of arterial catheters: A double blind randomized clinical trial. *Intensive Care Medicine, 34,* 339–343. doi:10.1007/s00134-007-0886-6

DeMoissac, D., & Jensen, L. (1998). Changing IV administration sets: Is 48 versus 24 hours safe for neutropenic patients with cancer? *Oncology Nursing Forum, 25,* 907–913.

Dickerman, R.D., & Eisenberg, M.B. (2005). Preassembled method for insertion of Ommaya reservoir. *Journal of Surgical Oncology, 89,* 36–38. doi:10.1002/jso.20174

Dickerson, N., Horton, P., Smith, S., & Rose, R. (1989). Clinically significant central venous catheter infections in a community hospital: Association with type of dressing. *Journal of Infectious Disease, 160,* 720–721.

Do, A.N., Ray, B.J., Banerjee, S.N., Illian, A.F., Barnett, B.J., Pham, M.H., ... Jarvis, W.R. (1999). Bloodstream infection associated with needleless device use and the importance of infection-control practices in the home health care setting. *Journal of Infectious Diseases, 179,* 442–448.

Dodd, S. (2007). Assessing patient preference for two types of elastomeric infusion device. *British Journal of Nursing, 16,* 1180–1185.

Donmez, A., Araz, C., & Kayhan, Z. (2005). Syringe pumps take too long to give occlusion alarm. *Pediatric Anesthesia, 15,* 293–296. doi:10.1111/ j.1460-9592.2005.01436.x

Douard, M.C., Arlet, G., Longuet, P., Troje, C., Rouveau, M., Ponscarme, D., & Eurin, B. (1999). Diagnosis of venous access port–related infections. *Clinical Infectious Diseases, 29,* 1197–1202. doi:10.1086/313444

Dumont, C.J., Keeling, A.W., Bourguignon, C., Sarembock, I.J., & Turner, M. (2006). Predictors of vascular complications post diagnostic cardiac catheterization and percutaneous coronary interventions. *Dimensions of Critical Care Nursing, 25,* 137–142. doi:10.1097/00003465 -200605000-00016

Dunser, M.W., Mayr, A.J., Hinterberger, G., Florl, C.L., Ulmer, H., Schmid, S., ... Hasibeder, W.R. (2005). Central venous catheter colonization in critically ill patients: A prospective, randomized, controlled study comparing standard with two antiseptic-impregnated catheters. *Anesthesia and Analgesia, 101,* 1778–1784. doi:10.1213/01. ANE.0000184200.40689.EB

Eggimann, P., Hugonnet, S., Sax, H., Harbarth, S., Chevrolet, J.C., & Pittet, D. (2005). Long-term reduction of vascular access–associated bloodstream infection [Letter to the editor]. *Annals of Internal Medicine, 142,* 875–876.

Eisenberg, S. (2009). Smart pumps help limit infusion errors. *ONS Connect, 24,* 19.

Elaraj, D.M., & Alexander, H.R. (2004). Current role of hepatic artery infusion and isolated liver perfusion for the treatment of colorectal cancer liver metastases. *Cancer Journal, 10,* 128–138. doi:10.1097/00130404 -200403000-00008

Elihu, A., & Gollin, G. (2007). Complications of implanted central venous catheters in neutropenic children. *American Surgeon, 73,* 1079–1082.

Elvy, J., Porter, D., & Brown, E. (2008). Treatment of external ventricular drain-associated ventriculitis caused by *Enterococcus faecalis* with intraventricular daptomycin. *Journal of Antimicrobial Chemotherapy, 61,* 461–462. doi:10.1093/jac/dkm501

Emergency Care Research Institute. (2008a). Infusion pump criteria. *Health Devices, 37,* 52–58.

Emergency Care Research Institute. (2008b). Syringe infusion pumps with dose error reduction systems. *Health Devices, 37,* 33–51.

Ensminger, W.D. (2008). Intraarterial chemotherapy. In M.C. Perry (Ed.), *The chemotherapy source book* (4th ed., pp. 88–98). Philadelphia, PA: Lippincott Williams & Wilkins.

Enzon Pharmaceuticals, Inc. (2007). *Diagnosis and treatment of lymphomatous meningitis.* Bridgewater, NJ: Author.

Esteve, F., Pujol, M., Limon, E., Saballs, M., Argerich, M.J., Verdaguer, R., ... Gudiol, F. (2007). Bloodstream infection related to catheter connections: A prospective trial of two connection systems. *Journal of Hospital Infection, 67,* 30–34. doi:10.1016/j.jhin.2007.05.021

Ethans, K.D., Schryvers, O.I., Nance, P.W., & Casey, A.R. (2005). Intrathecal drug therapy using the Codman Model 3000 constant flow implantable infusion pumps: Experience with 17 cases. *Spinal Cord, 43,* 214–218. doi:10.1038/sj.sc.3101684

Falagas, M.E., Fragoulis, K., Bliziotis, I.A., & Chatzinikolaou, I. (2007). Rifampicin-impregnated central venous catheters: A meta-analysis of randomized controlled trials. *Journal of Antimicrobial Chemotherapy, 59,* 359–369. doi:10.1093/jac/dkl522

Falagas, M.E., Kazantzi, M.S., & Bliziotis, I.A. (2008). Comparison of utility of blood cultures from intravascular catheters and peripheral veins: A systematic review and decision analysis. *Journal of Medical Microbiology, 57*(Pt. 1), 1–8. doi:10.1099/jmm.0.47432-0

Field, K., McFarlane, C., Cheng, A.C., Hughes, A.J., Jacobs, E., Styles, K., ... Athan, E. (2007). Incidence of catheter-related bloodstream infection among patients with a needleless, mechanical valve-based intravenous connector in an Australian hematology-oncology unit. *Infection Control and Hospital Epidemiology, 28,* 610–613. doi:10.1086/516660

Fink, R.M., Hjort, E., Wenger, B., Cook, P.F., Cunningham, M., Orf, A., ... Zwink, J. (2009). The impact of dry versus moist heat on peripheral IV catheter insertion in a hematology-oncology outpatient population [Online exclusive]. *Oncology Nursing Forum, 36,* E198–E204. doi:10.1188/09.ONF.E198-E204

Fisher, A., Deffenbaugh, C., Poole, R., Garcia, M., & Kerner, J. (2004). The use of alteplase for restoring patency to occluded central venous access devices in infants and children. *Journal of Infusion Nursing, 27,* 171–174. doi:10.1097/00129804-200405000-00006

Fonzo-Christe, C., Vukasovic, C., Wasilewski-Rasca, A.-F., & Bonnabry, P. (2005). Subcutaneous administration of drugs in the elderly: Survey of practice and systematic literature review. *Palliative Medicine, 19,* 208–219. doi:10.1191/0269216304pm1006oa

Fraenkel, D., Rickard, C., Thomas, P., Faoagali, J., George, N., & Ware, R. (2006). A prospective, randomized trial of rifampicin-minocycline-coated and silver-platinum-carbon-impregnated central venous catheters. *Critical Care Medicine, 34,* 668–675. doi:10.1097/01 .CCM.0000201404.05523.34

Frey, A.M. (2003). Drawing blood samples from vascular access devices: Evidence-based practice. *Journal of Infusion Nursing, 26,* 285–293. doi:10.1097/00129804-200309000-00004

Frey, A.M., & Schears, G.J. (2006). Why are we stuck on tape and suture? *Journal of Infusion Nursing, 29,* 34–38. doi:10.1097/00129804 -200601000-00007

Frolich, M.A., & Caton, D. (2001). Pioneers in epidural needle design. *Anesthesia and Analgesia, 93,* 215–220. doi:10.1097/00000539 -200107000-00043

Fung-Kee-Fung, M., Provencher, D., Rosen, B., Hoskins, P., Rambout, L., Oliver, T., ... Covens, A. (2007). Intraperitoneal chemotherapy for patients with advanced ovarian cancer: A review of the evidence and standards for the delivery of care. *Gynecologic Oncology, 105,* 747–756. doi:10.1016/j.ygyno.2007.02.015

Gabriel, J. (2008). Infusion therapy part one: Minimizing the risks. *Nursing Standard, 22*(31), 51–56.

Gallieni, M., Pittiruti, M., & Biffi, R. (2008). Vascular access in oncology patients. *CA: A Cancer Journal for Clinicians, 58,* 323–346. doi:10.3322/CA.2008.0015

Galloway, S., & Bodenham, A. (2004). Long-term central venous access. *British Journal of Anaesthesia, 92,* 722–734. doi:10.1093/bja/aeh109

Galpern, D., Guerrero, A., Tu, A., Fahoum, B., & Wise, L. (2008). Effectiveness of a central line bundle campaign on line-associated infections in the intensive care unit. *Surgery, 144,* 492–495. doi:10.1016/j.surg.2008.06.004

Ganeshan, A., Upponi, S., Hon, L., Warakaulle, D., & Uberoi, R. (2008). Hepatic arterial infusion of chemotherapy: The role of diagnostic and interventional radiology. *Annals of Oncology, 19,* 847–851. doi:10.1093/annonc/mdm528

Garland, J.S., Alex, C.P., Mueller, C.D., Otten, D., Shivpuri, C., Harris, M.C., … Maki, D.G. (2001). A randomized trial comparing povidone-iodine to a chlorhexidine gluconate-impregnated dressing for prevention of central venous catheter infections in neonates. *Pediatrics, 107,* 1431–1436. doi:10.1542/peds.107.6.1431

Geerts, W.H., Bergqvist, D., Pineo, G.F., Heit, J.A., Samama, C.M., Lassen, M.R., & Colwell, C.W. (2008). Prevention of venous thromboembolism: American College of Chest Physicians Evidence-Based Clinical Practice Guidelines (8th Edition). *Chest, 133,* 381S–453S. doi:10.1378/chest.08-0656

Geerts, W.H., Pineo, G.F., Heit, J.A., Bergqvist, D., Lassen, M.R., Colwell, C.W., & Ray, J.G. (2004). Prevention of venous thromboembolism. The Seventh ACCP Conference on Antithrombotic and Thrombolytic Therapy. *Chest, 126*(Suppl. 3), 338S–400S. doi:10.1378/chest.126.3_suppl.338S

Ghafoor, V.L., Epshteyn, M., Carlson, G.H., Terhaar, D.M., Charry, O., & Phelps, P.K. (2007). Intrathecal drug therapy for long-term pain management. *American Journal of Health-System Pharmacy, 64,* 2447–2461. doi:10.2146/ajhp060204

Gholz, R., Whitehill, N., & Franer, K. (2009). Fact or fiction: An implanted venous access device when not in use must be flushed monthly to maintain patency [Abstract No. 3956]? *Oncology Nursing Forum, 36,* 64.

Gibbins, J., Steeds, C., Greenslade, G.L., Tunstall, S.R., Patel, N.K., & Stannard, C.F. (2008). To replace or not to replace? Partial coning and a sixth nerve palsy secondary due to displacement of a tunnelled intrathecal catheter for pain control. *Palliative Medicine, 22,* 668–670. doi:10.1177/0269216308091558

Gillies, D., O'Riordan, E., Carr, D., O'Brien, I., Frost, J., & Gunning, R. (2003). Central venous catheter dressings: A systematic review. *Journal of Advanced Nursing, 44,* 623–632. doi:10.1046/j.0309-2402.2003.02852.x

Glass, M., & Spitrey, J. (2009). Heparin-induced thrombocytopenia: Your questions answered. *Advanced Critical Care, 20,* 5–9.

Goetz, A.M., Wagener, M.M., Miller, J.M., & Muder, R.R. (1998). Risk of infection due to central venous catheters: Effect of site of placement and catheter type. *Infection Control and Hospital Epidemiology, 19,* 842–845. doi:10.1086/647742

Gokal, R., Alexander, S., Ash, S., Chen, T.W., Danielson, A., Holmes, C., … Vas, S. (1998). *Peritoneal catheters and exit-site practices toward optimum peritoneal access: 1998 update* (Official report from the International Society for Peritoneal Dialysis). Retrieved from http://www.ispd.org/media/pdf/Optimum.pdf

Goossens, G.A., Verbeeck, G., Moons, P., Sermeus, W., De Wever, I., & Stas, M. (2008). Functional evaluation of conventional 'Celsite®' venous ports versus 'Vortex®' ports with a tangential outlet: A prospective randomised pilot study. *Supportive Care in Cancer, 16,* 1367–1374. doi:10.1007/s00520-008-0436-y

Gorski, L., Perucca, R., & Hunter, M.R. (2010). Central venous access devices: Care, maintenance, and potential complications. In M. Alexander, A. Corrigan, L. Gorski, J. Hankins, & R. Perucca (Eds.), *Infusion nursing: An evidence-based approach* (3rd ed., pp. 495–515). St. Louis, MO: Elsevier Saunders.

Gorski, L.A. (2007). Standard 53: Phlebitis. *Journal of Infusion Nursing, 30,* 265–266. doi:10.1097/01.NAN.0000292567.17022.53

Gorski, L.A. (2009). Standard 14: Documentation. *Journal of Infusion Nursing, 32,* 19–20. doi:10.1097/NAN.0b013e3181924fe4

Gorski, L.A., & Czaplewski, L.M. (2004). Peripherally inserted central catheters and midline catheters for the homecare nurse. *Journal of Infusion Nursing, 27,* 399–409. doi:10.1097/00129804-200411000-00005

Green, J. (2008). Care and management of patients with skin-tunnelled catheters. *Nursing Standard, 22*(42), 41–48.

Guth, A.A. (2001). Routine chest x-rays after insertion of implantable long-term venous catheters: Necessary or not? *American Surgeon, 67,* 26–29.

Gynecologic Oncology Group. (2007). *GOG nursing manual.* Philadelphia, PA: Author.

Hadaway, L. (2006). Technology of flushing vascular access devices. *Journal of Infusion Nursing, 29,* 137–145.

Hadaway, L.C. (2004). Preventing and managing peripheral extravasation. *Nursing, 34,* 66–67.

Hadaway, L.C. (2010). Infusion therapy equipment. In M. Alexander, A. Corrigan, L. Gorski, J. Hankins, & R. Perucca (Eds.), *Infusion nursing: An evidence-based approach* (3rd ed., pp. 391–436). St. Louis, MO: Elsevier Saunders.

Hagle, M. (2007). Central venous access. In S.M. Weinstein (Ed.), *Plumer's principles and practice of intravenous therapy* (8th ed., pp. 277–330). Philadelphia, PA: Lippincott Williams & Wilkins.

Halaby, T., Leyssius, A., & Veneman, T. (2007). Fatal bacterial meningitis after spinal anaesthesia. *Scandinavian Journal of Infectious Diseases, 39,* 280–283. doi:10.1080/00365540600951309

Hall, K.F., Bennetts, T.M., Whitta, R.K., Welman, L., & Rawlins, P. (2006). Effect of heparin in arterial line flushing solutions on platelet count: A randomized double-blind study. *Critical Care and Resuscitation, 8,* 294–296.

Hamilton, C.A., Maxwell, G.L., Chernofsky, M.R., Bernstein, S., Farley, J.H., & Rose, G.S. (2008). Intraperitoneal bevacizumab for the palliation of malignant ascites in refractory ovarian cancer. *Gynecologic Oncology, 111,* 520–532. doi:10.1016/j.ygyno.2008.04.028

Hamilton, H. (2006). Complications associated with venous access devices: Part two. *Nursing Standard, 20,* 59–65.

Hanna, H., Benjamin, R., Chatzinikolaou, I., Alakech, B., Richardson, D., Mansfield, P., … Raad, I. (2004). Long-term silicone central venous catheters impregnated with minocycline and rifampin decrease rates of catheter-related bloodstream infection in cancer patients: A prospective randomized clinical trial. *Journal of Clinical Oncology, 22,* 3163–3171. doi:10.1200/JCO.2004.04.124

Harney, D., & Victor, R. (2004). Traumatic syrinx after implantation of an intrathecal catheter. *Regional Anesthesia and Pain Medicine, 29,* 606–609.

Harter, C., Salwender, H.J., Bach, A., Egerer, G., Goldschmidt, H., & Ho, A.D. (2002). Catheter-related infection and thrombosis of the internal jugular vein in hematologic-oncologic patients undergoing chemotherapy: A prospective comparison of silver-coated and uncoated catheters. *Cancer, 94,* 245–251. doi:10.1002/cncr.10199

Hayden, B., & Goodman, M. (2005). Chemotherapy: Principles of administration. In C.H. Yarbro, M.H. Frogge, & M. Goodman (Eds.), *Cancer nursing: Principles and practice* (6th ed., pp. 351–411). Sudbury, MA: Jones and Bartlett.

Heard, S.O., Wagle, M., Vijayakumar, E., McLean, S., Brueggemann, A., Napolitano, L.M., … Doern, G.V. (1998). Influence of triple-lumen central venous catheters coated with chlorhexidine and silver sulfadiazine on the incidence of catheter-related bacteremia. *Archives of Internal Medicine, 158,* 81–87.

Heath, J., & Jones, S. (2001). Utilization of an elastomeric continuous infusion device to maintain catheter patency. *Journal of Intravenous Nursing, 24,* 102–106.

Hebl, J.R. (2006). The importance and implications of aseptic techniques during regional anesthesia. *Regional Anesthesia and Pain Medicine, 31,* 311–323.

Heran, M.K.S., Smith, A.D., & Legiehn, G.M. (2008). Spinal injection procedures: A review of concepts, controversies, and complications. *Radiologic Clinics of North America, 46,* 487–514. doi:10.1016/j.rcl.2008.02.005

Herts, B.R., O'Malley, C.M., Wirth, S.L., Lieber, M.L., & Pohlman, B. (2001). Power injection of contrast media using central venous catheters: Feasibility, safety, and efficacy. *American Journal of Roentgenology, 176,* 447–453.

Hesdorffer, M.E., Chabot, J., DeRosa, C., & Taub, R. (2008). Peritoneal mesothelioma. *Current Treatment Options in Oncology, 9,* 180–190. doi:10.1007/s11864-008-0072-2

Hibbard, J.S., Mulberry, G.K., & Brady, A.R. (2002). A clinical study comparing the skin antisepsis and safety of ChloraPrep, 70% isopropyl alcohol, and 2% aqueous chlorhexidine. *Journal of Infusion Nursing, 25,* 244–249. doi:10.1097/00129804-200207000-00007

Higuchi, K.A.S., Edwards, N., Danseco, E., Davies, B., & McConnell, H. (2007). Development of an evaluation tool for a clinical practice guideline on nursing assessment and device selection for vascular access. *Journal of Infusion Nursing, 30,* 45–54. doi:10.1097/00129804-200701000-00007

Hind, D., Calvert, N., McWilliams, R., Davidson, A., Paisley, S., Beverley, C., & Thomas, S. (2003). Ultrasonic locating devices for central venous cannulation: Meta-analysis. *BMJ, 327,* 361–367. doi:10.1136/bmj.327.7411.361

Hinds, P.S., Quargnenti, A., Gattuso, J., Srivastava, D.K., Tong, X., Penn, L., ... Head, D. (2002). Comparing the results of coagulation tests on blood drawn by venipuncture and through heparinized tunneled venous access devices in pediatric patients with cancer [Online exclusive]. *Oncology Nursing Forum, 29,* E26–E34. doi:10.1188/02.ONF.E26-E34

Ho, K.M., & Litton, E. (2006). Use of chlorhexidine-impregnated dressing to prevent vascular and epidural catheter colonization and infection: A meta-analysis. *Journal of Antimicrobial Chemotherapy, 58,* 281–287. doi:10.1093/jac/dkl234

Hockenhull, J.C., Dwan, K., Boland, A., Smith, G., Bagust, A., Dundar, Y., ... Dickson, R. (2008). The clinical effectiveness and cost-effectiveness of central venous catheters treated with anti-infective agents in preventing bloodstream infections: A systematic review and economic evaluation. *Health Technology Assessment, 12*(12), 1–154.

Hockenhull, J.C., Dwan, K.M., Smith, G.W., Gamble, C.L., Boland, A., Walley, T.J., & Dickson, R.C. (2009). The clinical effectiveness of central venous catheters treated with anti-infective agents in preventing catheter-related bloodstream infections: A systematic review. *Critical Care Medicine, 37,* 702–712. doi:10.1097/CCM.0b013e3181958915

Hoffmann, K.K., Weber, D.J., Samsa, G.P., & Rutala, W.A. (1992). Transparent polyurethane film as an intravenous catheter dressing. *JAMA, 267,* 2072–2076.

Holmes, K.R. (1998). Comparison of push-pull versus discard method from central venous catheters for blood tested. *Journal of Intravenous Nursing, 21,* 282–285.

Holmfred, A., Vikerfors, T., Berggren, L., & Gupta, A. (2006). Intrathecal catheters with subcutaneous port systems in patients with severe cancer-related pain managed out of hospital: The risk of infection. *Journal of Pain and Symptom Management, 31,* 568–572. doi:10.1016/j.jpainsymman.2005.11.010

Homer, L., & Holmes, K. (1998). Risks associated with 72- and 96-hour peripheral intravenous catheter dwell times. *Journal of Intravenous Nursing, 21,* 301–305.

Homsi, J., & Garrett, C.R. (2006). Hepatic arterial infusion of chemotherapy for hepatic metastases from colorectal cancer. *Cancer Control, 13,* 42–47. Retrieved from http://www.medscape.com/viewarticle/525586_print

Horne, M.K., III, McCloskey, D.J., Calis, K., Wesley, R., Childs, R., & Kasten-Sportes, C. (2006). Use of heparin versus lepirudin flushes to prevent withdrawal occlusion of central venous access devices. *Pharmacotherapy, 26,* 1262–1267. doi:10.1592/phco.26.9.1262

Hunter, J. (2008). Subcutaneous injection technique. *Nursing Standard, 22*(21), 41–44.

Hydzik, C. (2007). Implementation of intraperitoneal chemotherapy for the treatment of ovarian cancer. *Clinical Journal of Oncology Nursing, 11,* 221–225. doi:10.1188/07.CJON.221-225

Inan, I., De Sousa, S., Myers, P.O., Bouclier, B., Dietrich, P.-Y., Hagen, M.E., & Morel, P. (2008). Management of malignant pleural effusion and ascites by a triple access multi perforated large diameter catheter port system. *World Journal of Surgical Oncology, 6,* 85. doi:10.1186/1477-7819-6-85

Infusion Nurses Society. (2006). *Policies and procedures for infusion nursing* (3rd ed.). Norwood, MA: Author.

Infusion Nurses Society. (2008). *Flushing protocols.* Norwood, MA: Author.

InfuSystem, Inc. (2008). *InfuSystem pump* [Brochure]. Madison Heights, MI: Author.

Institute for Healthcare Improvement. (n.d.). Implement the central line bundle. Retrieved from http://www.ihi.org/IHI/Topics/CriticalCare/IntensiveCare/Changes/ImplementtheCentralLineBundle.htm

Jaeger, K., Osthaus, A., Heine, J., Ruschulte, H., Kuhlmann, C., Weissbrodt, H., ... Karthaus, M. (2001). Efficacy of a benzalkonium chloride-impregnated central venous catheter to prevent catheter-associated infection in cancer patients. *Chemotherapy, 47,* 50–55. doi:10.1159/000048501

Jaeger, K., Zenz, S., Juttner, B., Ruschulte, H., Kuse, E., Heine, J., ... Karthaus, M. (2005). Reduction of catheter-related infections in neutropenic patients: A prospective controlled randomized trial using a chlorhexidine and silver sulfadiazine-impregnated central venous catheter. *Annals of Hematology, 84,* 258–262. doi:10.1007/s00277-004-0972-6

James, H.E., & Bradley, J.S. (2008). Aggressive management of shunt infection: Combined intravenous and intraventricular antibiotic therapy for twelve or less days. *Pediatric Neurosurgery, 44,* 104–111. doi:10.1159/000113111

Jansen, N.C.A.J., Kingma, A., Schuitema, A., Bouma, A., Veerman, A.J.P., & Kamps, W.A. (2008). Neuropsychological outcome in chemotherapy-only-treated children with acute lymphoblastic leukemia. *Journal of Clinical Oncology, 26,* 3025–3030. doi:10.1200/JCO.2007.12.4149

Jensen, M.O. (2008). Anatomical basis of central venous catheter fracture. *Clinical Anatomy, 21,* 106–110. doi:10.1002/ca.20605

Jhas, S., & Tuli, S. (2008). Intrathecal catheter-tip inflammatory masses: An intraparenchymal granuloma. *Journal of Neurosurgery: Spine, 9,* 196–199.

Joint Commission. (2005, July 14). Preventing vincristine administration errors [Issue 34]. *Sentinel Event Alert.* Retrieved from http://www.jointcommission.org/SentinelEvents/SentinelEventAlert/sea_34.htm

Joint Commission. (2006, April 3). Tubing misconnections—A persistent and potentially deadly occurrence [Issue 36]. *Sentinel Event Alert.* Retrieved from http://www.jointcommission.org/SentinelEvents/SentinelEventAlert/sea_36.htm

Jones, P.M. (1987). Indwelling central venous catheter-related infections and two different procedures of catheter care. *Cancer Nursing, 10,* 123–130. doi:10.1097/00002820-198706000-00001

Justad, M. (2009). Continuous subcutaneous infusion: An efficacious, cost-effective analgesia alternative at the end of life. *Home Healthcare Nurse, 27,* 140–147. doi:10.1097/01.NHH.0000347677.15617.ff

Kaler, W., & Chinn, R. (2007). Successful disinfection of needleless access ports: A matter of time and friction. *Journal of the Association for Vascular Access, 12,* 140–142. doi:10.2309/java.12-3-9

Kalfon, P., de Vaumas, C., Samba, D., Boulet, E., Lefrant, J.-Y., Eyraud, D., ... Riou, B. (2007). Comparison of silver-impregnated with standard multi-lumen central venous catheters in critically ill patients. *Critical Care Medicine, 35,* 1032–1039. doi:10.1097/01.CCM.0000259378.53166.1B

Kannan, A. (2008). Heparinised saline or normal saline? *Journal of Perioperative Practice, 18,* 440–441.

Karakaya, C., Baris, S., Geidogus, F., Incesu, L., Sarihasan, B., & Ter, A. (2000). Brachial plexus injury during subclavian vein catheterization for hemodialysis. *Journal of Clinical Anesthesia, 12,* 220–223. doi:10.1016/S0952-8180(00)00144-6

Kasuda, H., Fukuda, H., Togashi, H., Hotta, K., Hirai, Y., & Hayashi, M. (2002). Skin disinfection before epidural catheterization: Comparative study of povidone-iodine versus chlorhexidine ethanol. *Dermatology, 204*(Suppl. 1), 42–46. doi:10.1159/000057724

Kefeli, U., Dane, F., Yumuk, P.F., Karamanoglu, A., Iyikesici, S., Basaran, A., & Turhal, N.S. (2009). Prolonged interval in prophylactic heparin flushing for maintenance of subcutaneous implanted port care in patients with cancer. *European Journal of Cancer Care, 18,* 191–194. doi:10.1111/j.1365-2354.2008.00973.x

Kelly, C., Dumenko, L., McGregor, S.E., & McHutchion, M.E. (1992). A change in flushing protocols of central venous catheters. *Oncology Nursing Forum, 19,* 599–605.

Kerner, J.A., Jr., Garcia-Careaga, M.G., Fisher, A.A., & Poole, R.L. (2006). Treatment of catheter occlusion in pediatric patients. *Journal of Parenteral and Enteral Nutrition, 30*(Suppl. 1), S73–S81. doi:10.1177/01486071060300S1S73

Khan, M., & Younger, G. (2007). Promoting safe administration of subcutaneous infusions. *Nursing Standard, 21*(31), 50–56.

Khare, M.D., Bukhari, S.S., Swann, A., Spiers, P., McLaren, I., & Myers, J. (2007). Reduction of catheter-related colonisation by the use of a silver zeolite-impregnated central vascular catheter in adult critical care. *Journal of Infection, 54,* 146–150. doi:10.1016/j.jinf.2006.03.002

Kinirons, B., Mimoz, O., Lafendl, L., Naas, T., Meunier, J., & Nordmann, P. (2001). Chlorhexidine versus povidone iodine in preventing colonization of continuous epidural catheters in children. *Anesthesiology, 94,* 239–244. doi:10.1097/00000542-200102000-00012

Knight, K.H., Brand, F.M., Mchaourab, A.S., & Veneziano, G. (2007). Implantable intrathecal pumps for chronic pain: Highlights and updates. *Croatian Medical Journal, 48,* 22–34.

Knutstad, K., Hager, B., & Hauser, M. (2003). Radiologic diagnosis and management of complications related to central venous access. *Acta Radiologica, 44,* 508–516. doi:10.1034/j.1600-0455.2003.00115.x

Koff, M.D., Loftus, R.W., Burchman, C.C., Schwartzman, J.D., Read, M.E., Henry E.S., & Beach, M.L. (2009). Reduction in intraoperative bacterial contamination of peripheral intravenous tubing through the use of a novel device. *Anesthesiology, 110,* 978–985. doi:10.1097/ALN.0b013e3181a06ec3

Kolaski, K., & Logan, L.R. (2007). A review of the complications of intrathecal baclofen in patients with cerebral palsy. *NeuroRehabilitation, 22,* 383–395.

Krach, L.E., Nettleton, A., & Klempka, B. (2006). Satisfaction of individuals treated long-term with continuous infusion of intrathecal baclofen by implanted programmable pump. *Pediatric Rehabilitation, 9,* 210–218. doi:10.1080/13638490500138678

Krzywda, E.A., & Edmiston, C.E. (2002). Central venous catheter infections: Clinical aspects of microbial etiology and pathogenesis. *Journal of Infusion Nursing, 25,* 29–35. doi:10.1097/00129804-200201000-00006

Kuizon, D., Gordon, S.M., & Dolmatch, B.L. (2001). Single-lumen subcutaneous ports inserted by interventional radiologists in patients undergoing chemotherapy: Incidence of infection and outcome of attempted catheter salvage. *Archives of Internal Medicine, 161,* 406–410. doi:10.1001/archinte.161.3.406

Kuo, Y.S., Schwartz, B., Santiago, J., Anderson, P.S., Fields, A.L., & Goldberg, G.L. (2005). How often should a Port-A-Cath be flushed? *Cancer Investigation, 23,* 582–585. doi:10.1080/07357900500276923

Kuter, D. (2004). Thrombotic complications of central venous catheters in cancer patients. *Oncologist, 9,* 207–216. doi:10.1634/theoncologist.9-2-207

Lafay-Cousin, L., & Strother, D. (2009). Current treatment approaches for infants with malignant central nervous system tumors. *Oncologist, 14,* 433–444. doi:10.1634/theoncologist.2008-0193

Lai, K.K. (1998). Safety of prolonging peripheral cannula and i.v. tubing use from 72 hours to 96 hours. *American Journal of Infection Control, 26,* 66–70. doi:10.1016/S0196-6553(98)70063-X

Lapum, J.L. (2006). Patency of arterial catheters with heparinized solutions versus non-heparinized solutions: A review of the literature. *Canadian Journal of Cardiovascular Nursing, 16,* 64–70.

Laura, R., Degl'Innocenti, M., Mocali, M., Alberani, F., Boschi, S., Giraudi, A., … Peron, G. (2000). Comparison of two different time interval protocols for central venous catheter dressing in bone marrow transplant patients: Results of a randomized, multicenter study. The Italian Nurse Bone Marrow Transplant Group (GITMO). *Haematologica, 85,* 275–279.

Lavery, I., & Smith, E. (2007). Peripheral vascular access devices: Risk prevention and management. *British Journal of Nursing, 16,* 1379–1383.

Leeper, B. (2006). What is the standard regarding isotonic sodium chloride solution versus heparin in pressure monitoring systems? *Critical Care Nurse, 26,* 137–138.

Leon, C., Ruiz-Santana, S., Rello, J., de la Torre, M.V., Valles, J., Alvarez-Lerma, F., … Alvarez-Salgado, F. (2004). Benefits of minocycline and rifampin-impregnated central venous catheters. *Intensive Care Medicine, 30,* 1891–1899. doi:10.1007/s00134-004-2378-2

Levy, I., Katz, J., Solter, E., Samra, Z., Vidne, B., Birk, E., … Dagan, O. (2005). Chlorhexidine-impregnated dressing for prevention of colonization of central venous catheters in infants and children: A randomized controlled study. *Pediatric Infectious Disease Journal, 24,* 676–679. doi:10.1097/01.inf.0000172934.98865.14

Lin, R.Z., Fowler, S., Dise, C.A., & Bustami, R. (2009). Venous access devices: Obtaining coagulation tests in adult inpatients with cancer. *Clinical Journal of Oncology Nursing, 13,* 347–349. doi:10.1188/09.CJON.347-349

Linenberger, M.L. (2006). Catheter-related thrombosis: Risks, diagnosis, and management. *Journal of the National Comprehensive Cancer Network, 4,* 889–901.

Liu, C.Y., Jain, V., Shields, A.F., & Heilbrun, L.K. (2004). Efficacy and safety of reteplase for central venous catheter occlusion in patients with cancer. *Journal of Vascular and Interventional Radiology, 15,* 39–44.

Lok, C.E., Stanley, K.E., Hux, J.E., Richardson, R., Tobe, S.W., & Conly, J. (2003). Hemodialysis infection prevention with polysporin ointment. *Journal of the American Society of Nephrology, 14,* 169–179. doi:10.1097/01.ASN.0000038688.76195.A4

Longuet, P., Douard, M.C., Arlet, G., Molina, J.M., Benoit, C., & Leport, C. (2001). Venous access port–related bacteremia in patients with acquired immunodeficiency syndrome or cancer: The reservoir as a diagnostic and therapeutic tool. *Clinical Infectious Diseases, 32,* 1776–1783. doi:10.1086/320746

Lopez, J.L.G., del Palacio, E.F., Marti, C.B., Corral, J.O., Portal, P.H., & Vilela, A.A. (2009). COSMOS—a study comparing peripheral intravenous systems. *British Journal of Nursing, 18,* 844–853.

Lorente, L., Santacreu, R., Martin, M.M., Jimenez, A., & Mora, M.L. (2006). Arterial catheter-related infection of 2,949 catheters. *Critical Care, 10*(3), R83. doi:10.1186/cc4930

Lucas, A.D., & Brown, R.P. (2005, April). *Release of the plasticizer di-2-ethylhexyl phthalate (DEHP) into normal saline stored in heated and nonheated PVC bags.* Presented at the 11th Annual FDA Science Forum, Washington, DC. Retrieved from http://www.accessdata.fda.gov/scripts/oc/scienceforum/sf2005/Search/preview.cfm?abstract_id=102&backto=category

Lybarger, E.H. (2009). Hypodermoclysis in the home and long-term care settings. *Journal of Infusion Nursing, 32,* 40–44. doi:10.1097/NAN.0b013e3181922552

Lyons, A., Given, M., & Marshall, N. (2008). Interventional radiology in the provision and maintenance of long-term central venous access. *Journal of Medical Imaging and Radiation Oncology, 52,* 10–17. doi:10.1111/j.1440-1673.2007.01904.x

Maaskant, J.M., De Boer, J.P., Dalesio, O., Holtkamp, M.J., & Lucas, C. (2009). The effectiveness of chlorhexidine-silver sulfadiazine impregnated central venous catheters in patients receiving high-dose chemotherapy followed by peripheral stem cell transplantation. *European Journal of Cancer Care, 18,* 477–482. doi:10.1111/j.1365-2354.2008.00964.x

Maaz, D.E. (2004). Troubleshooting non-infectious peritoneal dialysis issues. *Nephrology Nursing, 31,* 521–532, 545.

Macklin, D.C. (2005). Developing a patient-centered approach to vascular access device selection. *Topics in Advanced Practice Nursing eJournal, 5.* Retrieved from http://medscape.com/viewarticle/508093_print

Madeo, M., Martin, C., & Nobbs, A. (1997). A randomized study comparing IV 3000 (transparent polyurethane dressing) to gauze dressing for peripheral intravenous catheter sites. *Journal of Intravenous Nursing, 20,* 253–256.

Magagnoli, M., Masci, G., Castagna, L., Pedicini, V., Poretti, D., Morenghi, E., … Santoro, A. (2006). Prophylaxis of central venous catheter-related thrombosis with minidose warfarin in patients treated with high-dose chemotherapy and peripheral-blood stem cell transplantation: Retrospective analysis of 228 cancer patients. *American Journal of Hematology, 81,* 1–4. doi:10.1002/ajh.20512

Maki, D.G., & Crnich, C.J. (2003). Line sepsis in the ICU: Prevention, diagnosis, and management. *Seminars in Respiratory and Critical Care Medicine, 24,* 23–36. doi:10.1055/s-2003-37914

Maki, D.G., Kluger, D.M., & Crnich, C.J. (2006). The risk of bloodstream infection in adults with different intravascular devices: A systematic review of 200 published prospective studies. *Mayo Clinic Proceedings, 81,* 1159–1171. doi:10.4065/81.9.1159

Mann, T.J., Orlikowski, C.E., Gurrin, L.C., & Keil, A.D. (2001). The effect of the Biopatch, a chlorhexidine impregnated dressing on bacterial colonization of epidural catheter exit sites. *Anaesthesia and Intensive Care, 29,* 600–603.

Maragakis, L.L., Bradley, K.L., Song, X., Beers, C., Miller, M.R., Cosgrove, S.E., & Perl, T.M. (2006). Increased catheter-related bloodstream infection rates after the introduction of a new mechanical valve intravenous access port. *Infection Control and Hospital Epidemiology, 27,* 67–70. doi:10.1086/499166

Marin, K., Oleszewski, K., & Muehlbauer, P. (2007). Intraperitoneal chemotherapy: Implications beyond ovarian cancer. *Clinical Journal of Oncology Nursing, 11,* 881–889. doi:10.1188/CJON.07.881-889

Markman, M. (2007). The current status of intraperitoneal therapy in the management of ovarian cancer. *Cancer Therapy, 6,* 1023–1030.

Markman, M., & Walker, J.L. (2006). Intraperitoneal chemotherapy of ovarian cancer: A review, with a focus on practical aspects of treatment. *Journal of Clinical Oncology, 24,* 988–994. doi:10.1200/JCO.2005.05.2456

Marschall, J., Mermel, L., Classen, D., Arias, K. Podgorny, K. Deverick, J., ... Yokoe, D.S. (2008). Strategies to prevent central line–associated bloodstream infections in acute care hospitals. *Infection Control and Hospital Epidemiology, 29*(Suppl. 1), S22–S30. doi:10.1086/591059

Martinez, E., Mensa, J., Rovira, M., Martinez, J.A., Marcos, A., Almela, M., & Carreras, E. (1999). Central venous catheter exchange by guidewire for treatment of catheter-related bacteraemia in patients undergoing BMT or intensive chemotherapy. *Bone Marrow Transplantation, 23,* 41–44. doi:10.1038/sj.bmt.1701538

Matthews, E., Snell, K., & Coats, H. (2006). Intra-arterial chemotherapy for limb preservation in patients with osteosarcoma: Nursing implications. *Clinical Journal of Oncology Nursing, 10,* 581–588. doi:10.1188/06.CJON.581-589

McDonald, L.C., Banerjee, S.N., & Jarvis, W.H. (1998). Line-associated bloodstream infections in pediatric intensive care unit patients associated with a needleless device and intermittent intravenous therapy. *Infection Control and Hospital Epidemiology, 19,* 772–777. doi:10.1086/647722

McGee, D.C., & Gould, M.K. (2003). Preventing complications of central venous catheterization. *New England Journal of Medicine, 348,* 1123–1133. doi:10.1056/NEJMra011883

McGill, R., Spero, J., Sysak, J., Sandoni, S., & Marcus, R. (2008). Tissue plasminogen activator as a hemodialysis catheter locking solution. *Hemodialysis International, 12,* 348–351. doi:10.1111/j.1542-4758.2008.00280.x

Medtronic, Inc. (2005). SynchroMed II implant manual. Retrieved from http://professional.medtronic.com/downloads/itb/synchromed-II-8637-implant-manual-221311_b_0041.pdf.

Mentz, H.A., Ruiz-Razura, A., Newall, G., & Patronella, C.K. (2005). Use of a regional infusion pump to control postoperative pain after an abdominoplasty. *Aesthetic Plastic Surgery, 29,* 415–421. doi:10.1007/s00266-005-0062-8

Menyhay, S.Z., & Maki, D.G. (2006). Disinfection of needleless catheter connectors and access ports with alcohol may not prevent microbial entry: The promise of a novel antiseptic-barrier cap. *Infection Control and Hospital Epidemiology, 27,* 23–27. doi:10.1086/500280

Menyhay, S.Z., & Maki, D.G. (2008). Preventing central venous catheter-associated bloodstream infections: Development of an antiseptic barrier cap for needleless connectors. *American Journal of Infection Control, 36,* 1–5. doi:10.1016/j.ajic.2008.10.006

Mermel, L.A. (2007). Prevention of central venous catheter-related infections: What works other than impregnated or coated catheters? *Journal of Hospital Infection, 65*(Suppl. 2), 30–33. doi:10.1016/S0195-6701(07)60011-5

Mermel, L.A., Allon, M., Bouza, E., Craven, D.E., Flynn, P., O'Grady, N.P., ... Warren, D.K. (2009). Clinical practice guidelines for the diagnosis and management of intravascular catheter-related infection: 2009 update by the Infectious Diseases Society of America. *Clinical Infectious Diseases, 49,* 1–45. doi:10.1086/599376

Mickler, P.A. (2008). Neonatal and pediatric perspectives in PICC placement. *Journal of Infusion Nursing, 31,* 282–285. doi:10.1097/01.NAN.0000336182.77656.4e

Middleton, R. (2006). Suturing as an advanced skill for registered nurses in the emergency department. *Australian Journal of Rural Health, 15,* 258–262. doi:10.1111/j.1440-1584.2006.00826.x

Milstone, A.M., Passaretti, C.L., & Perl, T.M. (2008). Chlorhexidine: Expanding the armamentarium for infection control and prevention. *Clinical Infectious Diseases, 46,* 274–281. doi:10.1086/524736

Mimoz, O., Villeminey, S., Ragot, S., Dahyot-Fizelier, C., Laksiri, L., Petitpas, F., & Debaene, B. (2007). Chlorhexidine-based antiseptic solution vs. alcohol-based povidone-iodine for central venous catheter care. *Archives of Internal Medicine, 167,* 2066–2072. doi:10.1001/archinte.167.19.2066

Minassian, V.A., Sood, A.K., Lowe, P., Sorosky, J.I., Al-Jurf, A.S., & Buller, R.E. (2000). Long-term central venous access in gynecologic cancer patients. *Journal of the American College of Surgeons, 191,* 403–409. doi:10.1016/S1072-7515(00)00690-6

Mirski, M., Lele, A., Fitzsimmons, L., & Toung, T. (2007). Diagnosis and treatment of vascular air embolism. *Anesthesiology, 106,* 164–177. doi:10.1097/00000542-200701000-00026

Mirza, B., Vanek, V., & Kupensky, D. (2004). Pinch-off syndrome case report and collective review of the literature. *American Surgeon, 70,* 635–644.

Misset, B., Timsit, J.-F., Dumay, M.-F., Garrouste, M., Chalfine, A., Flouriot, I., ... Carlet, J. (2004). A continuous quality-improvement program reduces nosocomial infection rates in the ICU. *Intensive Care Medicine, 30,* 395–400. doi:10.1007/s00134-003-2096-1

Molinari, A.C., Haupt, R., Saracco, P., Di Marco, M., Castagnola, E., & Fratino, G. (2004) Urokinase for restoring patency in blocked central venous catheters in children with hemato-oncologic diseases. *Supportive Care in Cancer, 12,* 840–843. doi:10.1007/s00520-004-0616-3

Moore, A., Espeleta, J., & McMenamin, E. (2008). Implementation of the continuous ambulatory drug delivery (CADD) pump in the inpatient oncology setting for the safe delivery of high dose opioid infusions in cancer patients [Abstract No. 3026]. *Oncology Nursing Forum, 35,* 543–544.

Moran, A.B., & Camp-Sorrell, D. (2002). Maintenance of venous access devices in patients with neutropenia. *Clinical Journal of Oncology Nursing, 6,* 126–130. doi:10.1188/02.CJON.126-130

Moran, J.E., & Ash, S.R. (2008). Locking solutions for hemodialysis catheters: Heparin and citrate—a position paper by ASDIN. *Seminars in Dialysis, 21,* 490–492. doi:10.1111/j.1525-139X.2008.00466.x

Morris, W., & Tay, M.H. (2008). Strategies for preventing peripheral intravenous cannula infection. *British Journal of Nursing, 17,* S14–S21.

Moss, H.A., Tebbs, S.E., Faroqui, M.H., Herbst, T., Isaac, J.L., Brown, J., & Elliott, T.S. (2000). A central venous catheter coated with benzalkonium chloride for the prevention of catheter-related microbial colonization. *European Journal of Anaesthesiology, 17,* 680–687.

Moureau, N.L. (2008). Tips for inserting an I.V. device in an older adult. *Nursing, 38*(12), 12. doi:10.1097/01.NURSE.0000342005.69106.d7

Murphy, E.M., Sexton, R., & Moran, B.J. (2007). Early results of surgery in 123 patients with *Pseudomyxoma peritonei* from a perforated appendiceal neoplasm. *Diseases of the Colon and Rectum, 50,* 37–42. doi:10.1007/s10350-006-0741-9

Narouze, S.N., Yonan, S., Kapural, L., & Malak, O. (2007). Erosion of the inferior epigastric artery: A rare complication of intrathecal drug delivery systems. *Pain Medicine, 8,* 468–470. doi:10.1111/j.1526-4637.2006.00166.x

National Cancer Institute. (2006, January 5). NCI clinical announcement: Intraperitoneal chemotherapy for ovarian cancer. Retrieved from http://ctep.info.nih.gov/highlights/docs/clin_annc_010506.pdf

National Institutes of Health. (2007a, October). Phase I study of intraperitoneal chemotherapy in patients with gastric adenocarcinoma with peritoneal seeding. Retrieved from http://www.clinicaltrials.gov/ct2/show/NCT00539877?term=Intraperitoneal+for+gastric+cancer&rank=10

National Institutes of Health. (2007b, April). Safety study of phIL-12-005/PPC to treat recurrent ovarian cancer. Retrieved from http://www.clinicaltrials.gov/ct2/show/NCT00137865?term=phIL-12-005%2FPPC+to+treat+recurrent+%09ovarian+%09cancer.&rank=1

Navilyst Medical, Inc. (n.d.). *Implantable ports with PASV® valve technology.* Retrieved from http://www.navilystmedical.com/Products/index.cfm/9

Naylor, C.L. (2007). Reduction of malposition in peripherally inserted central catheters with tip location system. *Journal of the Association for Vascular Access, 12,* 29–31. doi:10.2309/java.12-1-8

Ng, R, Li, X., Tu, T., & Semba, C.P. (2004). Alteplase for treatment of occluded peripherally inserted central catheters: Safety and efficacy in 240 patients. *Journal of Vascular and Interventional Radiology, 15,* 45–49.

Niel-Weise, B.S., Stijnen, T., & van den Broek, P.J. (2007). Anti-infective-treated central venous catheters: A systematic review of randomized controlled trials. *Intensive Care Medicine, 33,* 2058–2068. doi:10.1007/s00134-007-0897-3

Nikoletti, S., Leslie, G., Gandossi, S., Coombs, G., & Wilson, R. (1999). A prospective, randomized, controlled trial comparing transparent polyurethane and hydrocolloid dressings for central venous catheters. *American Journal of Infection Control, 27,* 488–496. doi:10.1016/S0196-6553(99)70026-X

Nuss, R., Cole, L., Le, T., Orsini, E., & Harned, R. (2008). Pinch-off syndrome in patients with sickle cell disease receiving erythrocytapheresis. *Pediatric Blood and Cancer, 50,* 354–356. doi:10.1002/pbc.21058

O'Neill, W.C., Wasse, H., Asif, A., & Ash, S.R. (2007). Diagnostic and interventional nephrology. In J. Feehally, J. Floege, & R.J. Johnson (Eds.), *Comprehensive clinical nephrology* (3rd ed., pp. 941–952). Philadelphia, PA: Elsevier Mosby.

Olson, K., Rennie, R., Hanson, J., Ryan, M., Gilpin, J., Falsetti, M., … Gaudet, S. (2004). Evaluation of a no-dressing intervention for tunneled central venous catheter exit sites. *Journal of Infusion Nursing, 27,* 37–44. doi:10.1097/00129804-200401000-00006

Ommaya, A.K. (1963). Subcutaneous reservoir and pump for sterile access to ventricular cerebrospinal fluid. *Lancet, 2,* 983–984. doi:10.1016/S0140-6736(63)90681-0

Opilla, M. (2008). Epidemiology of bloodstream infection associated with parenteral nutrition. *American Journal of Infection Control, 36,* S173.e5–S173.e8.

Osborne, D., Pappas, E., Alexander, G., Boe, B., Cantor, A.B., Rosemurgy, A., & Zervos, E. (2006). A complication-free course ensures a survival advantage in patients after regional therapy for metastatic colorectal cancer. *American Surgeon, 72,* 505–510.

Osma, S., Kahveci, S.F., Kaya, F.N., Akalin, H., Ozakin, C., Yilmaz, E., & Kutlay, O. (2006). Efficacy of antiseptic-impregnated catheters on catheter colonization and catheter-related bloodstream infections in patients in an intensive care unit. *Journal of Hospital Infection, 62,* 156–162. doi:10.1016/j.jhin.2005.06.030

Otto, S. (2005). *Mosby's pocket guide series: Infusion therapy* (5th ed.). St. Louis, MO: Elsevier Mosby.

Ozdemir, N.Y., Abali, H., Oksuzoglu, B., Budakoglu, B., Akmangit, I., & Zengin, N. (2009). It appears to be safe to start chemotherapy on the day of implantation through subcutaneous venous port catheters in inpatient setting. *Supportive Care in Cancer, 17,* 399–403. doi:10.1007/s00520-008-0498-x

Paice, J.A., DuPen, A., & Schwertz, D. (1999). Catheter port cleansing techniques and the entry of povidone-iodine into the epidural space. *Oncology Nursing Forum, 26,* 603–605.

Penel, N., & Yazdanpanah, Y. (2008). Vancomycin flush as antibiotic prophylaxis for early catheter-related infections: A cost-effectiveness analysis. *Supportive Care in Cancer, 17,* 285–293.

Penwarden, L.M., & Montgomery, P.G. (2002). Developing a protocol for obtaining blood cultures from central venous catheters and peripheral sites. *Clinical Journal of Oncology Nursing, 6,* 268–270. doi:10.1188/02.CJON.268-270

Perucca, R. (2010). Peripheral venous access devices. In M. Alexander, A. Corrigan, L. Gorski, J. Hankins, & R. Perucca (Eds.), *Infusion nursing: An evidence-based approach* (3rd ed., pp. 456–479). St. Louis, MO: Elsevier Saunders.

Petrosino, B., Becker, H., & Christian, B. (1988). Infection rates in central venous catheter dressings. *Oncology Nursing Forum, 15,* 709–717.

Pettit, J. (2007). Technological advances for PICC placement and management. *Advances in Neonatal Care, 7,* 122–131.

Pian-Smith, M., & Nishida, T. (2007). Spinal, epidural, and caudal anesthesia. In P.F. Dunn (Ed.), *Clinical anesthesia procedures of the Massachusetts General Hospital* (7th ed., pp. 247–272). Philadelphia, PA: Lippincott Williams & Wilkins.

Pieger-Mooney, S. (2005). Innovations in central vascular access device insertion. *Journal of Infusion Nursing, 28*(Suppl. 3), S7–S12. doi:10.1097/00129804-200505001-00002

Pikwer, A., Baath, L., Davidson, B., Perstoft, I., & Akeson, J. (2008). The incidence and risk of central venous catheter malpositioning: A prospective cohort study in 1619 patients. *Anaesthesia and Intensive Care, 36,* 30–37.

Poage, E., Singer, M., Armer, J., Poundall, M., & Shellabarger, J. (2008). Demystifying lymphedema: Development of the lymphedema Putting Evidence Into Practice card. *Clinical Journal of Oncology Nursing, 12,* 951–964. doi:10.1188/08.CJON.951-964

Polovich, M., Whitford, J.M., & Olsen, M. (Eds.). (2009). *Chemotherapy and biotherapy guidelines and recommendations for practice* (3rd ed.). Pittsburgh, PA: Oncology Nursing Society.

Porzionato, A., Montisci, M., & Manani, G. (2003). Brachial plexus injury following subclavian vein catheterization: A case report. *Journal of Clinical Anesthesiology, 15,* 582–586. doi:10.1016/j.jclinane.2003.02.009

Potter, K.L., & Held-Warmkessel, J. (2008). Intraperitoneal chemotherapy for women with ovarian cancer: Nursing care and considerations. *Clinical Journal of Oncology Nursing, 12,* 265–271. doi:10.1188/08.CJON.265-271

Powell, J., Tarnow, K.G., & Perucca, R. (2008). The relationship between peripheral intravenous catheter indwell time and the incidence of phlebitis. *Journal of Infusion Nursing, 13,* 39–45. doi:10.1097/01.NAN.0000308544.67744.50

Pratt, R.J., Pellowe, C.M., Wilson, J.A., Loveday, H.P., Harper, P.J., Jones, S., … Wilcox, M.H. (2007). epic2: National evidence-based guidelines for preventing healthcare-associated infections in NHS hospitals in England. *Journal of Hospital Infection, 65*(Suppl. 1), S1–S59. doi:10.1016/S0195-6701(07)60002-4

Pronovost, P. (2008). Interventions to decrease catheter-related bloodstream infections in the ICU: The Keystone Intensive Care Unit Project. *American Journal of Infection Control, 36,* S171.e1–S171.e5.

Prue-Owens, K.K. (2006). Use of peripheral venous access devices for obtaining blood samples for measurement of activated partial thromboplastin times. *Critical Care Nurse, 26,* 30–38.

Prunet, B., Meaudre, E., Montcriol, A., Asencio, Y., Bordes, J., Lacroix, G., & Kaiser, E. (2008). A prospective randomized trial of two safety peripheral intravenous catheters. *Anesthesia and Analgesia, 107,* 155–158. doi:10.1213/ane.0b013e318174df5f

Putigna, F., & Solenberger, R. (2009). Central venous access. Retrieved from http://emedicine.medscape.com/article/940865-overview

Raad, I., & Bodey, G.P. (1992). Infectious complications of indwelling vascular catheters. *Clinical Infectious Diseases, 15,* 197–210.

Raad, I., Hanna, H., & Maki, D. (2007). Intravascular catheter-related infections: Advances in diagnosis, prevention, and management. *Lancet Infectious Diseases, 7,* 645–657. doi:10.1016/S1473-3099(07)70235-9

Raad, I., Hanna, H.A., Alakech, B., Chatzinikolaou, I., Johnson, M.M., & Tarrand, J. (2004). Differential time to positivity: A useful method for diagnosing catheter-related bloodstream infections. *Annals of Internal Medicine, 140,* 18–25.

Raad, I., Hanna, H.A., Awad, A., Alrahwan, A., Bivins, C., Khan, A., … Mansour, G. (2001). Optimal frequency of changing intravenous administration set: Is it safe to prolong use beyond 72 hours? *Infection Control and Hospital Epidemiology, 22,* 136–139. doi:10.1086/501879

Ragni, M., Journeycake, J., & Brambilla, D. (2008). Tissue plasminogen activator to prevent central venous access device infections: A systematic review of central venous access catheter thrombosis, infection and thrombophylaxis. *Haemophilia, 14,* 30–38.

Ramritu, P., Halton, K., Collignon, P., Cook, D., Fraenkel, D., Battistutta, D., ... Graves, N. (2008). A systematic review comparing the relative effectiveness of antimicrobial-coated catheters in intensive care units. *American Journal of Infection Control, 36,* 104–117. doi:10.1016/j.ajic.2007.02.012

Rawson, K.M., & Newburn-Cook, C.V. (2007). The use of low-dose warfarin as prophylaxis for central venous catheter thrombosis in patients with cancer: A meta-analysis. *Oncology Nursing Forum, 34,* 1037–1043. doi:10.1188/07.ONF.1037-1043

Reddy, A., Lang, E., Cutts, J., Loh, S., & Rosen, M. (2007). Fibrin sheath removal from central venous catheters: An internal snare maneuver. *Nephrology, Dialysis, Transplantation, 22,* 1762–1765. doi:10.1093/ndt/gfm154

Redmond, A., & Doherty, E. (2005). Peritoneal dialysis. *Nursing Standard, 19*(40), 55–65.

Remerand, F., Vuitton, A.S., Palud, M., Buchet, S., Pourrat, X., Baud, A., ... Fusciardi, J. (2008). Elastomeric pump reliability in postoperative regional anesthesia: A survey of 430 consecutive devices. *Anesthesia and Analgesia, 107,* 2079–2084. doi:10.1213/ane.0b013e318187c9bb

Remington, R., & Hultman, T. (2007). Hypodermoclysis to treat dehydration: A review of the evidence. *Journal of the American Geriatrics Society, 55,* 2051–2055. doi:10.1111/j.1532-5415.2007.01437.x

Renard, E. (2008). Clinical experience with an implanted closed-loop insulin delivery system. *Arquivos Brasileiros de Endocrinologia e Metabologia, 52,* 349–354. doi:10.1590/S0004-27302008000200023

Rhinehart, E., & McGoldrick, M. (2005). *Infection control in home care and hospice* (2nd ed.). Sudbury, MA: Jones and Bartlett.

Richard, C.J. (1980). Peritoneal dialysis—a nursing update Part I. *Nephrology Nurse, 2,* 38–40.

Rijnders, B.J., Van Wijngaerden, E., Vandecasteele, S.J., Stas, M., & Peetermans, W.E. (2005). Treatment of long-term intravascular catheter-related bacteraemia with antibiotic lock: Randomized, placebo-controlled trial. *Journal of Antimicrobial Chemotherapy, 55,* 90–94. doi:10.1093/jac/dkh488

Rippe, B. (2007). Peritoneal dialysis: Principles, techniques, and adequacy. In J. Feehally, J. Floege, & R.J. Johnson (Eds.), *Comprehensive clinical nephrology* (3rd ed., pp. 979–990). Philadelphia, PA: Elsevier Mosby.

Rondina, M.T., Markewitz, B., Kling, S.J., Nohavec, R., & Rodgers, G.M. (2007). The accuracy of activated partial thromboplastin times when drawn through a peripherally inserted central catheter. *American Journal of Hematology, 82,* 738–739. doi:10.1002/ajh.20900

Rosenthal, K. (2002). Optimal infusion therapy? Overcome occlusions. *Nursing Management, 33*(2), 49–50.

Rosenthal, K. (2006). When your patient develops phlebitis. *Nursing, 36*(2), 14.

Rosenthal, K. (2007). Reducing the risks of infiltration and extravasation. *Nursing, 37*(Suppl.), 4–8. doi:10.1097/01.NURSE.0000298011.91516.98

Rosot Enterprises, Inc. (n.d.). Cruz® catheters for peritoneal dialysis. Retrieved from http://rosot.com/ingle/peritoneal.dialysis.php

Rosovsky, R.P., & Kuter, D.J. (2005). Catheter-related thrombosis in cancer patients: Pathophysiology, diagnosis, and management. *Hematology/Oncology Clinics of North America, 19,* 183–202. doi:10.1016/j.hoc.2004.09.007

Rubin, L.G., Shih, S., Shende, A., Karayalcin, G., & Lanzkowsky, P. (1999). Cure of implantable venous port-associated bloodstream infections in pediatric hematology-oncology patients without catheter removal. *Clinical Infectious Diseases, 29,* 102–105. doi:10.1086/520135

Rummel, M.A., Donnelly, P.J., & Fortenbaugh, C.C. (2001). Clinical evaluation of a positive pressure device to prevent central venous catheter occlusion: Results of a pilot study. *Clinical Journal of Oncology Nursing, 5,* 261–265.

Rupp, M.E., Lisco, S.J., Lipsett, P.A., Perl, T.M., Keating, K., Civetta, J.M., ... Sherertz, R. (2005). Effect of a second-generation venous catheter impregnated with chlorhexidine and silver sulfadiazine on central catheter-related infections: A randomized, controlled trial. *Annals of Internal Medicine, 143,* 570–580.

Ruschulte, H., Franke, M., Gastmeier, P., Zenz, S., Mahr, K.H., Buchholz, S., ... Piepenbrock, S. (2009). Prevention of central venous catheter related infections with chlorhexidine gluconate impregnated wound dressings: A randomized controlled trial. *Annals of Hematology, 88,* 267–272. doi:10.1007/s00277-008-0568-7

Safdar, N., & Maki, D.G. (2005). Risk of catheter-related bloodstream infection with peripherally inserted central venous catheters used in hospitalized patients. *Chest, 128,* 489–495. doi:10.1378/chest.128.2.489

Safdar, N., & Maki, D.G. (2006). Use of vancomycin-containing lock or flush solutions for prevention of bloodstream infection associated with central venous access devices: A meta-analysis of prospective, randomized trials. *Clinical Infectious Diseases, 43,* 474–484. doi:10.1086/505976

Saladow, J. (2004). Trends in ambulatory infusion pumps. *Infusion Magazine, 10*(4), 16–19.

Saladow, J. (2007). Ambulatory infusion pump technologies: New development and how they might affect alternate site care. *Infusion Magazine, 13*(4), 17–22.

Salgado, C.D., Chinnes, L., Paczesny, T.H., & Cantey, J.R. (2007). Increased rate of catheter-related bloodstream infection associated with use of a needleless mechanical valve device at a long-term acute care hospital. *Infection Control and Hospital Epidemiology, 28,* 684–688. doi:10.1086/516800

Salis, A.I., Eclavea, A., Johnson, M.S., Patel, N.H., Wong, D.G., & Tennery, G. (2004). Maximal flow rates possible during power injection through currently available PICCs: An in vitro study. *Journal of Vascular and Interventional Radiology, 15,* 275–281. doi:10.1097/01.RVI.0000116195.44877.88

Sanelli, P.C., Deshmukh, M., Ougorets, I., Caiati, R., & Heier, L.A. (2004). Safety and feasibility of using a central venous catheter for rapid contrast injection rates. *American Journal of Roentgenology, 183,* 1829–1834.

Sariosmanoglu, N., Ugurlu, B., Turgut, N.H., Demirkan, F., Ozsan, H., Ergor, G., ... Oto, O. (2008). Use of tunnelled catheters in haematological malignancy patients with neutropenia. *Journal of International Medical Research, 36,* 1103–1111.

Sattler, B. (2006). Nursing alert: Warming i.v. bags. *Alabama Nurse, 33*(2), 1, 7.

Sauerland, C., Engelking, C., Wickham, R., & Corbi, D. (2006). Vesicant extravasation part I: Mechanisms, pathogenesis, and nursing care to reduce risk. *Oncology Nursing Forum, 33,* 1134–1141. doi:10.1188/06.ONF.1134-1141

Scales, K. (2008). Intravenous therapy: A guide to good practice. *British Journal of Nursing, 17*(Suppl. 19), S4–S12.

Schilling, S., Doellman, D., Hutchinson, N., & Jacobs, B.R. (2006). The impact of needleless connector device design on central venous catheter occlusion in children: A prospective, controlled trial. *Journal of Parenteral and Enteral Nutrition, 30,* 85–90. doi:10.1177/014860710603000285

Schulmeister, L. (2007). Extravasation management. *Seminars in Oncology Nursing, 23,* 184–190. doi:10.1016/j.soncn.2007.05.003

Schulmeister, L. (2008). Managing vesicant extravasations. *Oncologist, 13,* 284–288. doi:10.1634/theoncologist.2007-0191

Schulmeister, L., & Camp-Sorrell, D. (2000). Chemotherapy extravasation from implanted ports. *Oncology Nursing Forum, 27,* 531–538.

Sethna, N.F., Verghese, S.T., Hannallah, R.S., Solodiuk, J.C., Zurakowski, D., & Berde, C.B. (2005). A randomized controlled trial to evaluate S-Caine Patch™ for reducing pain associated with vascular access in children. *Anesthesiology, 102,* 403–408. doi:10.1097/00000542-200502000-00025

Seymour, V.M., Dhallu, T.S., Moss, H.A., Tebbs, S.E., & Elliott, T.S.J. (2000). A prospective clinical study to investigate the microbial contamination of a needleless connector. *Journal of Hospital Infection, 45,* 165–168. doi:10.1053/jhin.2000.0726

Shah, P.S., & Shah, N. (2007). Heparin-bonded catheters for prolonging the patency of central venous catheters in children. *Cochrane Database of Systematic Reviews* 2007, Issue 4. Art. No.: CD005983. doi:10.1002/14651858.CD005983.pub2

Shivnan, J.C., McGuire, D., Freedman, S., Sharkazy, E., Bosserman, G., Larson, E., & Grouleff, P. (1991). A comparison of transparent adherent and dry sterile gauze dressings for long-term central catheters in patients undergoing bone marrow transplant. *Oncology Nursing Forum, 18,* 1349–1356.

Simhi, E., Kachko, L., Bruckheimer, E., & Katz, J. (2008). A vein entry indicator device for facilitating peripheral intravenous cannulation in children: A prospective, randomized, controlled trial. *Anesthesia and Analgesia, 107,* 1531–1535. doi:10.1213/ane.0b013e318185cdab

Skryabina, E.A., & Dunn, T.S. (2006). Disposable infusion pumps. *American Journal of Health-System Pharmacy, 63,* 1260–1268. doi:10.2146/ajhp050408

Smith, B. (2006). Peripheral intravenous catheter dwell times: A comparison of 3 securement methods for implementation of a 96-hour scheduled change protocol. *Journal of Infusion Nursing, 29,* 14–17. doi:10.1097/00129804-200601000-00004

Smith, L.H. (2008). Alteplase for the management of occluded central venous access devices: Safety considerations. *Clinical Journal of Oncology Nursing, 12,* 155–157. doi:10.1188/08.CJON.155-157

Smith, P.B., Benjamin, D.K., Jr., Cotten, C.M., Schultz, E., Guo, R., Nowell, L., ... Thornburg, C.D. (2008). Is an increased dwell time of a peripherally inserted catheter associated with an increased risk of bloodstream infection in infants? *Infection Control and Hospital Epidemiology, 29,* 749–753. doi:10.1086/589905

Smith, T.J., & Coyne, P.J. (2005). Implantable drug delivery systems (IDDS) after failure of comprehensive medical management (CMM) can palliate symptoms in the most refractory cancer pain patients. *Journal of Palliative Medicine, 8,* 736–742. doi:10.1089/jpm.2005.8.736

Smiths Medical. (2005a). *P.A.S. port systems implantable venous access systems: Instructions for use.* St. Paul, MN: Author.

Smiths Medical. (2005b). Port-A-Cath® peritoneal implantable access system: Instructions for use. Retrieved from http://www.smiths-medical.com/Upload/products/product_relateddocs/access/PORT-A-CATH-Access-Systems/40-2300-24B(19425).pdf

Smiths Medical. (2008). CADD®-Solis [Brochure]. Retrieved from http://www.smiths-medical.com/plugins/news/2008/mar/cadd-solis-launched.html

Stephens, L.C., Haire, W.D., Tarantolo, S., Reed, E., Schmit-Pokorny, K., Kessinger, A., & Klein, R. (1997). Normal saline versus heparin flush for maintaining central venous catheter patency during apheresis collection of peripheral blood stem cells (PBSC). *Transfusion Science, 18,* 187–193. doi:10.1016/S0955-3886(97)00008-8

Stevens, B., Barton, S.E., Brechbill, M., Moenter, S., Piel, A.L., & Shankle, D. (2000). A randomized, prospective trial of conventional vascular ports versus the Vortex 'clear-flow' reservoir port in adult oncology patients. *Journal of Vascular Access Devices, 5*(2), 37–40. Retrieved from http://www.angiodynamics.com/uploads/pdf/10-08-09-10-43-15-Vortex%20Clinical%20Study.pdf

Stuart, O.A., Knight, C., & Sugarbaker, P.H. (2005). Avoiding carcinogen exposure with intraperitoneal paclitaxel. *Oncology Nursing Forum, 32,* 44–48. doi:10.1188/05.ONF.44-48

Sugarbaker, P.H. (2006). New standard of care for appendiceal epithelial neoplasms and pseudomyxoma peritonei syndrome. *Lancet Oncology, 7,* 69–76. doi:10.1016/S1470-2045(05)70539-8

Sugarbaker, P.H. (2009). Cytoreductive surgery and perioperative intraperitoneal chemotherapy for the treatment of advanced primary and recurrent ovarian cancer. *Current Opinion in Obstetrics and Gynecology, 21,* 15–24. doi:10.1097/GCO.0b013e32831f8f32

Surov, A., Buerke, M., John, E., Kosling, S., Spielmann, R.P., & Behrmann, C. (2008). Intravenous port catheter embolization: Mechanisms, clinical features, and management. *Angiology, 59,* 90–97. doi:10.1177/0003319707303883

Svoboda, P., Barton, R.P., Barbarash, O.L., Butylin, A.A., Jacobs, B.R., Lata, J., ... El-Shahawy, M.A. (2004). Recombinant urokinase is safe and effective in restoring patency to occluded central venous access devices: A multiple-center, international trial. *Critical Care Medicine, 32,* 1990–1996. doi:10.1097/01.CCM.0000142706.01717.EB

Tanguy, M., Seguin, P., Laviolle, B., Desbordes, L., & Malledant, Y. (2005). Hub qualitative blood culture is useful for diagnosis of catheter-related infections in critically ill patients. *Intensive Care Medicine, 31,* 645–648. doi:10.1007/s00134-005-2600-x

Thalhammer, A., Jacobi, V., Balzer, J., & Vogl, T.J. (2002). Repositioning of malpositioned or flipped central venous catheters. *European Radiology, 12,* 698–700.

Thibodeau, S., Riley, J., & Rouse, K.B. (2007). Effectiveness of a new flushing and maintenance policy using peripherally inserted central catheters for adults: Best practice. *Journal of Infusion Nursing, 30,* 287–292. doi:10.1097/01.NAN.0000292571.62763.76

Tilton, D. (2006). Central venous access device infections in the critical care unit. *Critical Care Nursing Quarterly, 29,* 117–122.

Timoney, J.P., Malkin, M.G., Leone, D.M., Groeger, J.S., Heaney, M.L., Keefe, D.L., ... Saltz, L.B. (2002). Safe and cost effective use of alteplase for the clearance of occluded central venous access devices. *Journal of Clinical Oncology, 20,* 1918–1922. doi:10.1200/JCO.2002.07.131

Timsit, J.F., Schwebel, C., Bouadma, L., Geffroy, A., Garrouste-Orgeas, M., Pease, S., ... Lucet, J.C. (2009). Chlorhexidine-impregnated sponges and less frequent dressing changes for prevention of catheter-related infections in critically ill adults: A randomized controlled trial. *JAMA, 301,* 1231–1241. doi:10.1001/jama.2009.376

Toscano, C.M., Bell, M., Zukerman, C., Shelton, W., Novicki, T.J., Nichols, W.G., ... Jarvis, W.R. (2009). Gram-negative bloodstream infections in hematopoietic stem cell transplant patients: The roles of needleless device use, bathing practices, and catheter care. *American Journal of Infection Control, 37,* 327–334. doi:10.1016/j.ajic.2008.01.012

Trerotola, S.O., Thompson, S., Chittams, J., & Vierregger, K.S. (2007). Analysis of tip malposition and correction in peripherally inserted central catheters placed at bedside by a dedicated nursing team. *Journal of Vascular and Interventional Radiology, 18,* 513–518. doi:10.1016/j.jvir.2007.01.020

Treston-Aurand, J., Olmsted, R.N., Allen-Bridson, K., & Craig, C.P. (1997). Impact of dressing materials on central venous catheter infection rates. *Journal of Intravenous Nursing, 20,* 201–206.

Tripepi-Bova, K.A., Woods, K.D., & Loach, M.C. (1997). A comparison of transparent polyurethane and dry gauze dressings for peripheral i.v. catheter sites: Rates of phlebitis, infiltration, and dislodgment by patients. *American Journal of Critical Care, 6,* 377–381.

Trope, C., & Kaern, J. (2006). Primary surgery for ovarian cancer. *European Journal of Surgical Oncology, 32,* 844–852.

Tu, T.M., & Tremmel, J.A. (2007, November). Management of femoral arterial access: To close or hold pressure? *Endovascular Today,* pp. 38–42.

Tuten, S.H., & Gueldner, S.H. (1991). Efficacy of sodium chloride versus dilute heparin for maintenance of peripheral intermittent intravenous devices. *Applied Nursing Research, 4,* 63–71. doi:10.1016/S0897-1897(05)80057-6

Twardowski, Z.J. (2004). History and development of the access for peritoneal dialysis. In C. Ronco & N.W. Levin (Eds.), *Hemodialysis vascular access and peritoneal dialysis access* (pp. 387–401). Basel, Switzerland: S. Karger AG.

Udy, A., Senthuran, S., & Lipman, J. (2009). Airway obstruction due to a pre-vertebral haematoma following difficult central line insertion—Implications for ultrasound guidance and review of the literature. *Anaesthesia and Intensive Care, 37,* 309–313.

U.S. Food and Drug Administration. (2002). FDA public health notification: PVC devices containing the plasticizer DEHP. Retrieved from http://www.fda.gov/MedicalDevices/Safety/AlertsandNotices/PublicHealthNotifications/UCM062182

U.S. Food and Drug Administration. (2009, April 30). Reminders from FDA regarding ruptured vascular access devices from power injection. Retrieved from http://www.fda.gov/MedicalDevices/Safety/AlertsandNotices/TipsandArticlesonDeviceSafety/ucm070193.htm

Vahid, B. (2006). Chylothorax secondary to SVC syndrome treated successfully with SVC stent placement and anticoagulation therapy. *Internet Journal of Thoracic and Cardiovascular Surgery, 8.* Retrieved from http://www.ispub.com/journal/the_internet_journal_of_thoracic_and_cardiovascular_surgery.html

Valles, J., Fernandez, I., Alcaraz, R., Chacon, E., Cazorla, A., Canals, M., … Moron, A. (2008). Prospective randomized trial of 3 antiseptic solutions for prevention of catheter colonization in an intensive care unit for adult patients. *Infection Control and Hospital Epidemiology, 29,* 847–853. doi:10.1086/590259

van de Wetering, M.D., & van Woensel, J.B.M. (2007). Prophylactic antibiotics for preventing early central venous catheter Gram positive infections in oncology patients. *Cochrane Database of Systematic Reviews* 2007, Issue 1. Art. No.: CD003295. doi:10.1002/14651858.CD003295.pub2

Veenstra, D.L., Saint, S., Saha, S., Lumley, T., & Sullivan, S.D. (1999). Efficacy of antiseptic-impregnated central venous catheters in preventing catheter-related bloodstream infection: A meta-analysis. *JAMA, 284,* 261–267. doi:10.1001/jama.281.3.261

Venkatram, S., Rachmale, S., & Kanna, B. (2009). Study of device use adjusted rates in health care–associated infections after implementation of "bundles" in a closed-model medical intensive care unit. *Journal of Critical Care, 25,* 174.e11-174.e18. doi:10.1016/j.jcrc.2009.06.016

Verso, M., Agnelli, G., Bertoglio, S., Di Somma, F.C., Paoletti, F., Ageno, W., … Mosca, S. (2005). Enoxaparin for the prevention of venous thromboembolism associated with central vein catheter: A double-blind, placebo-controlled, randomized study in cancer patients. *Journal of Clinical Oncology, 23,* 4057–4062. doi:10.1200/JCO.2005.06.084

Verso, M., Agnelli, G., Kamphuisen, P.W., Ageno, W., Bazzan, M., Lazzaro, A., … Bertoglio, S. (2008). Risk factors for upper limb deep vein thrombosis associated with the use of central vein catheter in cancer patients. *Internal and Emergency Medicine, 3,* 117–122. doi:10.1007/s11739-008-0125-3

Vescia, S., Baumgartner, A.K., Jacobs, V.R., Kiechle-Bahat, M., Rody, A., Loibl, S., & Harbeck, N. (2008). Management of venous port systems in oncology: A review of current evidence. *Annals of Oncology, 19,* 9–15. doi:10.1093/annonc/mdm272

Waki, F., Ando, M., Takashima, A., Yonemori, K., Nokihara, H., Miyake, M., … Tamura, T. (2008). Prognostic factors and clinical outcomes in patients with leptomeningeal metastasis from solid tumors. *Journal of Neuro-Oncology, 93,* 205–212. doi:10.1007/s11060-008-9758-3

WalkMed Infusion LLC. (2009). WalkMed 350VL [Brochure]. Retrieved from http://www.walkmed.net/site/pumps-ambulatory.php

Walker, J.L., Armstrong, D.K., Huang, H.Q., Fowler, J., Webster, K., Burger, R.A., & Clarke-Pearson, D. (2006). Intraperitoneal catheter outcomes in a phase III trial of intravenous versus intraperitoneal chemotherapy in optimal stage III ovarian and primary peritoneal cancer: A Gynecologic Oncology Group study. *Gynecologic Oncology, 100,* 27–32. doi:10.1016/j.ygyno.2005.11.013

Walsh, G. (2005). Hypodermoclysis: An alternate method for rehydration in long-term care. *Journal of Infusion Nursing, 28,* 123–129. doi:10.1097/00129804-200503000-00006

Watanabe, M., Takita, W., Nakazaki, H., Tanemura, H., Kaneko, H., & Kobayashi, K. (2004). Hepatic arterial catheterization combining interventional radiological and laparotomic approaches. *Journal of Surgical Oncology, 88,* 256–260. doi:10.1002/jso.20160

Weigand, D.. & Carlson, K. (Eds.). (2005). *AACN procedure manual for critical care* (5th ed.). St. Louis, MO: Elsevier Saunders.

White, S.A. (2001). Peripheral intravenous therapy–related phlebitis rates in an adult population. *Journal of Intravenous Nursing, 24,* 19–24.

Whitta, R.K., Hall, K.F., Bennetts, T.M., Welman, L., & Rawlins, P. (2006). Comparison of normal or heparinised saline flushing on function of arterial lines. *Critical Care and Resuscitation, 8,* 205–208.

Williamson, E.E., & McKinney, J.M. (2001). Assessing the adequacy of peripherally inserted central catheters for power injection of intravenous contrast agents for CT. *Journal of Computer Assisted Tomography, 25,* 932–937. doi:10.1097/00004728-200111000-00016

Winkelman, L. (2004). Malignant ascites. In C.H. Yarbro, M.H. Frogge, & M. Goodman (Eds.), *Cancer symptom management* (3rd ed., pp. 399–419). Sudbury, MA: Jones and Bartlett.

Wolf, H.H., Leithauser, M., Maschmeyer, G., Salwender, H., Klein, U., Chaberny, I., … Mousset, S. (2008). Central venous catheter-related infections in hematology and oncology: Guidelines of the Infectious Diseases Working Party (AGIHO) of the German Society of Hematology and Oncology (DGHO). *Annals of Hematology, 87,* 863–876. doi:10.1007/s00277-008-0509-5

Worth, L.J., Seymour, J.F., & Slavin, M.A. (2009). Infective and thrombotic complications of central venous catheters in patients with hematological malignancy: Prospective evaluation of nontunneled devices. *Supportive Care in Cancer, 17,* 811–818. doi:10.1007/s00520-008-0561-7

Worthington, T., & Elliott, T.S.J. (2005). Diagnosis of central venous catheter related infection in adult patients. *Journal of Infection, 51,* 267–280. doi:10.1016/j.jinf.2005.06.007

Yahav, D., Rozen-Zvi, B., Gafter-Gvili, A., Leibovici, L., Gafter, U., & Paul, M. (2008). Antimicrobial lock solutions for the prevention of infections associated with intravascular catheters in patients undergoing hemodialysis: Systematic review and meta-analysis of randomized, controlled trials. *Clinical Infectious Diseases, 47,* 83–93. doi:10.1086/588667

Yebenes, J.C., & Serra-Prat, M. (2008). Clinical use of disinfectable needle-free connectors. *American Journal of Infection Control, 36,* S175.e1–S175.e4.

Yebenes, J.C., Vidaur, L., Serra-Prat, M., Sirvent, J.M., Batlle, J., Motje, M., … Palomar, M. (2004). Prevention of catheter-related bloodstream infection in critically ill patients using a disinfectable, needle-free connector: A randomized controlled trial. *American Journal of Infection Control, 32,* 291–295. doi:10.1016/j.ajic.2003.12.004

Yoshida, J., Ishimaru, T., Fujimoto, M., Hirata, N., Matsubara, N., & Koyanagi, N. (2008). Risk factors for central venous catheter-related bloodstream infection: A 1073-patient study. *Journal of Infection and Chemotherapy, 14,* 399–403. doi:10.1007/s10156-008-0637-9

Young, A.M., Billingham, L.J., Begum, G., Kerr, D.J., Hughes, A.I., Rea, D.W., … Wheatley, K. (2009). Warfarin thromboprophylaxis in cancer patients with central venous catheters (WARP): An open-label randomised trial. *Lancet, 373,* 567–574. doi:10.1016/S0140-6736(09)60205-1

Yucel, N., Lefering, R., Maegele, M., Max, M., Rossaint, R., Koch, A., … Neugebauer, E.A.M. (2004). Reduced colonization and infection with miconazole-rifampicin modified central venous catheters: A randomized controlled clinical trial. *Journal of Antimicrobial Chemotherapy, 54,* 1109–1115. doi:10.1093/jac/dkh483

Yung, X.-J., Li, Y., Al-shammaa Hassan, A.H., Yang, G.-L., Liu, S.-Y., Lu, Y.-L., … Yonemura, Y. (2009). Cytoreductive surgery plus hyperthermic intraperitoneal chemotherapy improves survival in selected patients with peritoneal carcinomatosis from abdominal and pelvic malignancies: Results of 21 cases. *Annals of Surgical Oncology, 16,* 345–351. doi:10.1245/s10434-008-0226-2

Zamos, D.T., Emch, T.M., Patton, H.A., D'Amico, F.J., & Bansal, S.K. (2007). Injection rate threshold of triple-lumen central venous catheters: An in vitro study. *Academic Radiology, 14,* 574–578. doi:10.1016/j.acra.2007.01.026

Appendix 1. Internet Resources for Information About Access Devices

American Association of Critical-Care Nurses: www.aacn.org

American College of Chest Physicians: www.chestnet.org

Association for Professionals in Infection Control and Epidemiology: www.apic.org

Association for Vascular Access: www.avainfo.org

Centers for Disease Control and Prevention: www.cdc.gov

Centers for Medicare and Medicaid Services: www.cms.hhs.gov

ECRI Institute (formerly Emergency Care Research Institute): www.ecri.org (A nonprofit organization that applies evidence-based research to discover which medical procedures, devices, drugs, and processes are best to improve patient care)

Gynecologic Oncology Group education materials: www.gog.org/ipchemoed/ipchemoed.html

Infectious Diseases Society of America: www.idsociety.org

Infusion Nurses Society: www.ins1.org

International Society for Peritoneal Dialysis Guidelines: www.ispd.org/lang-en/treatmentguidelines/guidelines

National Cancer Institute Cancer Therapy Evaluation Program clinical announcement regarding intraperitoneal chemotherapy for ovarian cancer: http://ctep.info.nih.gov/highlights/docs/clin_annc_010506.pdf

Oncology Nursing Society: www.ons.org

Vascular Access Society: www.vascularaccesssociety.com

Appendix 2. Peripheral/Midline IV Practicum

Skill	Met	Not Met
A. Patient preparation		
1. Performs preplacement assessment of patient		
2. Explains procedure to patient and/or significant others		
B. Inserting catheter		
1. Organizes equipment		
2. Examines veins on both extremities		
3. Washes hands; dons gloves		
4. Applies local anesthetic, if ordered		
5. Applies tourniquet; cleanses site		
6. Stabilizes vein below venipuncture site with nondominant hand		
7. Observes for blood return; advances catheter into vein; pushes catheter off stylet		
8. Releases tourniquet		
9. Occludes tip of catheter by pressing fingers of nondominant hand over vein to prevent retrograde bleeding		
10. Attaches to appropriate device for IV therapy		
11. Discards all equipment appropriately		
C. Blood drawing		
1. Washes hands; accesses system appropriately		
2. Removes at least 0.5 ml of blood (or twice the catheter and add-on device volume) and discards		
3. Withdraws appropriate amount for laboratory test		
4. Flushes catheter with 1–3 ml of normal saline		
5. Caps catheter or connects to appropriate solution		
D. Injection cap change		
1. Washes hands		
2. Prepares appropriate equipment		
3. Applies gloves		
4. Changes injection cap at appropriate frequency		
E. Insertion-site care		
1. Washes hands		
2. Prepares appropriate equipment		
3. Applies gloves		
4. Removes old dressing carefully and discards dressing and gloves		
5. Washes hands		
6. Applies new gloves		
7. Cleanses exit site and allows to dry		
8. Applies appropriate dressing		
F. Documentation/patient education		
1. Documents all procedures		
2. Teaches patient and/or significant others signs and symptoms of phlebitis, infiltration, or other anticipated complications		
Comments:		

Appendix 3. Nontunneled Central Venous Catheter (CVC) Practicum		
Skill	**Met**	**Not Met**
A. Patient preparation		
1. Performs preplacement assessment of patient		
2. Explains procedure to patient and/or significant others		
3. Ensures that informed consent is obtained for CVC insertion		
B. Assisting with placement		
1. Obtains necessary equipment and prepares IV solutions as ordered		
2. Obtains pump for all continuous infusions		
3. Positions patient in 15° Trendelenburg position with head turned away from insertion side and rolled towel under the shoulders if needed		
4. Washes hands (applies mask per institutional policy) and puts on gloves		
5. Assists practitioner placing line as requested, maintaining strict aseptic technique; supports and reassures patient		
6. Confirms proper tip placement with chest x-ray before beginning IV therapy		
7. Evaluates patient for post-insertion complications		
C. Accessing the short-term venous catheter		
1. Organizes CVC care to minimize entry into the system		
2. Explains procedure to patient		
3. Assembles equipment and washes hands		
4. Unless CVC has a valved distal tip, ensures the catheter is clamped whenever the line is opened; uses only smooth-edged clamps or latex- or plastic-covered clamps		
5. If therapy is continuous, vigorously scrubs injection cap with cleansing agent, removes cap, and attaches syringe with normal saline to flush		
6. Opening clamp, if necessary, flushes catheter and verifies positive blood return, then removes syringe and attaches IV tubing directly to catheter hub		
7. If therapy is intermittent IV push, inserts needleless needle through injection cap using the SASH (saline, administer medication, saline, heparin) method, scrubbing the injection port between each access; may alternately attach syringes directly to the hub, maintaining strict asepsis and utilizing new injection cap when completed.		
D. Blood drawing (discard method)		
1. Explains procedure to patient		
2. Washes hands and prepares appropriate equipment		
3. Applies gloves		
4. Removes at least 1–2 ml of blood and discards		
5. Removes necessary blood for testing using additional syringes or Vacutainer® (Becton, Dickinson and Co.) system		
6. Flushes catheter with at least 10 ml normal saline (20 ml for valved catheters)		
7. Heparinizes catheter if appropriate		
E. Injection cap change		
1. Explains procedure to patient		
2. Washes hands and obtains necessary equipment		
3. Ensures catheter is clamped if necessary		
4. Vigorously scrubs injection cap and hub with cleansing agent		
5. Removes old cap and scrubs hub, minimizing time catheter is opened		
6. Attaches new cap to hub using aseptic technique		
7. Changes cap at least once weekly and PRN		

(Continued on next page)

Appendix 3. Nontunneled Central Venous Catheter (CVC) Practicum *(Continued)*		
Skill	**Met**	**Not Met**
F. Exit-site care		
1. Explains procedure to patient		
2. Washes hands and obtains necessary equipment		
3. Applies gloves		
4. Removes old dressing carefully to minimize tugging on the line and avoids the use of scissors near the catheter		
5. Inspects exit site for erythema, tenderness, edema, exudate, integrity of sutures if appropriate, length of catheter protruding from the skin, and integrity of external portion of catheter; removes gloves		
6. Applies new gloves		
7. Cleanses exit site and applies appropriate dressing per institutional policy		
8. Tapes catheter and/or tubing to the patient's skin to minimize traction on the catheter		
9. Changes dressing as often as required per institutional policy for dressing type and PRN if soiled or nonocclusive		
G. Removal of catheter		
1. Verifies order for catheter removal and reason		
2. Explains procedure to patient		
3. Washes hands and assembles necessary equipment		
4. Applies gloves		
5. Removes old dressing and discards		
6. Applies new gloves		
7. Removes sutures if necessary		
8. Instructs patient to perform the Valsalva maneuver		
9. Ensures all IV solutions are discontinued		
10. Grasps hub and gently and steadily pulls the catheter out until completely removed		
11. Applies pressure to the exit site until bleeding has stopped		
12. If catheter infection is suspected, ensures tip does not contact any surface, cuts tip off with sterile scissors and places in a sterile container for culture		
13. Applies dressing over exit site per institutional policy		
14. Measures catheter and compares to inserted length		
15. Inspects catheter for defects or jagged edges suggestive of breakage		
16. If length or appearance warrant, notifies healthcare provider and preserves line		
H. Documentation/patient education		
1. Documents all procedures, assessments, and patient response		
2. Teaches patient and/or significant others short-term venous catheter care and observation		
Comments:		

Appendix 4. Long-Term* Venous Catheter Practicum		
Skill	**Met**	**Not Met**
A. Patient preparation		
1. Performs preplacement assessment of patient		
2. Explains procedure to patient and/or significant others		
3. Performs preplacement preparation		
4. Ensures that informed consent is obtained		
5. Performs postoperative assessment of patient and catheter		
6. Confirms placement of catheter by radiographic imaging prior to initiating treatment		
B. Accessing the long-term venous catheter		
1. Organizes catheter care to minimize entry into system		
2. Maintains strict aseptic technique		
3. Never leaves catheter open to air		
4. Uses only smooth-edged clamps or latex- or plastic-covered clamps as appropriate		
5. Tapes catheter securely to patient's body as needed		
6. Washes hands		
7. Prepares appropriate equipment		
8. Applies gloves		
9. Cleanses injection cap or catheter; accesses catheter		
10. Flushes catheter at appropriate frequency		
C. Blood drawing (discard method)		
1. Follows procedure for accessing system		
2. Removes at least 3–5 ml of blood or solution and discards (PICC 1–2 ml)		
3. Clamps catheter at appropriate times		
4. Withdraws desired amount of blood		
5. Flushes catheter with 10–20 ml of normal saline after blood withdrawal		
D. Injection cap change		
1. Washes hands		
2. Prepares appropriate equipment		
3. Applies gloves		
4. Cleanses catheter and applies cap using aseptic technique		
5. Changes injection cap at appropriate frequency		
E. Exit-site care		
1. Washes hands		
2. Prepares appropriate equipment		
3. Applies gloves		
4. Carefully removes old dressing		
5. Inspects exit site		
6. Removes gloves		
7. Applies new gloves		
8. Cleanses exit site		
9. Applies appropriate dressing		
F. Documentation/patient education		
1. Documents all procedures		
2. Teaches patient and/or significant other long-term venous catheter care		
Comments:		

*Can be used for peripherally inserted central catheter, or tunneled, pheresis, and hemodialysis catheters

Appendix 5. Implanted Port Practicum		
Skill	**Met**	**Not Met**
A. Patient preparation		
1. Performs preplacement assessment of patient		
2. Explains procedure to patient and/or significant others		
3. Ensures that informed consent is obtained for port insertion		
4. With patient in sitting position, assesses two best locations for port and marks areas for surgeon		
B. Accessing the implanted port		
1. Explains procedure to patient		
2. Washes hands and obtains necessary equipment		
3. Chooses appropriate size and length noncoring needle for therapy planned		
4. Applies gloves		
5. Removes dressing if appropriate		
6. Palpates port and locates center of septum to be accessed		
7. Observes site for edema, erythema, tenderness, condition of the catheter tunnel, or swelling of ipsilateral chest or neck veins or extremity		
8. Discards used gloves and reapplies new gloves; applies topical anesthetic cream if ordered		
9. Cleanses the area over the septum; administers topical anesthetic, if ordered		
10. Grasps the edges of the portal body firmly through the skin to stabilize, pushing the noncoring needle firmly through the skin and diaphragm, stopping when the bottom of the reservoir is reached		
11. Flushes saline into port and checks for blood return		
12. Applies dressing per institutional policy and planned length of infusion		
13. Attaches IV tubing directly to catheter hub if continuous infusion		
14. Attaches injection cap if intermittent infusion is planned		
15. If continuous infusion is planned, changes noncoring needle at least once every seven days and PRN		
C. Flushing an implanted port		
1. Explains procedure to patient		
2. Washes hands and assembles necessary equipment		
3. If port is not accessed, accesses per above procedure		
4. Flushes catheter with 10–20 ml normal saline for valved catheters and 5 ml 100 units/ml heparin lock flush for open-ended catheters		
5. If port does not need to be used, deaccesses per procedure below		
6. Accesses and flushes port every four to eight weeks when not in use		
D. Deaccessing an implanted port		
1. Explains procedure to patient		
2. Washes hands and assembles necessary equipment		
3. Applies gloves and removes dressing		
4. Discards used gloves and reapplies new gloves		
5. Stabilizing port through skin with one hand, grasps noncoring needle wings or hub with the other hand and administers flush		
6. While instilling the final 1 ml of flushing solution, simultaneously pulls the needle from the port septum, pushing down on the port edges to prevent tugging the port upward		
7. Applies pressure over the needle exit site, then applies adhesive bandage if needed		
E. Blood drawing from an implanted port		
1. Explains procedure to patient		
2. Washes hands and assembles necessary equipment		
3. Accesses port per above procedure if not accessed		

(Continued on next page)

Appendix 5. Implanted Port Practicum *(Continued)*		
Skill	**Met**	**Not Met**
4. Removes at least 5 ml of blood and discards		
5. Removes necessary blood for testing using additional syringes or Vacutainer® (Becton, Dickinson and Co.) system		
6. Flushes catheter per above procedure and either continues infusion, recaps, or deaccesses per above procedure		
F. Documentation/patient education		
1. Documents all procedures, assessments, and patient response		
2. Teaches patient and/or significant others implanted port care and observation		

Comments:

Appendix 6. Subcutaneous Infusion Practicum		
Skill	**Met**	**Not Met**
A. Patient preparation		
1. Performs preplacement assessment of patient		
2. Explains procedure to patient and/or significant others		
3. Performs preplacement preparation		
B. Inserting catheter, needle, or commercial device for subcutaneous infusion		
1. Organizes catheter care to minimize entry into system		
2. Maintains strict aseptic technique		
3. Washes hands		
4. Prepares appropriate equipment and primes set		
5. Cleanses intended access site and allows to dry		
6. Puts on gloves; stabilizes tissue with free hand, holding hand flat in a natural position or pinched lightly		
7. Supports tissue and inserts device appropriately		
8. Aspirates to check for blood		
9. If no blood, starts infusion and applies transparent dressing		
C. Infusion of fluids or medications		
1. States appropriate range for infusion rate		
2. States two possible complications and appropriate interventions		
D. Documentation/patient education		
1. Documents all procedures		
2. Teaches patient and/or significant others to report pain, burning, or leaking and any signs of redness, swelling, or other irritation		

Comments:

Appendix 7. Arterial Catheter Practicum		
Skill	**Met**	**Not Met**
A. Patient preparation		
1. Performs preplacement assessment of patient		
2. Explains procedure to patient and/or significant others		
3. Performs preplacement preparation of patient		
4. Ensures that informed consent is obtained		
5. Performs postoperative/post-procedure assessment of patient and catheter		
B. Accessing the arterial catheter		
1. Organizes catheter equipment/care to minimize entry into system		
2. Maintains strict aseptic technique		
3. Never leaves catheter open to air		
4. Uses only Luer-lock connections		
5. Administers all infusions through an infusion pump to maintain patency of catheter and prevent backflow and labels lines: arterial		
6. Tapes catheter securely to patient's body		
7. Washes hands		
8. Prepares appropriate equipment (including personal protective equipment)		
9. Applies gloves		
10. Accesses catheter		
11. Infuses infusate		
C. Maintaining patency		
1. Flushes catheter with normal saline before and after drug (unless drug not compatible with saline, then flush with dextrose 5% in water [D5W] after initial saline flush and again after D5W flush after drug infusion)		
2. Heparinizes catheter with correct dose of heparin at appropriate frequency		
D. Exit-site care		
1. Gathers and prepares appropriate equipment		
2. Washes hands and dons gloves; removes old dressing		
3. Inspects exit site. Washes hands; applies gloves		
4. Cleanses site as needed		
5. Applies appropriate dressing		
E. Documentation/patient education		
1. Documents all procedures		
2. Teaches patient and significant others arterial catheter care and/or signs and symptoms of complications		
3. Teaches patient and significant others precautions for bodily fluids required for 48 hours following chemotherapy		
Comments:		

Appendix 8. Intraventricular Reservoir Practicum		
Skill	**Met**	**Not Met**
A. Patient preparation		
1. Performs preplacement assessment of patient		
2. Explains procedure to patient and/or significant others		
3. Ensures informed consent is obtained for reservoir insertion		
B. Access of reservoir		
1. Explains procedure to patient		
2. Washes hands and assembles equipment		
3. Positions patient appropriately in a supine, semi-recumbent, or sitting position		
4. Prepares sterile field and opens equipment		
5. Shaves or clips hair over reservoir if necessary		
6. Palpates reservoir and checks for appropriate filling		
7. Applies sterile gloves		
8. Cleanses area over reservoir with three alcohol swabs in a circular manner from the center outward		
9. Repeats with three povidone-iodine swabs		
10. Allows povidone-iodine to air-dry for 30 seconds		
11. Accesses reservoir with 25-gauge butterfly needle at a 45° angle		
12. Allows 3 ml of cerebrospinal fluid (CSF) to flow into syringe and reserves for flush, maintaining sterility of syringe		
13. Reports abnormal-appearing CSF to physician and stops procedure if observed		
14. Withdraws additional CSF for testing, if ordered; withdraws equal amount of CSF to drug being infused		
15. Administers medication over 5–10 minutes		
16. Flushes reservoir with reserved CSF (3 ml) or preservative free-NS		
17. Removes needle and covers site with sterile 2 × 2 gauze		
18. Gently pumps reservoir three to five times to distribute the drug		
19. Assesses vital signs and neurologic status; contacts provider if abnormal		
C. Patient education/documentation		
1. Documents all procedures, assessments, and patient's responses		
2. Teaches patient and/or significant others implanted ventricular reservoir care and observation		

Comments:

Appendix 9. Epidural/Intrathecal Devices Practicum		
Skill	**Met**	**Not Met**
A. Patient preparation		
1. Performs preplacement assessment of patient		
2. Explains procedure to patient and/or significant others		
3. Performs preplacement preparation and ensures informed consent is obtained		
4. Performs postoperative assessment of patient and catheter		
B. Accessing epidural/intrathecal catheter		
1. Assesses patient's vital signs and neurologic status		
2. Assembles appropriate equipment		
3. Washes hands; applies sterile gloves and mask		
4. Cleans injection cap and allows to dry for one minute; uses a 25-gauge, 5/8-inch needle with an attached syringe; gently aspirates 1 ml; if blood or greater than 0.5 ml of clear fluid is aspirated from epidural catheter (normal to aspirate clear CSF from intrathecal catheter), gives no medication and notifies physician		
5. Injects medication slowly and steadily through 0.2 micron filter		
6. Flushes catheter with 1–2 ml of preservative-free normal saline and removes needle		
7. Places a label reading "epidural" or "intrathecal" around the tubing		
C. Accessing epidural/intrathecal port		
1. Assesses patient's vital signs and neurologic status		
2. Assembles appropriate equipment		
3. Washes hands and uses aseptic technique for accessing port		
4. Cleanses port site; allows to dry for one minute		
5. Puts on sterile gloves and mask		
6. Accesses port with a noncoring needle; gently aspirates 1 ml; if blood or greater than 0.5 ml of clear fluid is aspirated, medication is not given and physician is notified		
7. Injects medication slowly and steadily		
8. Flushes catheter with up to 3 ml of preservative-free normal saline and checks neurologic status		
D. Filter and injection cap change of epidural catheter		
1. Assembles appropriate equipment		
2. Washes hands		
3. Applies sterile gloves and mask		
4. Connects the new injection cap to the new filter and flushes the system with preservative-free normal saline using aseptic technique		
5. Cleans the connection between the catheter and the filter; allows to dry one minute		
6. Removes old filter and injection cap		
7. Screws on the new filter and injection cap securely		
E. Exit-site care of epidural/intrathecal catheter, procedure documentation, patient education, and response		
1. Assembles appropriate equipment		
2. Washes hands		
3. Applies gloves and mask		
4. Removes old dressing carefully		
5. Inspects exit site for redness, leakage, or swelling; removes gloves		
6. Applies sterile gloves		
7. Cleanses the site using friction; allows to dry for one minute		
8. Coils the catheter near exit site and applies a dressing over the area		
Comments:		

Appendix 10. Intraperitoneal Catheter Practicum		
Skill	**Met**	**Not Met**
A. Patient preparation		
1. Performs preplacement assessment of patient		
2. Explains procedure to patient and/or significant others		
3. Performs preplacement preparation		
4. Ensures informed consent is obtained		
5. Applies topical numbing medication as ordered 30 minutes before accessing implanted port		
6. Verifies orders; obtains medication from pharmacy, and with second RN, verifies patient, drug, dose, and route		
7. Performs postoperative assessment of patient, catheter, and surrounding skin		
8. Requests that patient void before starting treatment		
B. Accessing external peritoneal catheter		
1. Assembles appropriate equipment and washes hands		
2. Explains procedure to patient and ensures privacy		
3. Primes intraperitoneal tubing with normal saline (NS)		
4. Opens supplies onto sterile field; dons mask		
5. Puts on one sterile glove, usually on dominant hand		
6. Picks up sterile syringe in gloved hand and saline in nongloved hand, drawing up 20 ml NS		
7. Drops syringe onto sterile field and puts on second sterile glove		
8. Cleans catheter, connector, and catheter cap with povidone-iodine or 2% chlorhexidine gluconate/70% isopropyl alcohol swab, repeating the procedure three times and allowing the solution to air-dry at least one minute		
9. Maintains aseptic technique when disconnecting cap, attaches NS syringe, and flushes system to ensure patency		
10. Withdraws peritoneal fluid for sample if ordered		
11. Attaches infusion tubing and applies dressing		
12. Tapes tubing in a loop to minimize tension		
13. Assesses patient's response to treatment		
14. Documents procedure		
15. Ensures that dressing is changed three times a week; catheter cap and clamp changed once a week.		
C. Accessing implanted peritoneal port		
1. Washes hands and gathers supplies, including 19-gauge 1–1½ inch bent noncoring needle, 20 ml syringe, and NS		
2. Explains procedure to patient and ensures privacy		
3. Opens supplies, including syringe and noncoring needle, onto sterile field		
4. Puts on one sterile glove, usually on dominant hand		
5. Picks up sterile syringe in gloved hand and NS in nongloved hand, drawing up 20 ml NS		
6. Places syringe onto sterile field and puts on second glove		
7. Cleanses access site over port using 2% chlorhexidine gluconate/70% isopropyl alcohol swab and allows to dry for 30–60 seconds		
8. Attaches noncoring needle to syringe and flushes system to ensure patency, leaving syringe attached to extension tubing		
9. Palpates and grips the edge of the port through the skin with nondominant hand		
10. Places index finger of opposite hand over the bend of the noncoring needle, asks patient to take deep breath and hold, and firmly pushes through the skin and septum, advancing the needle slowly until the needle makes contact with the bottom of the septum		
11. Avoids rocking or twisting the needle once in the septum		

(Continued on next page)

Appendix 10. Intraperitoneal Catheter Practicum *(Continued)*

Skill	Met	Not Met
12. Flushes with 20 ml NS to ensure system patency, then applies occlusive dressing		
13. Is aware that a blood return is not expected as the catheter is not in a vein		
14. Attempts to withdraw peritoneal fluid if ordered; if unable to obtain fluid, flushes catheter with remaining NS		
15. If flush is successful, attaches infusion tubing or cap		
16. If resistance is felt with flushing, or if swelling or pain occurs, discontinues procedure and reaccesses using all-new sterile equipment; if resistance is felt again, and it is certain that needle is in right place, discontinues procedure and notifies provider		
17. Tapes the tubing in a loop to minimize tension on the needle		
18. Encourages the patient to stay in bed during infusion, dwell, and drain time to minimize potential for needle dislodgment		
19. Documents procedure, assessment of site, size of needle, appearance and amount of peritoneal fluid, and patient response		
20. Ensures that noncoring needle is changed every seven days		
D. Dressing peritoneal catheter (external or implanted)		
1. Original dressing remains in place for one week, unless it becomes soiled. Thereafter, the dressing is changed three times a week for the external catheter.		
2. Is aware that implanted port does not require dressing changes when not in use		
3. Assembles necessary supplies and washes hands		
4. Explains procedure to patient and ensures privacy		
5. Applies nonsterile gloves and removes old dressing, being careful not to touch exit site or needle		
6. Assesses site for infection or leakage		
7. Opens all supplies and puts on sterile gloves		
8. Cleans around catheter with povidone-iodine swab or 2% chlorhexidine gluconate/70% isopropyl alcohol swab, working in a circular motion from the catheter outward, being careful not to go over the same area twice, and repeats procedure three times		
9. Allows antiseptic to air-dry for at least one minute		
10. Applies either transparent dressing or gauze and tape, making sure the edges are occlusive		
11. Disposes of waste in a hazardous waste container		
12. Documents assessment and procedure		
E. Discontinuing intraperitoneal treatment		
1. Allows intraperitoneal treatment to dwell for the amount of time specified by physician order		
2. Drains fluid into sterile peritoneal drainage bag by opening clamp, if ordered		
3. Allows up to one hour for external catheters and two hours for implanted ports for fluid to drain off. Obtains as close to the amount infused as possible.		
4. To disconnect peritoneal therapy system, obtains supplies and empties onto sterile field		
5. Removes old dressing and assesses exit site		
6. For implantable port, removes the needle aseptically; cleanses exit-site area as described for accessing device. Applies pressure to exit site with sterile 2 × 2 gauze to prevent leakage. Applies sterile occlusive dressing.		
7. For external catheter, removes old dressing and cleanses exit site, catheter, and cap as described for accessing device		
8. Applies sterile dressing to exit site		
9. Is aware that dressing can be removed in 48 hours for implanted device and that external catheter dressing should be changed three times a week		
10. Documents patient response to treatment and procedure		
11. Disposes of all tubing and supplies into a hazardous waste container		

(Continued on next page)

Appendix 10. Intraperitoneal Catheter Practicum *(Continued)*		
Skill	**Met**	**Not Met**
F. Assesses and intervenes in catheter malfunction		
1. Differentiates between inflow and outflow problem, fibrin sheath formation, catheter kinking, and catheter migration		
2. Is aware of signs and symptoms of chemical versus bacterial peritonitis; exit-site versus tunnel-site infection		
3. Obtains orders for necessary flush medications if appropriate		
4. Reassures patient and prepares for diagnostic procedure to determine cause of problem if applicable		
5. Offers additional psychological support if catheter has to be removed		
G. Documentation		
1. Documents patient's and/or significant others' education and response to teaching, including return demonstration of technical tasks		
2. Documents procedures, assessments, and patient response		
3. Documents referrals to outside agencies		
Comments:		

Appendix 11. Implanted Pump Practicum		
Skill	**Met**	**Not Met**
A. Patient preparation		
1. Performs preplacement assessment of patient for appropriateness of implanted pump		
2. Educates patient and/or significant others regarding		
a. Purpose of implanted pump		
b. Patient's activity restrictions and maintenance schedule		
3. Obtains informed consent		
B. Accessing implanted pump		
1. Organizes and assembles equipment		
2. Explains procedure to patient and maintains privacy		
3. Maintains aseptic technique; applies gloves		
4. Determines site of pump and appropriate septum (template optional)		
5. Cleanses site		
6. Uses correct needle and maintains closed system; accesses pump		
C. Drug administration and pump fill		
1. Confirms and correctly calculates medication dosage and route		
2. Checks appropriate laboratory results		
3. Notes reservoir volume; takes appropriate action if pump is overfilled		
4. Flushes and injects appropriate solutions		
5. Applies pressure and bandage (as needed) after needle removal		
6. Follows agency procedure for waste disposal		
7. Monitors patient for complications and side effects		
D. Pump complications		
1. Describes major complications associated with implanted pump and measures to prevent or minimize complications		
2. Identifies two potential causes for no fluid return from pump reservoir		
3. Describes two possible consequences of accessing the incorrect port or septum		
E. Documentation		
1. Documents patient education and patient's and/or significant others' understanding		
2. Documents assessment, procedure, evaluation of interventions, and patient's response		
3. Documents pump refill information		
Comments:		

Appendix 12. Patient Education Handout on Vascular Access Devices

VASCULAR ACCESS DEVICE (VAD)
When to contact your healthcare professional

You have a vascular access device in place. It may be totally implanted under your skin, or you may have one or two tubings (lumens) on your chest or in your arm. The device will be used for your IV medications. Your nurse will let you know how he or she will use the device and will show you how to care for your device.

There are several things you will need to let your nurse or doctor know about if they should occur.

Fever of 100.5°F (38°C) or higher	The VAD is placed in a large vein in your chest. Bacteria can enter the bloodstream through the catheter and cause a bloodstream infection (sepsis). This is an <u>emergency call</u> to your healthcare professional. Phone # clinic: Phone # after hours:
Redness or tenderness at insertion site or up your arm	This can be a sign of infection or irritation of the vein. Notify your doctor's office as soon as possible, especially if you have a fever.
Inability to flush a lumen	If you are administering your IV therapy at home and are unable to flush the line, do not force it. If your catheter has clamps, make sure they are open. Try flushing again. If you are still unable to flush the line, you will need to contact your home healthcare nurse or your doctor's office immediately.
Breakage of your line	If you have tubing coming from your arm or your chest and the tubing breaks, <u>immediately clamp your tubing closest to your body</u> and contact your doctor's office or go to the nearest emergency room.

Index

The letter f after a page number indicates that relevant information appears in a figure; the letter t, in a table.